PEDIATRIC ORTHOPAEDICS
IN
PRIMARY CARE

PEDIATRIC ORTHOPAEDICS
IN
PRIMARY CARE

Vernon T. Tolo, M.D.
Chairman, Orthopaedic Surgery
Childrens Hospital Los Angeles
Los Angeles, California

Beverly Wood, M.D.
Chairman, Department of Radiology
Childrens Hospital Los Angeles
Los Angeles, California

Illustrations by
ROBERT S. AMARAL
Medical Illustrator
Childrens Hospital Los Angeles
Los Angeles, California

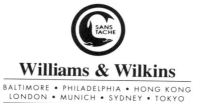

Williams & Wilkins
BALTIMORE • PHILADELPHIA • HONG KONG
LONDON • MUNICH • SYDNEY • TOKYO
A WAVERLY COMPANY

Editor: Jonathan Pine
Managing Editor: Molly Mullen
Copy Editor: Thomas Lehr
Designer: Norman W. Och
Illustration Planner: Wayne Hubbel
Production Coordinator: Barbara J. Felton

Accurate indications, adverse reactions, and dosage schedules for drugs are provided in this book, but it is possible that they may change. The reader is urged to review the package information data of the manufacturers of the medications mentioned.

Printed in the United States of America

Libary of Congress Cataloging-in-Publication Data

Tolo, Vernon T.
    Pediatric orthopaedics in primary care / Vernon T. Tolo, Beverly
Wood ; illustrations by Robert S. Amaral.
        p.   cm.
    Includes bibliographical references and index.
    ISBN 0-683-08330-9
    1. Pediatric orthopedics. 2. Primary care (Medicine)   I. Wood,
Beverly P.   II. Title.
    [DNLM: 1. Orthopedics—in infancy & childhood.   2. Primary Health
Care.   WS 270 T653p   1993]
RD732.3.C48T65   1993
617.3′083—dc20
DNLM/DLC
for Library of Congress   93-13960
                                                              CIP

                        93 94 95 96 97
                1   2   3   4   5   6   7   8   9   10

Foreword

It is a great privilege to contribute a foreword to this exceptional textbook on Pediatric Orthopaedics. During the last 25 years, pediatric orthopaedics has developed as an expert specialty within orthopaedics. However, most of the articles and texts that have been written on the subject have been on specific techniques and other topics primarily of interest to surgeons. Until now there has been very little comprehensive information available for the use of primary care physicians and, indirectly, the families of patients. We are therefore indebted to Dr. Tolo—an acknowledged expert in the field of pediatric orthopaedics—for developing such a clear yet concise textbook on the subject. The general consistency of the chapters is evident, as the majority of the work was done by Dr. Tolo himself, with the support of Dr. Beverly Wood in the area of radiologic imaging. Many of the chapters have already been presented to general practitioners and pediatricians in a lecture forum. In addition, each chapter that deals with a particular region of the body contains a section on the principles of the treatment of fractures.

I recommend this text to you for many reasons. It presents accurate information concisely and using a contemporary approach. There is also a moderately sized, up-to-date bibiliography, which serves as an excellent source for additional information on the subject. Dr. Tolo's attention to detail and his inclusion of all of the above components has resulted in the publication of an excellent comprehensive guide to Pediatric Orthopaedics.

G. Dean Mac Ewen, M.D.
Chairman, Pediatric Orthopaedic Surgery
Children's Hospital
New Orleans, Louisiana

Preface

This book is an excursion through the common muscular and skeletal disorders encountered in childhood and the teenage years. Musculoskeletal abnormalities account for approximately one-fifth of the office visits to primary-care physicians, following only respiratory infection in frequency. Increasingly, the responsibility for diagnosis and management of musculoskeletal conditions is being assumed by primary care providers, and it is essential for these physicians to possess the ability to recognize, evaluate, diagnose, and manage the many musculoskeletal problems encountered in childhood and adolescence.

The purpose of this book is to provide an introduction to the evaluation and initial management of musculoskeletal disorders in the pediatric age group and to serve as a quick reference text in the office or emergency room. Based on the authors' extensive clinical and teaching experience, this book is aimed toward helping the primary care physician arrive at the proper diagnosis by combining known anatomic features with physical examination findings and results of appropriate imaging studies. A particular emphasis is placed on sports injuries unique to the growing child.

As this book is intended to be inclusive of the pediatric orthopaedic conditions seen in everyday primary-care practice, exhaustive presentations of orthopaedic treatment have been avoided. Treatment appropriately provided by primary-care physicians has been emphasized. We have attempted to achieve inclusiveness and continuity of the text and subject material and to avoid overlapping.

Any undertaking such as this book involves considerable time away from our families. We thank them for their understanding and forbearance.

Contents

1

The Immature Skeletal System: How Is It Different?

The musculoskeletal system in a growing child is a dynamic one. Compared to bones in an adult, the child's skeletal system has the ability to heal fractures more quickly and to remodel bones after fracture healing is complete. These qualities in a growing child often make treating skeletal injury in the child easier than in a mature individual, provided the physician is able to recognize the limitations of this remodeling process.

Certain injuries that occur in children are not seen in normal adults. The long bones of children are more flexible due to a more porous cortex than in the adult. As a result, a child may present after an injury with a bent bone without an obvious fracture, and a bone scan showing increased tracer activity indicates that microfractures have occurred at the time of the plastic deformation of the injured bone. Residual bowing in the form of an acute plastic bowing fracture may be seen alone or accompanying a fracture of a paired bone (Fig. 1.1).

A further example is that of a torus or buckle fracture, an injury in which the cortex on the compression side of the bending bone buckles (Fig. 1.2), resembling the injury in an osteoporotic bone in an elderly patient. In the case of a buckle fracture, one must remember that substantial deformation of the bone has occurred prior to fracture. Accordingly, when one is casting the arm of a child with a buckle fracture, the cast needs to be applied in such a way as to prevent further displacement or angulation as the fracture heals.

The quintessential difference between immature and adult bone is the presence of the physis, or growth plate, at the ends of each long bone. The cartilage at the physis is the weak link in the skeletal system and is more liable to injury than the rest of the bone, adjacent ligaments, or tendons. When evaluating an injury to a growing child's extremity, the region that should be thoroughly assessed is the physis. Rather than a sprain or a ligamentous injury, there is more likely to be a physeal fracture, which may be nondisplaced.

The most widely used classification of fractures involving the growth plate is that developed by Salter and Harris. The Salter-Harris classification describes five types of physeal fractures (Fig. 1.3). The physis consists of several distinct zones that provide longitudinal bone growth (Figure 1.4). A type I fracture occurs primarily through the zone of hypertrophy of the growth plate cartilage. If the fracture is nondisplaced, the radiograph will appear normal or show slight growth plate widening (Fig. 1.5), but the child will have tenderness to palpation at the region of the growth plate. A type II fracture passes through the zone of hypertrophy of the physis but exits through the metaphysis, displacing a small fragment of metaphyseal bone that is visible on the radiographs (Fig. 1.6). Type III and IV frac-

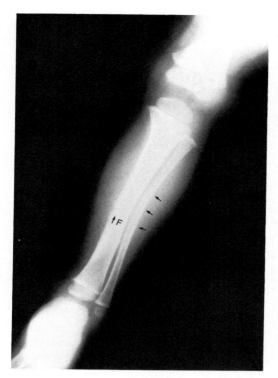

Figure 1.1.   Acute plastic bowing fracture of the fibula (*arrows*) and a transverse fracture (*F*) of the tibia secondary to deformation.

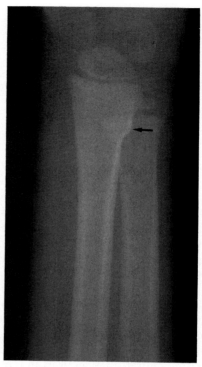

Figure 1.2.   Buckle fracture of the dorsal surface of the distal radius shows cortical buckling at the site of compression (*arrow*).

tures pass through the germinal layer or resting zone of the physis and exit through the articular cartilage in the adjacent joint. A type III fracture passes through a portion of the zone of hypertrophy of the physis before entering the joint (Fig. 1.7), while a type IV fracture begins at the articular surface, extends through the physis and exits out the metaphysis (Fig. 1.8). Both type III and IV injuries, if displaced at all, require surgical reduction to decrease the later likelihood of premature growth arrest and degenerative arthritis of the adjacent joint.

Type V physeal fractures are crush injuries and may not be detected at the time of the original injury. There is no displacement of the epiphysis or metaphysis in this injury, but later growth arrest at the site of the crush injury is commonplace. Any Salter fracture may later be found to have had a type V physeal injury (Fig. 1.9).

Children with physeal fractures need periodic follow-up for at least a year or two after the injury so that a growth arrest can be detected promptly, should one occur. Growth arrest may affect only a part of the

Figure 1.4.   The physis has several identifiable zones. The germinal cells reside on the epiphyseal side. As the growth cartilage cells proliferate, cell columns form. After passing through the hypertrophic stage, calcification begins in the septa between the cell columns. Finally, calcification continues to form bone on the metaphyseal side of the physis. Physeal fractures most commonly occur along the hypertrophic zone. If the fracture passes through the germinal layer, such as with Salter-Harris types III and IV, the potential for growth disturbance is greater.

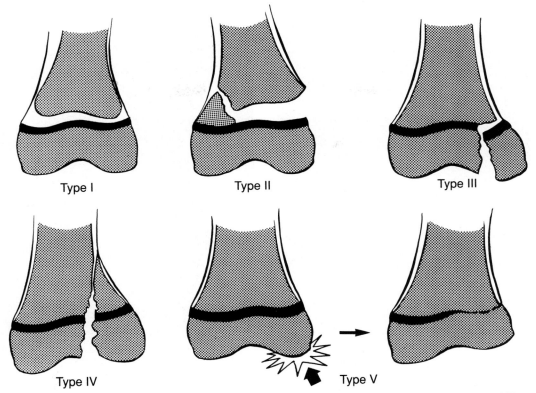

Figure 1.3. The Salter-Harris classification of physeal fractures contains five types. Types III, IV, and V are most likely to lead to growth disturbances and, if displaced, are best treated surgically.

Type I

Type II

Type III

Type IV

Type V

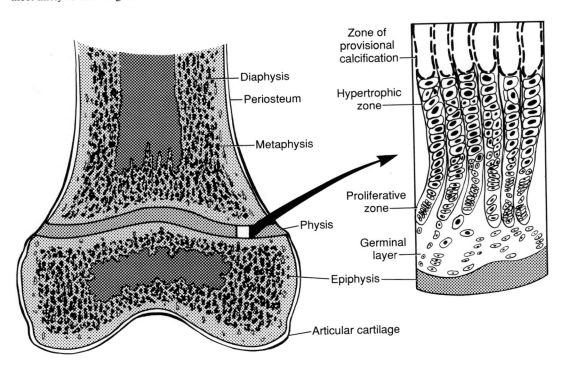

Diaphysis

Periosteum

Metaphysis

Physis

Epiphysis

Articular cartilage

Zone of provisional calcification

Hypertrophic zone

Proliferative zone

Germinal layer

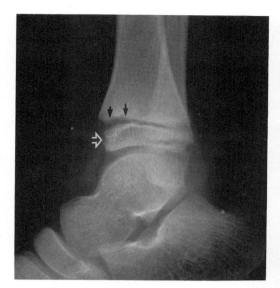

Figure 1.5. Salter-Harris type I fracture of the distal tibia shows widening of the anterior portion of the physis (*black arrows*) and posterior movement (*open white arrow*) of the epiphysis.

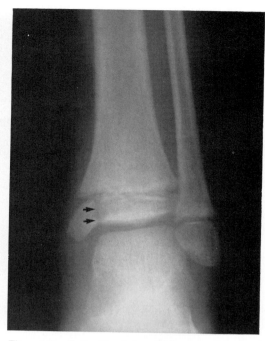

Figure 1.7. Salter-Harris type III fracture of the distal tibia (*arrows*) extends through the physis into the joint. There is medial angulation at the fracture site.

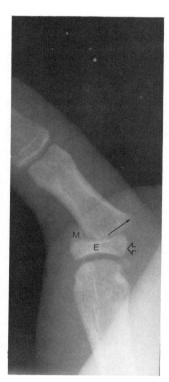

Figure 1.6. In this Salter-Harris type II fracture of the thumb, the epiphysis (*E*) is laterally located (*open arrow*). There is displacement of the shaft of the phalanx medially (*arrow*) as the result of a physeal fracture. Note the metaphyseal fragment (*M*).

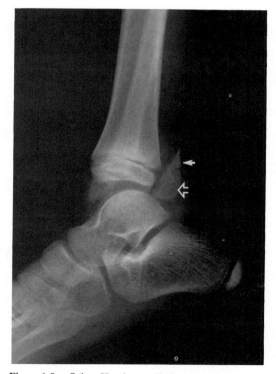

Figure 1.8. Salter-Harris type IV fracture of the ankle shows fragments of epiphysis (*open arrow*) and of metaphysis (*closed arrow*).

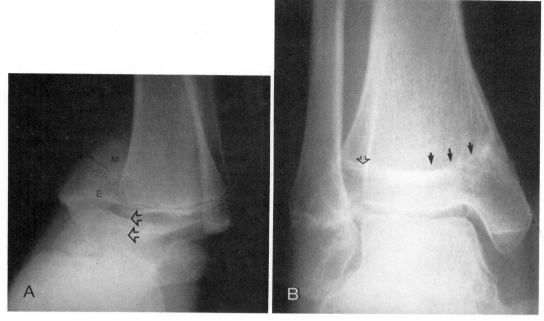

Figure 1.9. **A,** Salter-Harris type IV fracture of the distal tibia (*open arrows*) with marked medial displacement of the fragments of the epiphysis (*E*) and metaphysis (*M*). Physeal fracture of the distal fibula is also present. **B,** Eight months later the fracture has healed and the medial aspect of the physeal plate (*arrows*) has sealed. The lateral aspect of the physis (*open arrow*) remains open. (*Note:* Medial and lateral are reversed in **B.**)

physis, producing an angular deformity, or may stop all growth in the physis, resulting in a shortened extremity on the injured side.

Long-bone fractures in children between the ages of 2 and 12 years may affect leg length equality. In this age group, fractures of the femur or tibia usually produce growth stimulation of about 1 cm in the injured limb, reflecting accelerated growth as a response to hyperemia in the region of the fracture. This growth stimulation is largely complete by 18 months after a femur or tibia fracture, so follow-up of these fractures in the growing child should extend for approximately this period of time.

Many bones in the immature child have a secondary ossification center attached to the primary bone by cartilage, termed an apophysis, similar in cellular architecture to the growth plate or physis. These secondary ossification centers often serve as insertion sites for tendons and are as susceptible to

injury as the physis. Apophyseal injuries occur primarily at the elbow, pelvis, knee, and foot.

In nontraumatic disorders, the physis also plays a major role in the progression and resolution of many orthopaedic conditions. Nutritional deficiencies such as rickets will affect physeal formation and growth, leading to angular deformity or short bones. Skeletal dysplasias produce short stature largely from aberrations in the physeal growth. Since osteomyelitis usually begins adjacent to the physis, growth arrest is frequent if some infections are not diagnosed and treated quickly.

In evaluating children for musculoskeletal disorders, the dynamic nature of the child's bone must always be considered. As will be demonstrated in the chapters that follow, this capacity of the child's bone for growth and for remodeling, combined with the vulnerability of the growth plate to injury, will be key factors in assessing our young patients' musculoskeletal problems.

Suggested Readings

Brighton, C.T.: Longitudinal bone growth: The growth plate and its dysfunctions. In Griffin, P.P. (ed.): American Academy of Orthopaedic Surgeons *Instructional Course Lectures, XXXVI*. Park Ridge, IL, American Academy of Orthopaedic Surgeons, 1987, pp. 3-25.

Hensinger, R.N. and Jones, E.T.: Growth and early development of the musculoskeletal system. In *Neonatal Orthopaedics*, New York, Grune & Stratton, 1981, pp. 5-13.

Light, T.R., Ogden, D.A., and Ogden, J.A.: The anatomy of metaphyseal torus fractures. Clin. Orthop. 188:103-111, 1984.

Mabrey, J.D. and Fitch, R.D.: Plastic deformation in pediatric fractures: Mechanism and treatment. J. Pediatr. Orthop. 9:310-314, 1989.

Maroteaux, P.: *Bone Diseases of Children*. Philadelphia, J.B. Lippincott, 1979.

Ogden, J.A.: The uniqueness of growing bones. In Rockwood, C.A., Jr., Wilkins, K.E., and King, R.E. (eds.): *Fractures in Children*. Philadelphia, J.B. Lippincott, 1983, volume 3, pp. 1-86.

Ogden, J.A.: Development and maturation of the neuromusculoskeletal system. In Morrissy, R.T. (ed.): *Lovell and Winter's Pediatric Orthopaedics*, 3rd edition. Philadelphia, J.B. Lippincott, 1990.

Ogden, J.A.: Anatomy and physiology of skeletal development. In *Skeletal Injury in the Child*. Philadelphia, Lea & Febiger, 1982, pp. 16-40.

Salter, R.B. and Harris, W.R.: Injuries involving the epiphyseal plate. J. Bone Joint Surg. 45A:587-622, 1963.

Wilson, F.C. (ed.): *The Musculoskeletal System: Basic Processes and Disorders*, 2nd edition. Philadelphia, J.B. Lippincott, 1983.

2
Clinical Imaging in Pediatrics: The Musculoskeletal System

In the past decade imaging of the pediatric musculoskeletal system has improved remarkably, largely as a result of the advent of more sophisticated methods of body imaging. Structures previously invisible have become readily visible, and radiologists have learned specific imaging characteristics that allow tissue and lesion identification. Future developments in the use of contrast materials, the ability to evaluate biochemical processes in vivo, and three-dimensional and cine capabilities will eventuate in more sensitive spatial diagnosis of abnormalities and follow-up evaluation of therapy.

Imaging Techniques in Children

PLAIN FILM RADIOGRAPHY

The plain film radiograph remains the least expensive and the most sensitive and reliable predictor of a lesion. It is the initial study for virtually all patients with suspected musculoskeletal abnormality, and when paired with knowledge of the patient's age, sex, and clinical presentation it is a most reliable method of characterization in the diagnosis of musculoskeletal diseases. A minimum of two projections at right angles are required. Improvements in high detail and faster film-screen combinations, small focal spot size, and lower exposure times have resulted in studies of excellent quality with lower radiation doses to the patient. Special techniques used include the

use of a small focal spot (0.3 or 0.15 mm) with geometric magnification and various types of tomography.

FLUOROSCOPY AND ARTHROGRAPHY

Fluoroscopy is used to evaluate motion at a joint or relationships between bones. It is also helpful as a guide in aspiration of a joint or for biopsy of a lesion. Joint arthrography is used less frequently, since magnetic resonance imaging has proved to be valuable in the assessment of structures within and surrounding the joint. Nonetheless, this technique may be used when performance of magnetic resonance studies is not practical or when a dynamic study is needed to assess joint injury or function.

ULTRASONOGRAPHY

High-resolution real-time ultrasound, achieved with the use of high-frequency transducers, has resulted in enhanced workup of patients with lesions in the subcutaneous tissues, muscles, tendons, joint spaces, and cartilage. Real-time monitoring of joint motion is particularly useful in the infant hip, assessed for the early diagnosis of congenital dislocation. Joint effusions and acute injuries involving muscles and tendons can be diagnosed by the use of ultrasound. Subcutaneous or intramuscular foreign bodies are also visualized and localized by use of ultrasound. Ultrasound has proved to be helpful in identifying stress fractures, in which the cortical fracture and subperiosteal hematoma are visualized.

COMPUTED TOMOGRAPHY

Computed tomography (CT) is an excellent and accurate method for demonstration of bone involvement by an extrinsic soft tissue mass or infection, bone destruction from an extrinsic or intrinsic cause, reactive change, extent of infection and trauma, and secondary effects of trauma. Characterization of these lesions—including evaluation of their extent and margination, involvement of surrounding structures, necrosis, and calcification—is easily assessed by CT. CT is an excellent method for the evaluation of vertebral and paravertebral lesions and provides assessment of spinal canal involvement. In the evaluation of lesions of the flat bones such as the pelvis, scapula, and sternum, CT is the imaging method of choice, providing information not obtained by other means.

MAGNETIC RESONANCE

Magnetic resonance (MR) has proved to be extremely useful in the evaluation of many organ systems of the body. Musculoskeletal applications of MR are among the fastest growing uses of this modality. The multiplanar imaging capability, the ability to differentiate different tissue types, possible tissue characterization, blood flow evaluation, and some indication of the biochemistry and physiology of specific tissue have made magnetic resonance an imaging modality with enormous potential. Excellent musculoskeletal imaging is achieved with the use of magnets with high, mid, or low field strength. The use of surface radiofrequency coils that may receive, or transmit and receive, adapted to the body part to be imaged and new capabilities, including three-dimensional acquisition and fast scan sequences based on gradient reversals are important features in muscular and skeletal imaging. Cine MR is used to evaluate joint motion. Like CT and ultrasound, MR provides excellent resolution and sensitive differentiation of tissue types. Magnetic resonance is particularly helpful in identifying occult abnormalities that are not visualized by other imaging techniques and in identifying cartilage, muscle, tendon, and joint capsule, which are impossible or difficult to image by other techniques. Experimental investigation of the maturing bone marrow has led to bone marrow imaging of specific replacement or destructive processes and assessment of repopulation of the marrow.

Patient Sedation and Restraint

Plain film radiography and ultrasound are easily accomplished without the need for sedation. Careful patient restraint and positioning are required for optimum examination in both modalities. Perfect positioning and the removal of any overlying, possibly obscuring clothing are important. It is not acceptable for patients to be held during radiographic procedures; thus a number of effective restraining devices have been developed. These include boards with Velcro straps, sheets, tape, Ace bandages, and related materials. Ultrasound examination rarely requires restraint further than holding the child, sometimes with the help of a parent or an assistant and with bottle feeding of babies to quiet the infant. In any situation, it is obvious that obtaining the cooperation of the child is an ideal way of obtaining optimum examinations. Very young or agitated patients require sedation, particularly for the longer imaging times of MR and CT. Again, careful and perfect positioning, secure restraints, careful patient monitoring, and sometimes sedation are required. Sedation with chloral hydrate administered orally is sufficient for children below the age of 6 months or some older children who are anxious. Children between the ages of 6 months and 4 to 5 years are most effectively sedated by the intravenous route. Nembutal (pentobarbital) administered intravenously in a dosage that is titrated carefully over 5 to 15 minutes is administered for a total dose between 2 and 6 mg/kg of body weight. The length of sedation with pentobarbital is approximately 1 hour, which is sufficient for a good examination. Patient monitoring for possible hypoxemia is important. Other intravenous or rectal sedating pharmaceuticals, including Valium, fentanyl, and midazolam are favored by some radiologists.

Contrast Material

An intravenous bolus of contrast material is extremely helpful in CT examination for evaluation of specific vascular structures, vascular supply to a lesion, or the general vascular nature of a lesion. An enhancing rim is often the sign of an inflammatory lesion. Some tumors are hypervascular. Contrast material is less helpful and only occasionally required for bony lesions. Gadolinium (gadopentetate dimeglumine) is the MR contrast medium currently FDA-approved and utilized in inflammatory lesions, tumors, arthritis, and subtle soft tissue lesions. This contrast material enhancement is of great value in identifying soft tissue tumors, inflammation, and masses within the spinal canal.

Imaging Abnormalities

CONGENITAL ABNORMALITIES

Congenital dislocation of the hip, acetabular dysplasias, and skeletal deficiencies that are initially present as cartilaginous abnormalities require carefully planned intervention early in life. Diagnosis and evaluation of these entities are not easily achieved by plain film radiography because of the lack of ossification in the epiphyseal centers of the young child. In the infant with suspected congenital dislocation of the hip, plain film radiography is of little or no value, as the structures in question cannot be visualized. Real-time ultrasound is the method of choice for evaluation of the congenitally dislocated hip. The femoral head and acetabulum are mostly cartilaginous, and ultrasound examination allows visualization and multiplanar evaluation of these structures. Detection of changes in the position of the

femoral head and its relationship to the acetabulum are possible by assessment with real-time ultrasound. Performance of the ultrasound examination in the transverse neutral view and coronal view with flexion of the hip results in visualization of the location, and possible dislocation, of the femoral head. This examination is more sensitive than the physical examination and is also used to evaluate capsular laxity of the hip that is subluxing but not dislocating. Magnetic resonance examination of the hip in the coronal and axial planes is valuable in complex congenital dislocation of the hip—those that are not reducible or that dislocate again following closed reduction. In these patients the infolded labrum and inverted, infolded joint capsule as well as an interposed psoas muscle tendon may be detected and guide surgical intervention. CT examination of the hip in dislocation is of limited usefulness; however, in infants in casts, several axial sections through the femoral head are useful to evaluate the resultant alignment of the femoral head with the acetabulum.

Congenital anomalies of limbs may be difficult to define without obtaining specific information concerning cartilaginous structures and muscular attachments. Complete absence of bony structure or a portion of a structure, such as in proximal focal femoral deficiency, may be evaluated by ultrasound examination for identification of a cartilaginous femoral head or a cartilaginous portion of the bone. Such identification is helpful in planning therapy. Absence or duplications of rays, portions of paired bones, carpals, metacarpals, or tarsal bones is an important predictor for the orthopaedist, and magnetic resonance imaging is valuable in yielding information concerning the cartilaginous structures of the limb, the status of articulation, and the degree of development of muscles and tendons associated with that portion of the limb. Pseudarthrosis may have cartilage or no cartilage connecting the two portions of the bones, and delineation is of important predictive value. Absence of the growth plate or portions of the growth plate secondary to a congenital abnormality, trauma, or infection can be identified by careful high-resolution magnetic resonance studies of the growth plate.

INFECTION (Soft Tissue or Muscle Infection, Septic Arthritis, Osteomyelitis, Periostitis)

Children with musculoskeletal infections present with limitation of motion, irritability, and sometimes fever, an elevated white blood cell count, and an elevated erythrocyte sedimentation rate. Because the management of each of the above entities is different, radiologic imaging is of vital importance in determining patient management and predicting outcome. In the search for infection, the three-phase bone scan remains the most sensitive and specific method of identification of the nature and extent of infection. Children with suspected osteomyelitis on physical examination should initially be imaged with plain film examination, followed by laboratory evaluation, and then nuclear scintigraphy. (However, treatment should not be delayed until all these studies are obtained if they are not quickly available.) It may be important to obtain further studies for evaluation of the exact morphology and location of infection, the effect on surrounding structures or tissues, the long-term effects of infection, and specific complications. Ultrasound examination is helpful in the localization of cellulitis, the identification of deep soft tissue infection, and the detection of an abscess. Periostitis is seen as a thin layer of fluid beside the periosteum. Joint fluid may be indicative of septic arthritis and may be tapped for culture. Osteomyelitis itself is not easily discernible by ultrasound examination. CT examination is useful in the identification of chronic osteomyelitis, for localization of the nidus, and possible aspiration for culture. Osteomyelitis is readily identified by magnetic resonance examination. If chemical shift lipid suppression techniques

are used the intramedullary high signal (short T1) is identifiable within the bone marrow. Breakthrough of the cortex is easily identified and surrounding tissue inflammation is also seen. As with ultrasound, the presence of a joint effusion can be identified easily by using the arthrogram-like effect of fluid on T2-weighted imaging.

TRAUMA

Plain film radiography in two planes is the study of choice for evaluation of all skeletal trauma. In most cases, this is perfectly adequate for the diagnosis of trauma and guidance in treatment. In addition to fractures and dislocations, traumatic effusions may be visualized by plain film and suspected ligamentous or physeal injuries may be revealed by stress views. Subtle or occult trauma may be visualized by obtaining supplementary radiographs. Nuclear scintigraphy is extremely useful, with bone scanning brought into use in the diagnosis of subtle fractures or multiple unsuspected fractures such as occur in child abuse. Although it is not usually utilized for evaluation of subtle fractures, ultrasound examination will identify surrounding edema and hematoma, subperiosteal hemorrhage, and cortical breaks. Magnetic resonance imaging is also helpful, T1-weighted imaging being utilized to identify stress fractures or occult fractures not visible on biplanar radiography. These fractures are commonly seen as a linear area of low signal intensity surrounded by high signal intensity on T1-weighted images. Surrounding hematoma and edema are identified. Although MR is not usually utilized in such cases, it is helpful in differentiating fracture from infection or malignancy. In children who are extremely osteoporotic (such as those with underlying metabolic bone disease or osteogenesis imperfecta or who are undergoing chemotherapy for treatment of malignancy), a stress fracture may not be readily visible except by this means.

Injuries to the Achilles tendon are imaged using high-frequency linear array transducers in ultrasound. In the case of muscle hematoma, organized blood clot generates internal echoes, while clot lysis and unclotted blood produce an anechoic appearance. Hematomas may have well-defined or irregular margins and may contain internal septae. Muscular hemorrhage is usually associated with focal or diffuse muscle enlargement. Tears of the Achilles tendon are identified as transverse hypoechoic bands within the tendon.

MR imaging is particularly helpful in evaluating children with Salter-Harris fractures in whom growth plate interruption or unsuspected cartilaginous fracture is present. T1-weighted spin echo sequences or T2-weighted gradient echo images in the coronal plane will identify both types of fracture. Separation of the physis or injury to the physis with the potential of subsequent growth abnormality is identified by this technique. Improved imaging of injuries to the growth plate will lead to earlier intervention and perhaps better long-term results.

Post-traumatic osteochondral lesions are identified as occult subcortical fractures, a nidus of trauma, in the chondral epiphysis of children. These regions are seen on sagittal and coronal T1-weighted images, usually in the lateral joint compartment, and are present in patients with known hemarthrosis. These are occult osteochondral impaction fractures and may frequently be associated with significant meniscal or ligamentous injuries, though alone they rarely require treatment.

Nonopaque soft tissue or intracapsular foreign bodies are visualized by ultrasound examination using high-frequency transducers. A foreign body is easily identified as hyperechoic with clearly defined focus and acoustic shadowing. Only the proximal surface of the foreign body is evident, so the exact size cannot be determined. Sonographic guidance for removal is helpful.

Injuries to the menisci and tendons are well defined by magnetic resonance imaging using surface coils. Magnetic resonance imaging of the knee has obviated the need for arthrography in most patients for evaluation of meniscal tears and cruciate ligament tears as well as traumatic defects of the articular surface. Magnetic resonance imaging of the knee in children is helpful in evaluating co-existing congenital abnormalities of the menisci leading to early degenerative change and tears. Examination of injuries to the anterior and posterior cruciate ligaments are ideally performed with imaging planes that are exactly perpendicular and parallel to these ligaments. Thus, the sagittal and tilted coronal views are of major importance for evaluating the cruciate ligament. Collateral ligament injuries are also identified, as are muscle hematomas.

Suggested Readings

Adam, G., Dammer, M., Bohndoft, K., Christoph, R., Fenke, F., Gunther, RW.: Rheumatoid arthritis of the knee: Value of gadopentetate dimeglumine-enhanced MR imaging. AJR 156:125-129, 1991.

Beltran, J.: MRI of the musculoskeletal system. Appl. Radiol. 23-32, 1990.

Berquist, T.H., Ehman, R.L., King, B.F., Hodgman, C.G., Ilstrup, D.M.: Value of MR imaging in differentiating benign from malignant soft-tissue masses: Study of 95 lesions. AJR 155:1251-1255, 1990.

Dock, W., Happak, W., Grabenwoger, F., Toifl, K., et al.: Neuromuscular diseases: Evaluation with high-frequency sonography. Radiology 177:825-828, 1990.

Harcke, H.T., Grisson, L.E.: Performing dynamic sonography of the infant hip. AJR 155:837-844, 1990.

Jaramillo, D., Hoffer, F.A., Shapiro, F., Rand, F.: MR imaging of fractures of the growth plate. AJR 155:1261-1265, 1990.

Jelinek, J.S., Kransdorf, M.J., Moser, R.P., et al.: MR imaging findings in patients with bone-chip allografts. AJR 155:1257-1260, 1990.

Kaplan, P.A., Matamoros, A. Jr., Anderson, J.C.: Sonography of the musculoskeletal system. AJR 155:237-245, 1990.

Lee, J.K.T., Glazer, H.S.: Controversy in the MR imaging appearance of fibrosis. Radiology 177:21-22, 1990.

Mitchell, D.G.: Using MR imaging to probe the pathophysiology of osteonecrosis. Radiology 171:25-26, 1989.

Moore, S.G., Dawson, K.L.: Red and yellow marrow in the femur: Age-related changes in appearance at MR imaging. Radiology 175:219-223, 1990.

Negendank, W.G., Al-Katib, A.M., Karanes, C., Smith, M.R.: Lymphomas: MR imaging contrast characteristics with clinical-pathologic correlations. Radiology 177:209-216, 1990.

Okada, Y., Aoki, S., Barkovich, A.J., et al.: Cranial bone marrow in children: Assessment of normal development with MR imaging. Radiology 171:161-164, 1989.

Pay, N.T., Singer, W.S., Bartal, E.: Hip pain in three children accompanied by transient abnormal findings on MR images. Radiology 171:147-149, 1989.

Ricci, C., Cova, M., Kang, Y.S., et al.: Normal age-related patterns of cellular and fatty bone marrow distribution in the axial skeleton: MR imaging study. Radiology 177:83-88, 1990.

Stevens, S.K., Moore, S.G., Amylon, M.D.: Repopulation of marrow after transplantation: MR imaging with pathologic correlation. Radiology 175:213-218, 1990.

Sundaram, M., McLeod, R.A.: MR imaging of tumor and tumorlike lesions of bone and soft tissue. AJR 155:817-824, 1990.

Teele, R.L., Share, J.C.: Ultrasonography of Infants and Children. Philadelphia, W.B. Saunders, 1991.

Turner, D.A., Templeton, A.C., Selzer, P.M., Rosenberg, A.G., Petasnick, J.P.: Femoral capital osteonecrosis: MR finding of diffuse marrow abnormalities without focal lesions. Radiology 171:135-140, 1989.

Vellet, A.D., Marks, P.H., Fowler, P.J., Munro, T.G.: Occult posttraumatic osteochondral lesions of the knee: Prevalence, classification, and short-term sequelae evaluated with MR imaging. Radiology 178:271-276, 1991.

Vogler, J.B. III, Murphy, W.A.: Bone marrow imaging. Radiology 168:679-693, 1988.

Weinreb, J.C.: MR imaging of bone marrow: A map could help. Radiology 177:23-24, 1990.

3
Neck

Anatomy

The seven cervical vertebrae, the sterno-cleidomastoid and trapezius muscles, and the adjacent neurologic structures are the primary anatomic structures of concern in musculoskeletal evaluation of the neck.

The upper two cervical vertebrae are specialized, while the other five can be thought of as being similar to each other (Fig. 3.1). The atlas, or first cervical vertebra, has superior articulations that closely match the occipital condyles at the base of the skull. With solid support of the skull as the main role of this vertebra, there is little movement at this articulation in the normal child. Inferiorly, the atlas articulates with the axis facets and is bound to the anterior axis by strong ligamentous structures.

The anterior portion of the axis, or second cervical vertebra, is the odontoid process, which is formed embryologically by an amalgamation of the anlage of the vertebral bodies for the first and second cervical vertebrae as well as the fourth occipital level. This anatomic feature produces synchondroses between these three levels prior to final ossification in late childhood. The articulation between the first and second cervical vertebrae is normally quite mobile both in flexion and in rotation, accounting for almost half of the rotation of the head in normal movement.

The lower five cervical vertebrae are similar in size, shape, and function. The ma-jority of neck flexion takes place here and each articulation level contributes an equal share. The remainder of neck rotation is also distributed fairly equivalently.

While several small neck muscles are present throughout the neck, the two with the most orthopaedic relevance are the ster-nocleidomastoid and the trapezius muscles. The sternocleidomastoid, as its name im-plies, originates at the mastoid and has a dual insertion into the clavicle and the ster-num. Because of the mastoid attachment, shortening of this muscle leads to head rota-tion away from the contracted muscle and head tilt toward the side of shortening. The trapezius, innervated by the eleventh cra-nial nerve, runs from the base of the skull to its attachment on the scapula and upper thoracic spine. This muscle is important for efficient shoulder movement and is often the region to which pain from the cervical spine is referred.

While serving as a mobile but stable sup-port for the head, the neck also functions to protect the neural structures here. Nerve roots exit at each level to provide arm motor and sensory function. The first cervical nerve root exits between the skull and the atlas and all cervical nerve roots exit above the vertebra with the same number, except at the seventh cervical vertebra, where the C7 nerve root exits above and the C8 nerve root exits below the vertebra. While some overlap exists, the knowledge of the motor and sensory level for each nerve root level

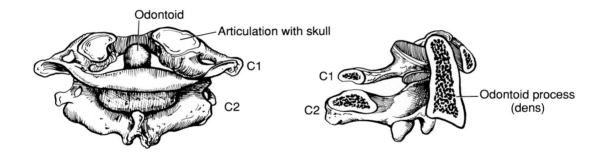

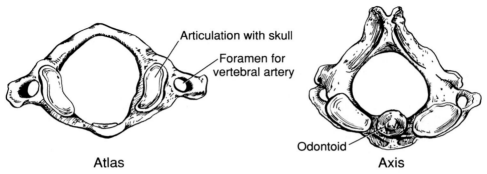

Figure 3.1. The upper two cervical vertebrae are the atlas and axis. The atlas supports the skull, and little movement takes place at the atlanto-occipital joint. The ring of the atlas or C1 surrounds the odontoid process of the axis; instability at this level may lead to spinal cord compression. Approximately 50% of the rotation of the head occurs at the atlantoaxial joint.

will enable a more clear-cut diagnosis of possible neural injury associated with neck trauma.

Physical Examination

The neck examination consists of observation of the surface features, evaluation of range of motion, palpation of the neck, and neurologic examination of the extremities.

OBSERVATION

Is the head held straight? Is the hairline low or does the neck appear short? Are skin markings (e.g., hemangiomata or café-au-lait spots) present to indicate some systemic condition? Is there facial asymmetry?

RANGE OF MOTION

Except in conditions of acute trauma, six planes of motion should be checked: lateral rotation to left and right, lateral flexion to left and right, and flexion and extension. Painless limitation of all neck motion should suggest a congenital abnormality of the cervical spine. Limitation of rotation alone might point to an atlantoaxial problem, while a deficit of lateral flexion most commonly occurs in torticollis and congenital cervical scoliosis. All motions of the neck should normally be painless.

In the case of acute trauma to the head or neck, the child should be kept supine with the head in a neutral position with lateral support. Flexion positions must be avoided. Because of the large head size relative to the body in children under 5 years old, care should be taken in using adult transport stretchers, since the neck can easily be placed in flexion, a position that is to be avoided with acute injury. Full range of motion should not be tested in the acute situation. Gentle range of motion testing may be appropriate after lateral cervical spine radiographs have demonstrated no unstable injury.

PALPATION

Manual examination of the paraspinous muscles and the sternocleidomastoids may demonstrate spasm or contracture to help make the definitive diagnosis. Point tenderness along the spinous processes should be sought, as this may indicate an interspinous ligament tear.

NEUROLOGIC EXAMINATION

Motor and sensory examinations, as well as reflex evaluation, of *both* the upper and lower extremities are essential as a part of the evaluation of the neck. Hyperreflexia may be the only early finding of spinal cord compression due to chronic neck instability, since muscle strength testing and sensory evaluation depend on strong patient cooperation for valid results.

Normal Radiologic Findings

In the newborn infant and during the first 6 months of life, the ossification of the cervical spine is slight compared to the bulk of cartilage within the vertebrae and their posterior elements. The ossification centers of the vertebral bodies are seen as small, ovoid osseous structures. With increasing maturity, the vertebral bodies develop a more trapezoidal shape than the expected rectangular configuration seen in older children and teenagers. The vertebral body size increases progressively and the amount of ossification increases proportionately.

In the infant and young child, there is considerably greater mobility of the cervical

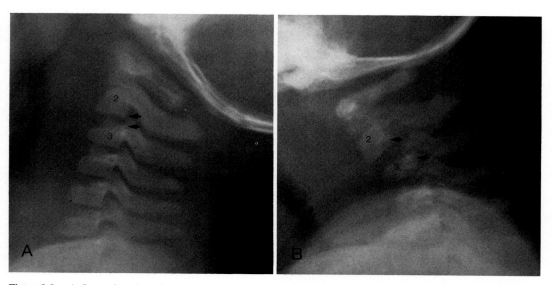

Figure 3.2. **A,** Lateral neck radiograph in neutral position with normal posterior alignment of the vertebral bodies of C2 and C3. Note also that the vertebral body ossification in the other cervical levels occurs last normally in the anterior superior aspect, a finding that may simulate a compression fracture. **B,** Lateral neck radiograph of normal child in flexion shows forward motion of C2 on C3 with an offset of the posterior borders (*arrows*). Up to 3 mm of forward motion with flexion is normal in the young child.

spine than is seen in the adult. This is reflected by increased motion of the arch of C1 upon the odontoid, with resultant wider spacing between the odontoid and C1 than is seen in the more mature spine; for this measurement up to 5 millimeters of space is considered normal. Increased flexibility of the cervical spine in the young child will often result in increased forward shift of the vertebral body of C2 on C3 of up to 3 mm, producing a "pseudosubluxation" appearance (Fig. 3.2).

Neck Disorders

CONGENITAL CONDITIONS

Klippel-Feil Syndrome

Described first in France in the mid 1800s, this inherited condition is most readily diagnosed by the radiologic finding of fusion of two or more cervical vertebrae due to lack of segmentation during embryologic development (Fig. 3.3). Pain is usually absent, and the primary concerns of the child or parents are the cosmetic appearance and the limitation of neck movement.

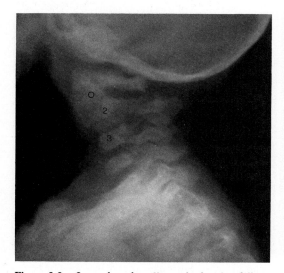

Figure 3.3. Lateral neck radiograph showing failure of vertebral segmentation with fusion of C2 and C3. There is only a vestigial disc space remaining and there is fusion of the laminae.

Physical examination will demonstrate a short neck and limitation of motion in all planes, with the stiffness of the neck dependent on the number of fused segments present. In about 20% of those affected, hearing may be impaired, and in many synkinesis or mirror movements of the hands will be seen. Shoulder evaluation is needed, as the child may have associated congenital elevation of the scapula (Sprengel's deformity) with limited shoulder abduction present on examination. An omovertebral bone is sometimes present, further limiting both neck and shoulder motion.

Aids in evaluating the seriousness of this condition in the individual child include flexion-extension cervical spine radiographs and magnetic resonance (MR) performed with the neck in a flexed position. Instability at the levels above and below the fused vertebrae occurs with increasing frequency as age increases. Flexion/extension lateral cervical radiographs will quantitate any instability present, and the flexion MR image will most clearly demonstrate any spinal cord compression present. As with all children with congenital spinal anomalies, a renal sonogram is essential to assess associated genitourinary anomalies, found in approximately one-third of these children.

The treatment of Klippel-Feil syndrome is often simple serial follow-up and re-evaluation, particularly if no neurological signs or symptoms are present. In fact, treatment of associated problems, such as the Sprengel's deformity, may take precedence. If neurologic abnormalities are noted, surgical fusion of the unstable level is generally needed.

This condition takes on special significance when evaluating a child for possible sports participation. Limited neck range of motion is a *contraindication* to sports participation in collision or high-contact sports that could lead to a sudden forceful flexion of the neck. This is particularly true here when latent instability may be present from hypermobility at the unfused cervical levels as the child ages. Non-contact sports are usually appropriate for these children. Since neck flexion is the position that may lead to neurologic injury, a towel or modified soft collar is sometimes worn during sports to limit neck flexion should a fall occur while playing.

Children with Klippel-Feil syndrome should be referred to an orthopaedist for follow-up, even though this may be needed only every year or two, primarily for initial assessment of associated orthopaedic conditions and for periodic evaluation of neck instability.

Down Syndrome

More scientifically called trisomy 21 syndrome, this generalized condition has asso-

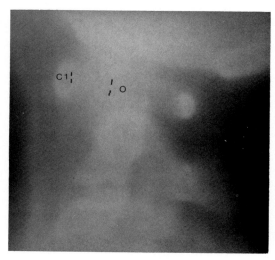

Figure 3.5. A lateral tomogram of C1 and C2 in an infant with Down syndrome shows abnormal anterior motion of the C1 ring. The *dotted lines* indicate the separation between the anterior arch of C1 and the odontoid (*O*).

ciated atlantoaxial instability in 20 to 30% of the children. This seems to cause no discernible neck pain, and the physical examination of the neck is normal. The parents may have noted some change in the child's ability to walk long distances. The first extremity finding on physical examination is usually hyperreflexia of either the upper or lower extremities.

All children with Down syndrome require screening with lateral flexion and extension cervical spine x-rays prior to participation in the Special Olympics program. Up to 30% of these children have greater than 5 mm of movement at the atlantoaxial level and about 10% have more than 10 mm of motion at this level (Figs. 3.4 and 3.5). An MR image will most clearly define spinal cord compression, particularly if the patient's neck is flexed when the lateral MR images are obtained.

If a child with Down syndrome has abnormal neurologic findings with any degree of atlantoaxial instability, surgical fusion is needed. If a child has 5 to 10 mm of atlantoaxial motion and is neurologically normal,

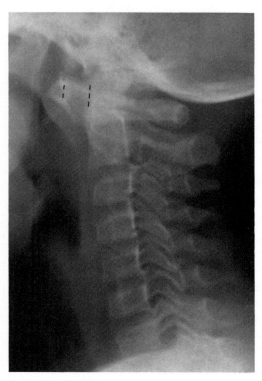

Figure 3.4. Lateral neck radiograph of a child with Down syndrome shows abnormal anterior motion of C1 on C2, indicating ligamentous laxity. *Dotted lines* indicate the posterior margin of the anterior C1 arch and the anterior aspect of the odontoid. If this space is greater than 5 mm, ligamentous laxity is present.

careful periodic neurologic evaluation appears appropriate. Instability greater than 10 mm should be treated with fusion even if the child is asymptomatic or free of neurologic deficits. Lateral flexion and extension x-rays of the cervical spine should be repeated periodically (about every 5 years) during growth in children with Down syndrome, as later cervical instability has been demonstrated in children who previously had normal flexion radiographs of the neck.

Hemivertebrae or Congenital Cervical Scoliosis

Failure of vertebral body formation or partial failure of disc segmentation may lead to scoliosis or angular deformity of the spine in the neck as well as in the thoracic and lumbar spines. Pain is rarely present and the primary parental concern is the head position.

Physical examination findings include a head tilt without tightness of the sternocleidomastoid and limited lateral flexion away from the side toward which the head is tilted. Associated facial findings may include branchial cleft defects in the mouth or ear regions (Goldenhar's syndrome). The thoracolumbar spine should be carefully assessed (Fig. 3.6).

The definitive diagnosis is made by an anteroposterior cervical spine radiograph. If a hemivertebra is seen here, a full spinal radiograph should be obtained because of the high incidence of other spinal abnormalities that occur with hemivertebrae. Over 30% of children with congenital scoliosis have anomalies of the genitourinary system, with unilateral renal agenesis being the most common; therefore all these children should be screened with a renal ultrasound. Since approximately 30% also have an abnormal MR of the spinal cord, careful ongoing neurologic assessment throughout growth is essential. A magnetic resonance imaging study of the spine is generally reserved for those with neurologic abnormalities on ex-

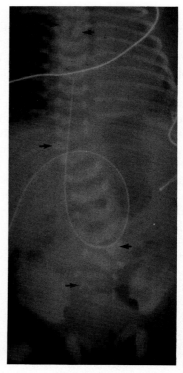

Figure 3.6. Anteroposterior radiograph of the spine of a newborn infant with multiple congenital anomalies, including anal atresia and esophageal atresia, shows multiple hemivertebrae (*arrows*).

amination or in children who have surgical spinal fusion planned.

The treatment for cervical hemivertebrae is periodic radiologic assessment in an attempt to detect worsening of this curvature. The child should be referred to a pediatric orthopaedist for this follow-up, which consists of careful evaluation of cervical x-rays at 1- to 2-year intervals. If worsening of 10° or more is noted, surgical fusion is indicated. Bracing has little or no role in the treatment of this type of scoliosis. If surgery is planned, an MR image should be obtained preoperatively to assess for possible spinal cord anomalies. Little correction can be obtained from surgery, but prevention of further deformity with continued growth can be anticipated following surgery.

If only one motion segment of the neck is involved with a hemivertebra, neck range of motion may appear normal on examination. In this case, sports participation is usually appropriate, though if the child has only one kidney, collision and contact sports are discouraged. If neck stiffness is seen from multiple cervical spine anomalies, restrictions from contact sports is advised.

TORTICOLLIS

Torticollis or "wry neck" may result from a number of causes. In this condition, the child will hold the head tilted laterally toward one shoulder, with the chin rotated away from that shoulder. Torticollis is the physical sign of an underlying problem, usually due to one of these causes: muscular fibrosis, the presence of a hemivertebra, or atlantoaxial rotatory subluxation.

In a newborn or an infant, the most common cause of torticollis is *fibrosis of the sternocleidomastoid muscle*. A fusiform swelling within this muscle may be present at birth or shortly thereafter. The etiology of the resultant fibrosis remains unclear, although various causes have been suggested, including birth trauma and ischemia due to the intrauterine position of the head and neck. Whether it is seen at birth or later, physical examination reveals enlargement of the sternocleidomastoid muscle on the side toward which the head is laterally tilted. Since the sternocleidomastoid muscle originates from the mastoid bone of the skull, contracture or shortening of this muscle will tilt the head toward the fibrotic muscle and rotate the chin and face away from this abnormal muscle. Facial asymmetry or plagiocephaly is present, being most noticeable in children not diagnosed until early childhood. Since there is a slightly higher incidence of developmental dysplasia of the hip in children with muscular torticollis, the hips need to be carefully evaluated in these children.

The role of imaging studies in the newborn or infant with torticollis is relatively small. Anteroposterior and lateral radiographs of the cervical spine should be normal except for the rotation at C1-C2 related to the torticollis position. A magnetic resonance scan or an ultrasound study (Fig. 3.7) will demonstrate evidence of fibrous tissue within the sternocleidomastoid muscle, but they are not generally needed to make this diagnosis.

If the diagnosis of muscular torticollis is

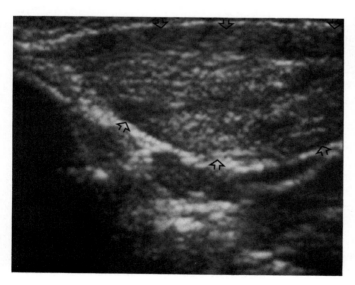

Figure 3.7. Ultrasound examination of an infant with torticollis from muscular fibrosis shows a mixed echogenic, bulbous sternomastoid muscle (*open arrows*).

made in the newborn or infant period, treatment consists of stretching exercises performed at home by the parents. It is generally useful to have a physical therapist instruct the parents in the proper stretching technique and then to review this with the parents a few months later. Often stretching exercises need to be continued for several months until the neck range of motion returns to normal. If normal range of motion is obtained by 1 year of age and maintained thereafter, the facial asymmetry should resolve. Bracing in this age group is not usually needed. Failure to regain a full range of neck motion will lead to persistent facial asymmetry, especially of the ears, eyes, and cheeks.

In older children with persistent or previously undiagnosed muscular torticollis, surgical lengthening of the affected sternocleidomastoid is indicated. Although some of the facial asymmetry will persist following surgery, improvement will occur in both appearance and cervical spine range of motion. If left untreated, visual disturbances may result.

Less commonly a cause of torticollis in the infant is the presence of a *cervical hemivertebra*, causing a tilting of the head. The sternocleidomastoid muscle is not enlarged and fibrotic. Before stretching exercises are begun for torticollis in the infant, anteroposterior and lateral radiographs should be obtained to evaluate for the presence of a cervical hemivertebra. If a hemivertebra is present, stretching exercises are of no use and may be harmful. Serial follow-up examination is needed and surgical fusion is used if the cervical scoliosis increases with growth.

In children more than a few years old, the most common cause of torticollis is *rotatory subluxation of C1 on C2*. This may result from trauma to the head and neck or may present following pharyngitis or an upper respiratory infection. In the immature child, inflammation in the posterior pharynx leads to edema in the C1-C2 region, which is located immediately dorsal to the pharynx. This edema is thought to lead to a rotatory shift of C1 on C2, which may resolve by itself or may become fixed in this position.

The child with rotatory subluxation will present with torticollis, holding the head in the "cocked-robin" position. Pain may be mild or absent, but limitation of cervical spine motion is noted. The sternocleidomastoid muscle is not enlarged or firm. Neurologic examination is usually normal in the extremities.

Radiographs may show mild anterior subluxation of C1 on C2 on the lateral view. The open-mouth odontoid radiograph will demonstrate asymmetry of the lateral masses of C2 relative to the odontoid (Fig. 3.8), but this same radiographic finding is present if a normal child turns the head to the side when the radiograph is obtained.

The key to establishing this diagnosis is to obtain a CT scan of C1 and C2, first with the head turned to the left and then with the head turned to the right. If rotatory subluxation is present, the atlas and axis are locked

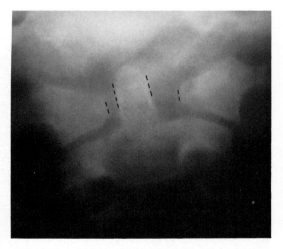

Figure 3.8. Anteroposterior tomogram of a child with torticollis after a fall shows asymmetry of the lateral masses of C1 in relation to the odontoid as the result of the atlas rotating on the axis. *Dotted lines* indicate the asymmetric widening of this space.

and the CT scan will show no change in the position of C1 on C2 with this change in head position (Fig. 3.9).

If the diagnosis of rotatory subluxation is established, the initial treatment consists of traction. If the torticollis has been present only a few days or a few weeks, head halter traction may be sufficient to reduce this subluxation; in these children, a neck brace can be used for a few weeks after reduction to maintain this position. If the torticollis has been present longer, halo traction followed by atlantoaxial fusion is usually needed.

Although approximately 40 to 50% of the rotation of the head on the neck takes place at the atlantoaxial level, fusion of this level in children seems to limit motion less than does a similar fusion procedure in the adult.

CERVICAL SPINE TRAUMA

Because of the potential for injury to the spinal cord, trauma to the cervical spine requires careful handling of the injured child and careful evaluation of the neck and neurologic system. Cervical spine injury should be suspected in any unconscious child even though the incidence of neck fractures is less in children than in adults with similar head injuries. The child's cervical spine is a flexible and elastic structure, but the spinal cord is less so. Experimental studies in stillborn children have shown that the spine can become four times more elongated before fracture occurs than the spinal cord can endure before tearing occurs.

As a general rule during transport of a child with a possible neck injury, it is safer to apply a soft or firm neck collar in the extended position rather than in flexion. In the emergency room, a lateral radiograph should be obtained to clear the cervical spine before head movement is instituted in an unconscious child with a head injury. Unstable cervical fractures or dislocations can generally be diagnosed on this one film, though more complete cervical radiographs are indicated later, after the child with polytrauma has been stabilized.

In the awake and cooperative child, palpation of the posterior spinous processes may serve to localize the site of cervical injury. Swelling here is usually absent but

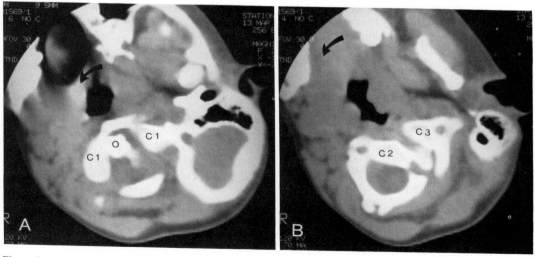

Figure 3.9. **A** and **B**, Sequential computed tomographic levels of a child with rotatory subluxation of C1 on C2 show counterclockwise rotation of the skull and C1 on the odontoid (*O*) of the body of C2, which rotates clockwise.

muscle spasm may be present. A thorough neurologic evaluation of both the upper and lower extremities is needed to establish baseline findings.

The initial imaging study used to evaluate for possible neck injury is a lateral and anteroposterior radiograph with the child supine. If these are normal and cervical spine injury is strongly suspected, flexion and extension lateral radiographs can be carefully obtained, either with the physician controlling the head or with the awake patient actively moving the head into these positions. While these flexion and extension lateral radiographs may demonstrate cervical instability from injury, the examiner needs to remember that the cervical spine in children under the age of 12 years is more lax than in adolescents or adults. In this age group, up to 3 mm of forward movement of C2 on C3 can be normal and this "pseudosubluxation" should not be overdiagnosed as an unstable injury (Fig. 3.2). Similarly, anterior movement of C1 on C2 of up to 5 mm is within a normal range in a child, while 3 mm is the upper limit in the mature patient. Care must be exercised in evaluating the cervical spine radiograph for prevertebral edema in a child; in this age group, unlike the adult, the apparent presence of prevertebral swelling may be produced by normal changes that occur with inspiration and expiration.

Jefferson Fracture of the Atlas

Usually resulting from a blow on the top of the head with the neck slightly flexed, this fracture of the ring of C1 most commonly occurs in teenagers, often being the result of an injury when playing football. Pain with neck motion is present. Neurologic deficits are uncommon. Radiographs demonstrate a fracture through the lamina of C1, and a CT scan will demonstrate fracture at two sites in the C1 ring. Halo-brace treatment for 3 months is needed, and surgery is usually not necessary unless there has been disruption of the atlanto-occipital joint as well.

Odontoid Fracture or Os Odontoideum

The odontoid portion of the axis or C2 vertebra is formed embryologically by portions of the fourth occipital level and the C1 and C2 vertebrae precursors. These three parts are joined initially by a synchondrosis, and fusion of these elements occurs as the child grows. As a result of a fall during early childhood, a fracture may occur through one of these cartilaginous synchondroses. If a displaced fracture occurs, radiographs will show displacement (usually anteriorly) of the proximal fracture fragment with the C1 vertebra. Children with this injury require fracture reduction and stabilization with either a halo brace or surgical fusion.

If, as a result of a fall, a nondisplaced fracture occurs through one of these synchondroses, the lateral radiograph will appear normal. Even though the diagnosis of a fracture is not made at the time of this nondisplaced fracture, it has been demonstrated that some of these children will develop instability at this level of the odontoid, and later lateral radiographs will show an "os odontoideum" or nonunion at the odontoid fracture site. The cephalad portion of the odontoid moves with the C1 vertebra on flexion radiographs, with the abnormal movement taking place at the nonunion site. The diagnosis of an os odontoideum may be an incidental finding, and neurologic injury is uncommon with this disorder. However, if there is more than 5 mm of forward movement of C1 on C2 with flexion, posterior atlantoaxial fusion is usually recommended. A MR image with the neck flexed may assist in deciding whether or not surgery is needed by demonstrating the presence or absence of spinal cord compression at this level.

Fracture of C2 Vertebra

If the posterior arch of C2 is fractured, usually from sudden forward flexion, a so-called "hangman's fracture" is present. This fracture does not generally cause spinal cord compression. Halo brace immobilization will allow healing and surgery can usually be avoided (Fig. 3.10).

Interspinous Ligament Injury with Chronic Instability

Particularly in the pre-adolescent and adolescent age groups, a flexion injury of the neck may produce a rupture of the interspinous ligament between two adjacent spinous processes. Tenderness can generally be well localized to the injured area on the dorsal aspect of the neck, and adjacent muscle spasm is present. No fracture is seen on radiographs and the diagnosis may initially be missed, though a lateral radiograph will usually show some increased distance between the injured spinous processes.

Because this diagnosis is difficult to make at the time of injury, many ligament injuries will go untreated. Neck pain will generally persist for several weeks or even months, particularly with flexion movements.

If a child has a history of neck injury and

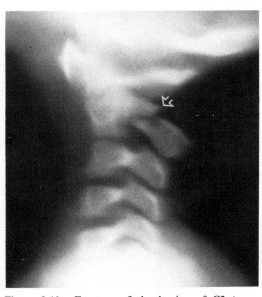

Figure 3.10. Fracture of the lamina of C2 (*open arrow*) has occurred after a sudden flexion injury. This type of fracture is called the "hangman's fracture," because it is the cause of death in judicial hangings.

has persistent neck pain, flexion and extension lateral radiographs after the neck spasm has resolved will help to make the diagnosis of interspinous ligament rupture. Instability in the flexed position is generally sufficient to warrant posterior cervical fusion at the injured level, which leads to pain resolution.

Fractures and Dislocations of C3 to C7

The primary cervical spine injuries that lead to spinal cord injury occur in the middle and lower cervical spine when force is applied to the top of the head with the neck in the flexed position. This injury most often occurs when the head is struck when diving into shallow water, in auto accidents, or in sports such as football. As the neck is hyperflexed, the anterior vertebral body may fracture, propulsing the posterior vertebral body into the spinal cord, or the vertebra may dislocate at the facet joints, pinching the spinal cord as the superior vertebra moves anteriorly. Both of these mechanisms may occur at the same time in some patients.

These fractures with spinal cord injury at C3 may lead to death from injury to the phrenic nerve (C4) with resultant cessation of breathing. At lower cervical levels, the neurologic deficit in the legs and arms will depend on the level and type of injury sustained. Initial stabilization of the cervical spine with traction, a halo brace, and/or surgery is needed and an accurate baseline neurologic examination must be well documented. If the neurologic deficit distal to the fracture site is complete, recovery is not expected. However, if this neurologic lesion is incomplete, substantial recovery can be expected, with recovery continuing for several months or even years after the child has been injured.

After a flexion injury, milder compression fractures of the anterior-superior aspect of the vertebral body may be present without instability or neurologic deficit. Especially in younger children, this diagnosis may be difficult to make, because the anterior-superior portion of the vertebral body is the last to ossify, thereby simulating a mild compression fracture. A bone scan may be useful a day or two after the injury to differentiate between a fracture and normal irregular ossification at this site. Computed tomography is helpful to diagnose sagittal or burst fractures of the vertebral body and to quantitate the spinal cord compression present (Fig. 3.11).

Spinal Cord Injury without Radiographic Abnormality (SCIWORA)

Particularly in the infant and young child, injury to the spinal cord may occur as a result of an accident without an apparent fracture of the cervical spine on radiographs. In the young child, the head is large relative to the remainder of the body, so a sudden force, such as to an unrestrained child in an automobile accident, may lead to a sudden stretch of the neck as the head is thrust forward. Since the cervical spine is more flexible than the spinal cord, the spine may demonstrate little injury while the spinal cord is disrupted, leading to severe neurologic deficits in the legs and arms.

In these children, even though the plain radiographs appear normal or nearly normal, other imaging studies are abnormal. A

myelogram will demonstrate extravasation of contrast material at the site of dural tear. An MR image will show the spinal cord injury (Fig. 3.12) and may also demonstrate a minimally displaced fracture at the ring apophysis of one of the cervical vertebrae, a condition analogous to a Salter-Harris type I physeal fracture in a long bone.

The neurologic injury in this setting is often complete and permanent. Stabilization of the spine with either a brace, a halo brace, or surgery is needed, with the choice of treatment dependent on the age of the child and the degree of instability present. Any child with paraplegia occurring before the age of 5 years is at high risk of develop-

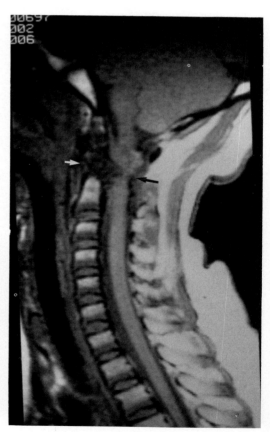

Figure 3.12. Magnetic resonance image following C1-occiput distraction injury in a young child shows ligamentous injury at C1 (*white arrow*) and spinal cord injury (*black arrow*). No fracture is seen.

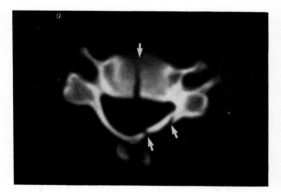

Figure 3.11. Axial computed tomogram of C3 from a child who was thrown from a bicycle onto the top of his head. The sagittal fracture of C3 was seen only in this image. There are also fractures of the posterior arch of C3. (*Arrows* indicate fractures.)

ing a progressive scoliosis as growth proceeds.

Suggested Readings

Cattell, H.S. and Filtzer, D.L.: Pseudosubluxation and other normal variations in the cervical spine in children. A study of one hundred and sixty children. J. Bone Joint Surg. 47A:1295-1309, 1965.

Davidson, R.G.: Atlantoaxial instability in individuals with Down syndrome. A fresh look at the evidence. Pediatrics 81:857-865, 1988.

Fielding, J.W., Hensinger, R.N. and Hawkins, R.J.: Os odontoideum. J. Bone Joint Surg. 62A:376-383, 1980.

Hensinger, R.N. and Fielding, J.W.: The cervical spine. In Morrissy, R.T. (ed): Pediatric Orthopaedics, 3rd edition. Philadelphia, J.B. Lippincott, 1990.

Herzenberg, J.E., Hensinger, R.N., Dedrick, D.K., et al.: Emergency transport and positioning of young children who have an injury of the cervical spine. J. Bone Joint Surg. 71A:15-22, 1989.

Hummer, C.D. and MacEwen, G.D.: The coexistence of torticollis and congenital dysplasia of the hip. J. Bone Joint Surg. 54A:1255-1256, 1972.

MacDonald, D.: Sternomastoid tumor and muscular torticollis. J. Bone Joint Surg. 51B:432-443, 1969.

Phillips, W.A. and Hensinger, R.N.: The management of rotatory atlanto-axial subluxation in children. J. Bone Joint Surg. 71A:664-668, 1989.

Pueschel, S.M., Findley, T.W., Furia, J., et.al.: Atlantoaxial instability in Down syndrome: Roentgenographic, neurologic, and somatosensory evoked potential studies. J. Pediatr. 110:515-521, 1987.

Roach, J.W., Duncan, D., Wenger, D.R., et.al.: Atlanto-axial instability and spinal cord compression in children: Diagnosis by computerized tomography. J. Bone Joint Surg. 66A:708-714, 1984.

Spierings, E.L. and Braakman, R.: The management of os odontoideum: Analysis of 37 cases. J. Bone Joint Surg. 64B:422-428, 1982.

Teng, M.M., Shoung, H.M., Chang, C.Y., et al.: CT and myelogram findings of os odontoideum. Comput. Med. Imaging Graphics 13:179-184, 1989.

Yngve, D.A., Harris, W.P., Herndon, W.A., et al.: Spinal cord injury without osseous spine fracture. J. Pediatr. Orthop. 8:153-159, 1988.

Yousefzadeh, D.K., El-Khoury, G.Y., and Smith, W.L.: Normal sagittal diameter and variation in the pediatric cervical spine. Radiology 144:319-325, 1982.

4
Shoulder

Anatomy

Anatomically, the shoulder is formed by three bones (scapula, clavicle, and proximal humerus), adjacent capsules and ligaments, and multiple muscles attaching to each of the bones. Motion of the shoulder occurs primarily at the articulation between the humerus and the glenoid portion of the scapula, but some motion also occurs at the scapular articulation with the thoracic wall and at the joint between the distal end of the clavicle and the acromial process of the scapula. This complex motion can most easily be demonstrated while abducting the arm at the shoulder, in which movement approximately two-thirds of the abduction is primarily at the glenohumeral joint, while one-third occurs at the scapulothoracic articulation, with some rotational movement at the acromioclavicular joint.

Numerous muscles attach to the scapula and influence its movement. On the medial side insert the rhomboids and the levator scapulae, which lead to scapular elevation and rotation together with the trapezius muscle, which inserts onto the scapular spine and acromion superiorly. The serratus anterior originates from the rib cage and inserts primarily on the inferior portion of the scapula, while the latissimus dorsi passes over the inferior scapular margin in its course from the spine and pelvis to the upper humerus. The pectoralis minor muscle also inserts onto the scapula anteriorly, passing from the chest wall to the coracoid process. These muscles work synchron-

ously to stabilize the scapula to facilitate glenohumeral movement, and also rotate the scapula in several different planes. If some of these scapular muscles are weak, winging of the scapula occurs, which will result in limited and inefficient glenohumeral movement.

In addition to serving as the insertion for several muscles, the scapula provides the origin for several muscles that arise from the scapular surface. The primary group of these muscles is the rotator cuff, consisting of four muscles: supraspinatus, infraspinatus, teres minor, and subscapularis, all of which insert into the proximal humerus and blend with the lateral shoulder capsule (Fig. 4.1). The final muscles originating from the scapula are the long head of the biceps, which runs from the glenoid rim to the proximal radius at the elbow, and the coracobrachialis and the short head of the biceps, which begin at the coracoid process.

Additional shoulder muscles insert into the proximal humerus. The pectoralis major begins on the anterior chest wall and clavicle and inserts into the proximal humerus, while the deltoid courses over the superior portion of the shoulder joint from the clavicle to the proximal humerus. Interposed between the deltoid muscle and the rotator cuff is the subacromial bursa (Fig. 4.2).

The principal ligaments in the shoulder girdle are the acromioclavicular and coracoclavicular ligaments, both of which assist in stabilizing the acromioclavicular joint as shoulder movement occurs.

The entire brachial plexus passes ante-

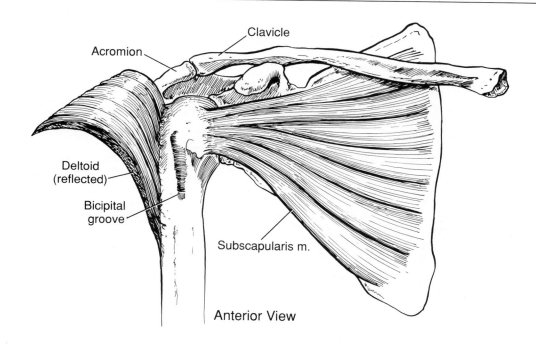

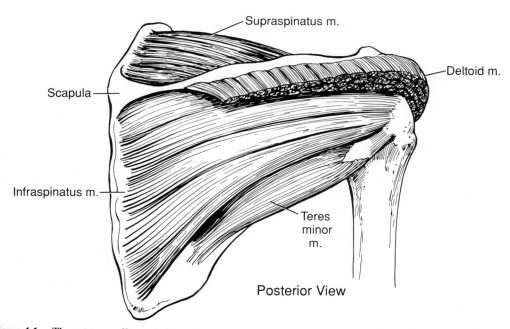

Figure 4.1. The rotator cuff, consisting of the supraspinatus, infraspinatus, teres minor, and subscapularis muscles, provides the power for glenohumeral abduction and rotation at the shoulder. Overuse injury to these muscles is common in throwing sports. If an acute tear of the rotator cuff occurs, surgical repair may be needed.

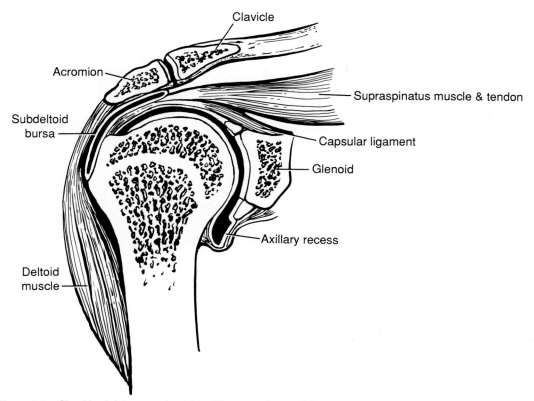

Figure 4.2. Shoulder joint, coronal section. The two primary abductors of the humerus at the shoulder are the deltoid and supraspinatus muscles. The subacromial or subdeltoid bursa lies between these two muscles and may develop inflammation in teenagers engaged in throwing sports. The acromioclavicular joint allows rotation to occur readily to facilitate shoulder movement.

romedial to the shoulder joint as the peripheral nerves to the more distal upper extremity are formed. While the details of the anatomy of the brachial plexus are better dealt with in standard anatomy texts, one must remember the proximity of these neural structures to the shoulder and routinely assess distal upper-extremity neurologic function following any injury to the shoulder area. In a similar location lies the brachial artery, which courses down the medial aspect of the upper arm before branching into the radial and ulnar arteries near the elbow.

PHYSICAL EXAMINATION

The shoulder girdle examination should include evaluation of multiple planes of shoulder motion, palpation to localize possible tenderness that will correlate with your anatomical knowledge of the shoulder, and neurovascular assessment of the more distal extremity. Always examine both shoulders, as one can generally use the unaffected side as a normal comparison.

Observation

Are the shoulder heights and scapular positions on both sides symmetrical? Is there deformity at the acromioclavicular joint? Are bruises or lacerations present? Is swelling present in the proximal or anterior shoulder area? Does the child prefer to hold the arm in a different position than the other arm?

Range of Motion

Because of the multiple planes of motion at the shoulder, accurate description of the motion planes can be confusing at times. Internal and external rotation can be best assessed with the arm at the side of the trunk, with the elbow flexed 90°. The arm should rotate inward to the trunk and outward to 60° to 90°, and should be symmetrical with the other shoulder. Forward elevation of the shoulder is termed flexion, while backward movement is shoulder extension. Abduction is measured with the arm moving from a position straight at the side outward and upward. It is generally possible to abduct the shoulder 180°, at which point the hand is pointed directly upward. If painless loss of motion is present, one should suspect either primary muscular weakness, a neurologic deficit, or a congenital abnormality. If pain is present with attempted movement, the point of maximal pain should be determined as clearly as possible.

Abduction of the shoulder is a complex motion that should be assessed by observing the posterior shoulder while *both* arms are abducted from the side of the trunk to above the child's head. The initial 90° to 110° of abduction should occur primarily at the glenohumeral joint, and during this portion of abduction the scapula should remain almost motionless. The final portion of abduction to place the arm overhead occurs at the scapulothoracic level and scapular movement is readily observed. If the scapula begins to move early in abduction, there is generally limitation of motion at the glenohumeral joint; if the scapula does not move in later abduction, abnormality at the scapulothoracic level can be diagnosed.

Careful attention to the plane of abduction of the shoulder can also help to detect weakness or injury of the deltoid or the rotator cuff, both of which are primary abductors of the shoulder. The rotator cuff attaches closely to the shoulder capsule and normally serves to initiate abduction, while the deltoid attaches more distally and is the stronger muscle to complete abduction after 40° to 60° of abduction is reached.

Palpation

Several regions should be screened for point tenderness to palpation, including the acromioclavicular joint, the bicipital tendon, and the rotator cuff. Instability of the shoulder may be detected by anterior prominence of the humeral head when the arm is externally rotated, abducted, and extended. Attempts to subluxate the shoulder joint manually may reveal latent instability.

Neurologic Examination

The distal upper extremity must be evaluated for neurologic function. If a neurologic deficit is detected, careful noting of the muscles that work normally and those that are weak allows determination of the lesion level, whether it is at a nerve root level or in a part of the brachial plexus.

NORMAL RADIOLOGIC FINDINGS

Radiographic features of a normal shoulder are clearly identified. A single ossification center of the proximal humeral head is present between 38 and 42 weeks of gestation and is identified with term birth. This center continues to enlarge with growth, and two ossification centers are present in the humeral head by 8 to 12 months of age. These then coalesce. There should be symmetry of the proximal humeri with their articulation at the glenoid fossa of the scapulae, and the medial border of the scapula (the vertebral border) parallels the long axis of the spine. The distal ends of the clavicle continue in a smooth line onto the superior aspect of the acromion. There is normally an open epiphyseal ossification center of the clavicle until the teens. An interesting feature of the distal or lateral end of the clavicle is the appearance of an open physis in this location until full skeletal maturity has been achieved in all other bones of the body. This feature may lead to increased uptake on technetium bone scans at an older age than for most other physeal areas. Ossification centers are also present at the acromion and the coracoid. Medial articulation of the clavicle to the body of the sternum manubrium is also a smooth articulation, and often the epiphyseal ossification center of the medial clavicle is visible.

Specific Shoulder Disorders

SPRENGEL'S DEFORMITY

Generally recognizable at birth, Sprengel's deformity presents with asymmetry of the superior aspect of the shoulder, often being accompanied by a bony prominence on the superior shoulder in the region of the trapezius muscle. This mass is nontender, and the child will move the rest of the extremity quite freely. Occasionally there is also an omovertebral bar, a bridge of bone that anchors the malrotated scapula to the posterior aspect of the cervical spine (Fig. 4.3).

This deformity is congenital, arising during fetal development. In an early stage of intrauterine development, the scapula is rotated laterally, with the glenoid directed caudally rather than laterally. As intrauterine development proceeds, the scapula gradually rotates medially and its vertebral border moves distally to assume its normal anatomic position. If this rotation and distal movement do not take place, the infant is born with Sprengel's deformity.

In addition to the asymmetrical shoulder appearance, asymmetrical shoulder motion is also present in this condition. Since there is essentially no scapulothoracic motion due to the scapular position, only glenohumeral motion is present. Also, since the glenoid is pointing caudally instead of laterally, glenohumeral motion is further impaired, with this impairment depending on the severity of the Sprengel's deformity. Internal and external shoulder rotation is only mildly affected, while forward elevation or flexion will demonstrate some limitation. The neurologic examination should be normal.

This diagnosis is most easily confirmed by an anteroposterior radiograph of both shoulders, in which the abnormal scapula can be seen to be rotated, with the superiormedial border of the scapula representing the bony mass palpable superiorly on examination. The radiograph should also be assessed for the presence of the omovertebral bone. Because Klippel-Feil syndrome (failure of complete cervical vertebral segmentation) can occur with Sprengel's deformity, a lateral radiograph of the cervical spine should be obtained.

The most important first step in treatment is to make an accurate diagnosis. Once the diagnosis is made, children with Sprengel's deformity should be referred for orthopaedic follow-up. While an initial exercise program may be helpful in improving motion to some degree, surgical treatment to change the scapular position may be beneficial if the child is unable to abduct the shoulder more than 90°.

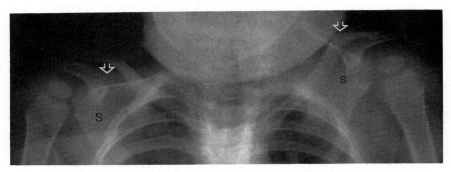

Figure 4.3. Sprengel's deformity of the shoulder is seen as elevation of the left scapula (*S*). The *open arrows* indicate the upper margins of the scapulae. Note the associated cervical spine abnormalities.

TRAUMATIC CONDITIONS

Clavicle Fracture

Fractures of the clavicle are among the most common fractures in children, particularly before adolescence. The mechanism of injury is from lateral compression of the shoulder. This usually occurs from a fall on the shoulder but may occur at the time of delivery. Most often the fracture involves the midportion of the clavicle.

In a newborn, the diagnosis should be suspected if the child is reluctant to move one arm as a result of pseudoparalysis from the pain associated with extremity movement. Confirmation of this diagnosis is completed by palpation of crepitance in the clavicle with arm movement and by a frontal radiograph of this area (Figs. 4.4 and 4.5).

Tenderness and clavicle deformity after a fall are the usual diagnostic features of this fracture after the newborn period. If the fracture is nondisplaced, there is no deformity and the pain often resolves quickly in the toddler or young child. If the diagnosis was not made at the time of injury, the parent or

physician may later note a hard lump on the clavicle. This bony lump, a result of the bone healing by the formation of a callus around the fracture site, will resolve over several months as bone remodeling occurs.

When displacement of the clavicular fracture is marked, injury to the brachial plexus or adjacent vessels may rarely occur. If there is also a fracture of the first or second ribs, neurovascular injury is more common. In each displaced clavicular fracture, neurovascular function of the distal upper extremity requires evaluation.

Clavicle fractures heal well, and nonunions are extremely rare. The time to healing is age dependent, ranging from 10 to 14 days in a newborn to 6 weeks in an adolescent. Casts are used infrequently, but splinting is useful to relieve pain and to prevent deformity as healing occurs. A figure-of-eight splint is tightened sufficiently to place the shoulders in a slightly extended position. Since the clavicle is an S-shaped bone, displaced fractures overlap, causing bone shortening. With shoulder girdle extension in this figure-of-eight splint, the clavicle is

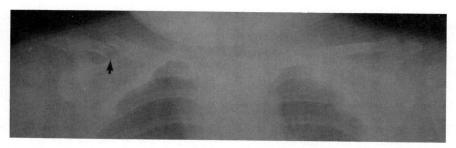

Figure 4.4. There is a clavicle fracture (*arrow*) on the right showing an inferiorly displaced distal fragment.

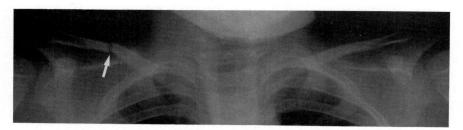

Figure 4.5. A nondisplaced fracture of the right clavicle (*arrow*) is shown.

held at normal length while healing occurs. Care must be exercised in tightening this splint to avoid excessive pressure on axillary vascular or neural structures, and the child must be assessed at regular intervals while wearing this splint.

Although the absence of tenderness to pressure at the fracture site and painless shoulder motion generally signify substantial fracture healing, despite the radiographic appearance adolescents may refracture the clavicle in the same location unless sports activities are restricted for at least 6 weeks.

Fractures at the lateral end of the clavicle less often have overlapping of the fracture ends. However, here it is necessary to assess the possibility of concurrent injury to the coracoclavicular ligament. If this is normal, the distal clavicle fracture may be treated with a sling to support the arm or with a figure-of-eight splint, whichever is more comfortable.

Later functional problems from a well-reduced clavicle fracture are almost nonexistent. Since the clavicle is located in a subcuticular position, a ball of healing bone will always be palpable at the fracture site. Reassurance of the child and parents is all that is needed, and bone remodeling as the child continues to grow will result in the gradual disappearance of this prominence over a period of several months.

Brachial Plexus Injury

If delivery of a newborn is difficult, particularly in instances of shoulder dystocia, the newborn child may not move one arm or shoulder. Although pain from a fractured clavicle is most often the reason for this lack of spontaneous movement, if a clavicle radiograph is normal, a stretching injury to the brachial plexus should be suspected. The site of nerve injury may be in the plexus itself or from an avulsion of nerve roots at the spinal cord level (Fig. 4.6).

If there is no fracture, the newborn is placed on an exercise program, in which the parents perform passive range of motion exercises to maintain joint motion, while one waits to see if the neural injury will recover within the first few months or is permanent. If the upper brachial plexus (C5-C6) is mainly involved, the condition is termed Erb's palsy, whereas the deficit is described as Klumpke's palsy if the lower roots (C7-C8) are injured. Surgical treatment to improve external rotation of the arm may be needed during mid-childhood.

Proximal Humeral Fractures

Fractures of the proximal humerus occur primarily either through the physis or in the proximal metaphysis. Curiously, fractures through the metaphysis seem to occur in childhood (Fig. 4.7), whereas physeal fractures (Fig. 4.8) are most common in early adolescence. The mechanism of injury involves a twisting injury to the arm, often in a position of external rotation-abduction-extension. If the growth plate is still open when the arm is forced into this position, a fracture occurs; if the growth plate is closed, an anterior glenohumeral shoulder dislocation occurs.

Both of these proximal humeral fractures are diagnosed by tenderness, swelling, and possible deformity in the upper arm just below the shoulder. The suspected diagnosis is confirmed by an anteroposterior radiograph of the shoulder. The distal fracture fragment is generally displaced laterally and superiorly (Fig. 4.8).

Nondisplaced fractures can be treated by the use of a sling and swathe for 3 weeks if the fracture occurs through the physis and 4 to 6 weeks if the fracture is in the proximal humeral metaphysis. If displacement is present, reduction is best obtained by abduction of the distal extremity with immobilization in an abduction cast or splint until healing occurs. In young children, remodeling at this fracture site is excellent (remember, the shoulder has multiple planes of motion and fracture angulation remodels well in the plane of motion of the adjacent joint),

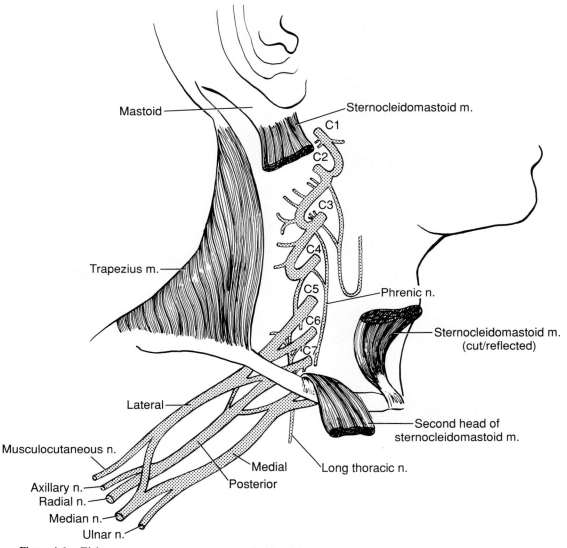

Figure 4.6. Eight nerve roots are present on each side of the cervical spine. The phrenic nerve is formed by the third and fourth roots and innervates the diaphragm. The lower four cervical nerve roots form the brachial plexus, which in turn forms the peripheral nerves of the upper extremity. Injury to the brachial plexus may occur from a clavicle fracture or from a shoulder injury.

and residual displacement can often be accepted with the expectation of later remodeling.

Anterior Dislocation of the Shoulder

Once the proximal humeral growth plate is closed, an anterior dislocation of the humeral head is the result of excessive ex-

ternal rotation-abduction-extension at the shoulder level. This commonly occurs during sports activities such as wrestling and gymnastics. As the humeral head dislocates anteriorly, the capsule is torn and the humeral head rests against the anterior rim of the glenoid and slightly inferiorly.

Physical examination demonstrates a

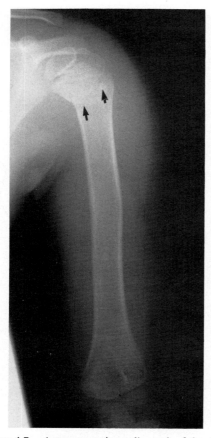

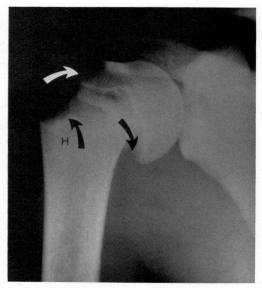

Figure 4.8. Shoulder radiograph in an older child shows a fracture through the physis with clockwise rotation of the humeral head (*arrows*) and lateral and superior displacement of the humeral shaft (*H, arrow*).

Figure 4.7. Anteroposterior radiograph of the shoulder demonstrates a fracture (*arrows*) of the proximal metaphysis of the humerus in a young child, with characteristic slight impaction at the fracture site and lateral displacement of the distal fragment.

palpable mass in the anterior aspect of the shoulder, with marked tenderness and pain on attempts at shoulder movement. Neurologic evaluation of the distal extremity is important, as the brachial plexus may be injured at the same time.

An anteroposterior radiograph of the shoulder may demonstrate the dislocation clearly. The humeral head overlies the glenoid and is slightly inferior. However, even with an anterior shoulder dislocation, the radiograph may appear relatively normal. If the physical findings suggest an anterior shoulder dislocation, an axillary view should be obtained to ascertain the relation of the humeral head to the glenoid. If too much pain is present to allow an axillary projection, a transthoracic lateral radiograph can be used to confirm the diagnosis of a dislocation.

Reduction of the initial anterior shoulder dislocation in an adolescent may be difficult, generally requiring substantial traction force. This is most easily effected by having the teenager lie prone with a weight attached to the dislocated arm for several minutes while intravenous analgesia is administered. Once reduction is obtained the arm is placed in a sling and swathe to allow soft tissue healing for about 3 weeks. Exercises to strengthen the subscapularis (internal rotator) are begun and continued for several weeks to try to prevent recurrent dislocation.

Because the force needed to cause a dislocation initially leads to significant soft tissue tearing, the chance of recurrent dislocation in a teenager is high, approaching 90 to

100%. If recurrent dislocation occurs, reduction is easier at the time of each dislocation, but surgical treatment is needed to regain stability if anterior shoulder dislocation occurs more than once.

Acromioclavicular Separation

Known commonly as a "shoulder separation," this injury results from a fall directly onto the tip of the shoulder. Instead of the clavicle breaking, as in a young child, the fall leads to disruption at the acromioclavicular joint. Injuries at this joint are classified into three grades: grade I—capsular tear but no displacement; grade II—tear of the acromioclavicular capsule with mild upward clavicle displacement, with the coracoclavicular ligament remaining intact (Fig. 4.9); and grade III--disruption of both the acromioclavicular joint and the coracoclavicular ligaments, resulting in marked superior displacement of the distal end of the clavicle (Fig. 4.10).

Physical findings depend on the degree of injury. In the grade I injury, the only positive finding is tenderness at the acromioclavicular joint on direct palpation. Similar tenderness is seen in higher grades of injury,

in addition to the deformity and pain on attempted shoulder motion. The patient generally holds the arm cradled at the side of the trunk, with the elbow flexed and the forearm supported by the opposite hand.

Treatment varies with the grade of injury. All sports activities should be avoided if any tenderness is present at the acromioclavicular joint. A sling is used for comfort. Grade II injury is also treated with a sling until pain and tenderness are absent. A grade III injury may be treated by surgical repair or by sling immobilization until pain is absent. The final functional results with surgical or conservative treatment of grade III injuries are the same.

Humeral Shaft Fractures

Though much less common than the metaphyseal fractures, fractures through the midshaft of the humerus have special considerations due to the possibility of radial nerve injury or residual angulation.

The radial nerve lies posterior to the humeral shaft in the proximal aspect of the humeral shaft, then curls around the midshaft in the radial groove to lie laterally in the lower third of the humerus. If an oblique

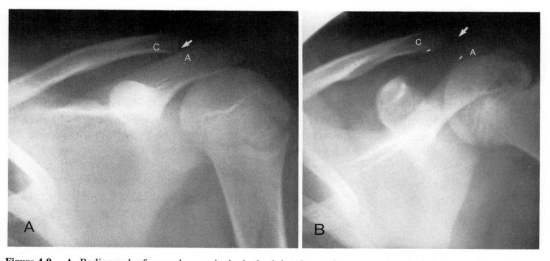

Figure 4.9. **A,** Radiograph of normal acromioclavicular joint shows close approximation of the tip of the clavicle to the acromion (*arrow*). **B,** This radiograph of the shoulder shows wide separation of the tip of the clavicle from the acromion (*A* and *arrow*). This acromioclavicular separation occurred from a fall on the shoulder when wrestling.

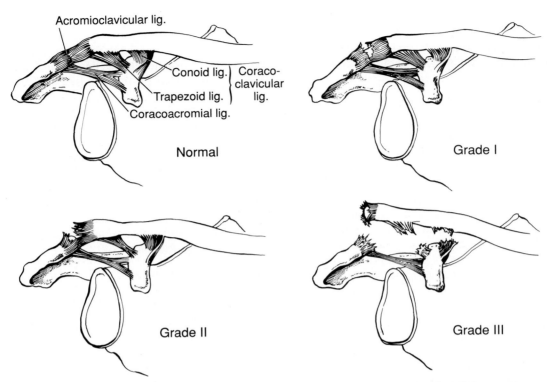

Figure 4.10. The primary ligaments connecting the normal clavicle to the acromial portion of the scapula are shown. Injury to one or more of these ligaments commonly results from a fall directly onto the tip of the shoulder during sports. Treatment differs for each injury, depending on the severity of the injury (grade I, II, or III).

fracture occurs at the mid-distal aspect of the humeral shaft, the radial nerve may become entrapped at this site and cause a neuropraxia of this nerve. Careful assessment of wrist and finger extension is needed when this fracture is seen.

Treatment of humeral shaft fractures does not require anatomical reduction, but all attempts of treatment should be directed to preventing angulation into a varus position. Treatment methods include a long arm cast or a long arm splint coursing over the shoulder. Fracture healing should be complete by 6 weeks after injury.

Myositis Ossificans of the Brachialis Muscle

Participants in contact sports, especially football, may develop a mass following trauma to the lateral distal upper arm, just above the elbow in the region of the brachialis muscle. Generally, a hematoma forms first, but instead of this hematoma resolving, pain and tenderness increase about 1 week after the formation of the hematoma, and the consistency of the mass becomes increasingly bony as the tenderness subsides. During the painful stage, exercises need to be avoided or the process of bleeding and recurrent inflammation will be repeated and recovery will be prolonged.

Radiographs of the hematoma region will initially be normal, but as the mass becomes increasingly hard, calcification will appear within the muscle, gradually forming mature-appearing bone. This bony mass is slightly separated from the humeral shaft, and radiographs with this finding help to differentiate this condition from osteosarcoma. Bone-scan imaging studies will show an increase in isotope uptake at the site of the bone formation within the hematoma.

Once this diagnosis is made, treatment is by rest with avoidance of both active and passive elbow exercises until pain is absent. Once the myositis ossificans matures, strengthening and range-of-motion exercises can be reinstituted. It is not usually necessary to remove this ectopic bone unless elbow function is significantly involved. Resection during the active stage of formation is contraindicated as the histologic appearance may mimic osteosarcoma and recurrence of bone formation will usually occur quickly. If resection is performed at a later stage, use of salicylates following surgery seems to prevent new bone formation at the excision site.

Suggested Readings

Eidman, D.K., Siff, S.J., and Tullos, H.S.: Acromioclavicular lesions in children. Am. J. Sports Med. 9:150-154, 1981.

Kohler, R. and Trillaud, J.M.: Fracture and fracture separation of the proximal humerus in children: Report of 136 cases. J. Pediatr. Orthop. 3:326-332, 1983.

Leibovic, S.J., Ehrlich, M.G., and Zaleske, D.J.: Sprengel deformity. J. Bone Joint Surg. 72A:192-197, 1990.

Rockwood, C.A., Jr.: Fractures and dislocations of the shoulder. Part III. Fractures and dislocations of the ends of the clavicle, scapula, and glenohumeral joint. In Rockwood, C.A., Jr., Wilkins, K.E., and King, R.E. (eds): Fractures in Children. Philadelphia, J.B. Lippincott, volume 3, pp. 624-682, 1984.

Wagner, K.T., Jr. and Lyne, E.D.: Adolescent traumatic dislocations of the shoulder with open epiphyses. J. Pediatr. Orthop. 3:61-62, 1983.

5
Elbow

Of all the musculoskeletal regions of the growing child's body, the elbow is the site of abnormalities and injuries that are the most difficult to diagnose accurately. This is primarily due to the presence of a large number of ossification centers that can confuse the examiner. Specific attention to examination and knowledge of the radiographic appearance of these diverse ossification centers is needed even more in this region than in other body regions.

Anatomy

Unlike the shoulder, which has multiple planes of motion, the elbow is a hinge joint, moving primarily in flexion and extension while allowing forearm rotation. The primary articulation needed for flexion and extension is that between the proximal ulna (olecranon) and the distal medial humerus (trochlea). The distal lateral humeral articulation (capitellum) with the radial head moves with flexion motion but is primarily responsible for allowing the radius to rotate around the ulna and produce pronation and supination of the forearm to facilitate positioning of the hand.

Muscles that cross the elbow affect flexion and extension of the elbow as well as rotation of the forearm. The biceps consists of two heads, a long head that crosses the anterior shoulder joint and a short head that arises from the acromion of the scapula. Inserting onto the bicipital tubercle of the proximal radius, the biceps flexes the elbow and supinates the forearm. The triceps is formed from three heads, joining to form a tendon that inserts on the olecranon of the ulna to provide elbow extension. The brachialis and brachioradialis muscles, located laterally on the distal upper arm, provide less elbow flexion force than the biceps.

The primary ligaments in the elbow are the lateral and medial collateral ligaments, which impart joint stability during flexion movements. The other ligament of clinical importance, particularly in children, is the annular ligament, which is wrapped circumferentially around the radial neck to stabilize the radial head against the capitellum (Fig. 5.1).

Numerous neurovascular structures pass across the elbow joint and are in positions that predispose to injury as a result of trauma in the elbow area. The brachial artery runs on the anterior aspect of the elbow joint with the median nerve. The ulnar nerve is positioned superficially in the medial aspect of the elbow, making it susceptible to injury (the "funny bone" of the elbow is caused by bumping the elbow over the ulnar nerve). The radial nerve passes laterally in the elbow before passing into the forearm. It is therefore essential to evaluate distal extremity function whenever examining the elbow to fully assess these neurovascular structures (Fig. 5.2).

Physical Examination

OBSERVATION

Is the elbow swollen? Is deformity apparent compared to the other elbow? Is full extension possible? Is hyperextension seen? The normal humeral-forearm angle (termed

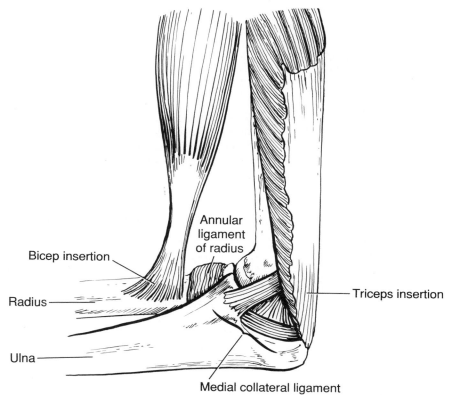

Figure 5.1. The primary elbow ligaments are the medial and lateral collateral ligaments and the annular ligament. Recurrent dislocation may occur if any of these ligaments are injured. The biceps, inserting on the bicipital tubercle of the proximal radius, produces elbow flexion and forearm rotation. The triceps is the prime extender of the elbow.

the carrying angle) with the elbow extended is 5° to 7° of valgus: is the carrying angle symmetrical on both arms?

PALPATION

Since the bones of the elbow are largely subcutaneous, identification of the point of maximal tenderness is fairly easy except when swelling is marked. Is the tenderness at the physis or at the joint itself? With one finger over the radiohumeral joint, rotate the forearm: is there displacement of the radial head with this movement?

RANGE OF MOTION

The normal range of motion of the elbow is from full extension to approximately 140°

of flexion and should be equal in both arms. This range of motion is generally recorded as 0° to 140° of flexion. If hyperextension of 10° to 15° is present bilaterally, this may be an indication of generalized joint laxity. Rotation of the forearm is normally 90° of pronation (with the forearm rotated so the palm of the hand is facing downward) and 90° of supination (with the palm facing upward).

NEUROVASCULAR

Accurate determination of hand motor and sensory function is the key to evaluating the peripheral nerves as they pass by the elbow. There are some autonomous areas of sensation where overlapping innervation from adjacent nerves seldom occurs: the tip of the index finger (median), the dorsal web

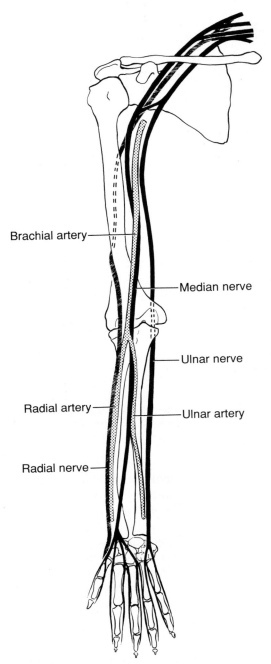

Brachial artery

Median nerve

Ulnar nerve

Radial artery

Ulnar artery

Radial nerve

Figure 5.2. Multiple important neurovascular structures pass adjacent to the elbow joint and may be injured with trauma to the elbow. Careful evaluation of the hand and wrist is needed in a child with a fracture around the elbow.

space between the thumb and index finger (radial), and the tip of the fifth finger (ulnar) are areas to be examined here. Similarly, motor function can be assessed quickly by evaluating flexion of the tip of the index finger (median), flexion of the fifth finger (ulnar), and extension of the wrist (radial). If these motor and sensory examinations are normal, the nerves at the elbow are grossly intact. Comparison of hand warmth and the presence of radial and ulnar artery pulses similar to the uninjured extremity complete this evaluation.

NORMAL RADIOGRAPHIC FEATURES

The appearance of numerous ossification centers in the elbow leads to potential confusion in the interpretation of radiographs of this region. At birth, the epiphyses of the distal humerus and the proximal radius are not ossified. During the first year of life, the capitellum ossification center of the humerus develops. The most common order for the appearance of the remaining ossification centers is as follows: radial head, medial epicondyle, trochlea, olecranon, and lateral epicondyle, at approximately ages 4, 5, 7, 9, and 10 years respectively (Fig. 5.3).

Since fractures can readily occur through nonossified cartilage and through the physis, it is imperative to differentiate between an ossification center and a fracture fragment. If there is any question on radiographic examination, the use of a comparison x-ray of the normal elbow is helpful to properly evaluate traumatic conditions.

In all projections of the elbow x-ray, whether properly positioned or not, a line should pass up the long axis of the radius and transect the epiphyseal ossification center of the capitellum. If this line does not intersect the capitellum, the radial head is dislocated (Fig. 5.4).

In evaluation for a supracondylar fracture of the humerus, on a lateral radiograph, a line drawn down the anterior shaft of the humerus will bisect the capitellar ossification center (Fig. 5.4). If this line passes anterior to the capitellum, a supracondylar

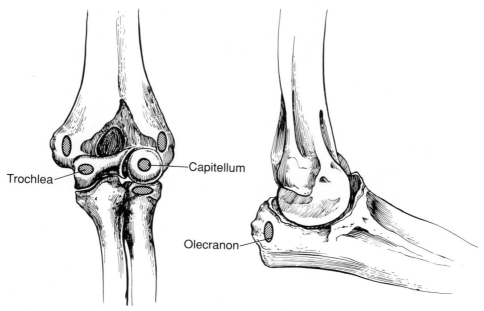

Figure 5.3. Secondary ossification centers of the elbow may be confused with fractures in the young child. As the child becomes older, these ossification centers typically appear in the following order: capitellum, radial head, medial humeral epicondyle, trochlea, olecranon, and lateral humeral epicondyle.

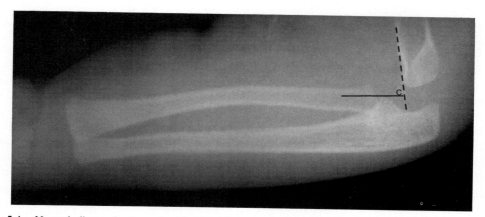

Figure 5.4. Normal elbow of a 6-month-old child. The *solid line* demonstrates the alignment of the axis of the radius with the capitellum (*C*). The *dashed line* shows the intersection of the anterior humeral line with the midcapitellum.

fracture dorsally angulated and requiring manipulation for reduction should be diagnosed (Fig. 5.5).

Disorders

Disorders specific to the elbow and forearm are either of a congenital or a traumatic cause, with trauma being the cause in the overwhelming majority of children.

CONGENITAL DISORDERS
Radial Head Dislocation

Dislocation of the radial head during intrauterine development may be seen in a

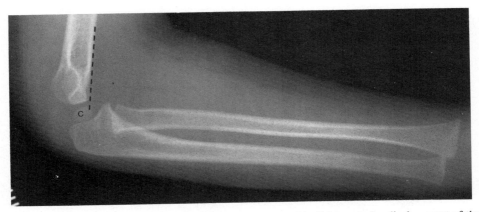

Figure 5.5. Subtle supracondylar fracture of the distal humerus with slight posterior displacement of the distal fragment shows that the anterior humeral line (*dashed line*) intersects the anterior portion of the capitellum (*C*) rather than the midcapitellum.

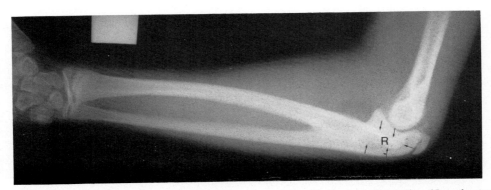

Figure 5.6. Congenital dislocation of the radial head (*R, arrows*), with posterior dislocation. Note the rounded appearance of the head; also a congenital radioulnar synostosis is present here but is usually not seen.

wide variety of genetic disorders and occasionally in an otherwise normal child.

The primary physical findings are a lack of full elbow extension and a palpable prominence on the lateral side of the elbow. An anteroposterior and lateral elbow radiograph will demonstrate that the line up the long axis of the radius does not bisect the capitellum, and the proximal radius bows posteriorly. The radial head is small and rounded.

Surgical procedures to attempt relocation of the radial head are not indicated if this dislocation is congenital. If the radial head and capitellum have not been in contact during development, the radial head remains convex and does not form the con-cave surface the capitellum requires for appropriate articulation. Surgical excision of the radial head may be appropriate in early adolescence if motion restriction, pain, or cosmetic concerns are sufficient to require treatment. If radial ulnar synostosis is associated with the congenital radial head dislocation, no treatment is usually indicated (Fig. 5.6).

TRAUMATIC CONDITIONS

Supracondylar Fracture of the Humerus

The most common fracture at the elbow occurs in the supracondylar region of the distal humerus. The fracture line generally passes transversely through the metaphysis and olecranon fossa of the humerus, just proximal to the physis, so growth disturbance following this fracture is unusual (Fig. 5.7).

A fall on the outstretched hand with the elbow extended is the means of fracture in about 99% of children. Because of this extension position of the elbow, the distal fracture fragment is displaced and angled posteriorly. Since this fracture fragment moves posteriorly, the brachial artery and median nerve may also be stretched over the end of the proximal fracture site, leading to neurovascular problems in the forearm and hand.

In the initial evaluation for a possible elbow fracture, observation of the elbow position is important even before palpation. If marked swelling and deformity are absent, palpation for maximal tenderness localization and careful testing of active (not passive) range of motion are performed. If obvious deformity is present, a fracture can be diagnosed and range of motion testing should not be attempted. In the case of obvious displacement, careful evaluation of the radial pulse and the neurologic function of the hand is completed. Whether this evaluation of a deformed, swollen elbow is done on the athletic field or in the office, the elbow should be splinted before transport for x-rays or for referral to an orthopaedist. Since the brachial artery may be caught in the fracture site of a supracondylar humeral fracture, the elbow should not be flexed but should be splinted in a position of relative extension, in which position there is a warm hand with a good radial pulse.

The diagnosis of a supracondylar fracture of the humerus is confirmed by anteroposterior and lateral radiographs of the elbow with the splint in place. If elbow deformity is obvious, it is not important to have perfect positioning for these x-rays, and these films should be obtained without much rotation of the arm at the shoulder, which will cause painful motion at the humeral fracture site. In nondisplaced or minimally angulated fractures with no gross deformity present, well-positioned radiographs are important for adequate assessment.

Supracondylar humeral fractures are generally classified into three types. Type I is a nondisplaced fracture. Type II has posterior angulation of the distal humeral condyles without displacement laterally or medially. Type III is a fracture with complete displacement of the fracture fragments.

Nondisplaced or type I fractures may be difficult to see on the radiographs. On the anteroposterior view, careful attention must be directed to the distal metaphysis of the humerus with particular attention to detecting a small discontinuity of either medial or lateral cortex. On the lateral radiograph, a positive ''fat pad'' sign (Fig. 5.8) strongly suggests that a supracondylar fracture is present. The ''fat pad'' sign consists of a crescentic lucency just posterior to the olecranon fossa. A fat pad is present in the olecranon fossa but is not visible on a lateral

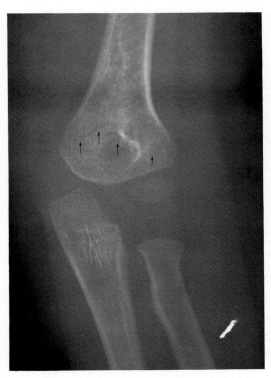

Figure 5.7. Nondisplaced supracondylar fracture (*arrows*) of the distal humerus interepicondylar region.

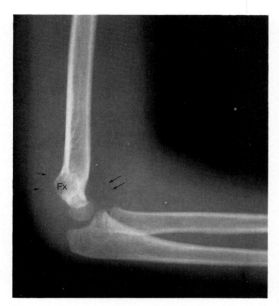

Figure 5.8.   Fracture (*Fx*) of the distal humeral shaft, supracondylar in location, shows slight posterior angulation of the distal fragment and displacement of the anterior and posterior fat pads of the humerus (*arrows*).

radiograph unless joint capsular distention from joint effusion forces it to extrude posteriorly. A second radiographic finding to look for here is a small linear radiolucency at the waist of the hourglass configuration in the humeral metaphysis (Fig. 5.9). The treatment of type I fractures consists of a long arm cast for 2 to 3 weeks with the elbow flexed 100°. When the cast is removed, the healing bone may make the fracture line more apparent than at the initial evaluation.

Type II fractures can be diagnosed by drawing a line down the anterior aspect of the humerus on the lateral radiograph of the elbow (Fig. 5.4). This line, which should pass through the middle of the capitellum, will pass anterior to the capitellum, indicating the distal fracture fragment has been significantly angulated posteriorly. Although posterior angulation alone would likely remodel with time, since this angulation is in the plane of motion of the elbow joint, there is often some varus angulation as well, a deformity that will not remodel and may worsen during cast treatment (Fig. 5.10).

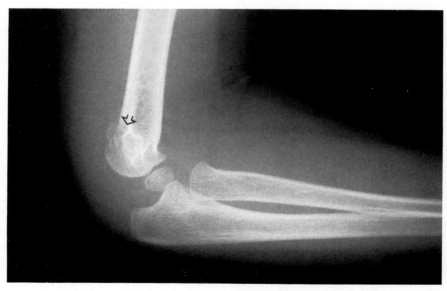

Figure 5.9.   Type I supracondylar humeral fracture (*open arrow*) with dorsal cortical impaction and slight dorsal angulation of the distal humeral fragment.

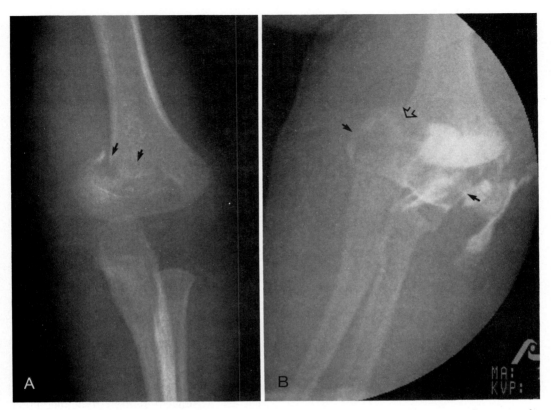

Figure 5.10. **A,** Oblique supracondylar fracture of the distal humerus with medial displacement and varus angulation of the fracture fragment. *Arrows* indicate the fracture line. **B,** Arthrogram of the elbow shows fracture (*open arrow*) and medial displacement of the entire distal fragment, which will result in a cubitus varus position.

Because of this, the type II fracture requires referral to an orthopaedist for reduction, often even requiring surgical treatment.

The principal role for the primary care physician in dealing with type III fractures (Fig. 5.11) is the initial careful assessment of neurovascular function of the distal extremity and the supervision of splinting of the arm until definitive orthopaedic care is available. Marked flexion is needed for the orthopaedist to obtain and maintain reduction of this fracture. Because of swelling in the elbow region with this fracture, casting the elbow in marked flexion will frequently impair brachial artery circulation, leading either to a forearm compartment syndrome or to an ischemic hand. Most commonly,

therefore, these fractures are reduced under general anesthesia and stabilized with percutaneous Kirschner wires, so that the long arm cast can be applied with sufficient elbow extension to allow maintenance of a radial pulse and a warm hand.

Both type II and type III fractures are maintained in a long arm cast for approximately 3 weeks. A radiograph 3 weeks after the injury may still show an apparent fracture line, but the cast can be safely removed at this time in almost every child. Longer periods of immobilization lead to more prolonged range of motion restriction. The child should be encouraged to actively exercise the injured elbow after cast removal, but passive stretching exercises should gen-

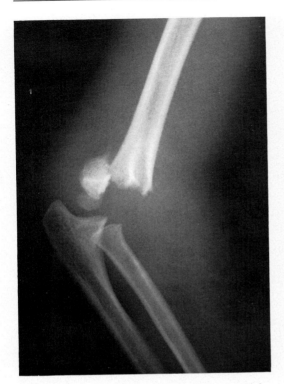

Figure 5.11. Type III distal humeral supracondylar fracture. There is complete dorsal displacement of the distal fragment.

erally be avoided initially in children. Although it may take several weeks to regain full motion, function should return to normal.

Complications. The two major complications associated with supracondylar humeral fractures are malunion (cubitus varus) and associated neurovascular injuries.

Cubitus varus is the term used to describe an abnormal carrying angle (humeral-forearm angle in full elbow extension) that normally measures 5 to 10° of valgus. If the supracondylar humeral fracture heals with residual varus deformity, usually as a result of comminution of the fracture on the medial side (Fig. 5.10), the arm will rest at the side abnormally, in a manner described as a "gunstock deformity." This abnormal arm

position is caused by the need to abduct the shoulder to hold the arm at the side, since the forearm below the elbow now points toward the trunk (varus) rather than away (valgus). Although concomitant physeal injury can occur with a supracondylar humeral fracture, this cubitus varus is nearly always a malunion from incomplete reduction. No matter what the type of treatment has been, all published series reporting results of treatment of supracondylar humeral fractures have some patients with cubitus varus. Since this varus deformity is not in the plane of joint motion, remodeling is not expected. If the deformity is mild, no treatment is needed. Although function is generally nearly normal, if the appearance of the arm is unacceptable, osteotomy of the humerus to realign the arm is possible and can be done even in the skeletally immature child.

Any of the peripheral nerves passing in the vicinity of the elbow may be injured in association with this fracture. The most commonly injured are the median and radial nerves. Absence of flexion of the distal phalanx of the index finger implies a median nerve injury. If the radial nerve is injured, active wrist extension will be absent. If the ulnar nerve is damaged, flexion of the fifth finger will be abnormal. These peripheral nerve injuries are generally the result of blunt trauma or stretch, and recovery is expected in the majority within a few days to several weeks after injury. If recovery is not present by 3 months following injury, surgical exploration of the nerve is indicated to determine if the nerve has been ruptured and will require microsurgical operative repair.

Vascular injury in association with supracondylar humeral fractures can lead to devastating permanent disability if it is not diagnosed in a timely manner. The injury occurs to the brachial artery at the fracture site, often being an intimal tear as a result of arterial stretch over the sharp proximal fracture fragment. If the radial pulse is absent and the hand is cool and pale, emergency arteriography and surgical exploration are needed to repair the brachial artery.

More often, however, the vascular injury with this fracture will lead to the development of a compartment syndrome in the forearm flexor muscles, usually in the first 24 to 72 hours following the injury. Even if an occlusion of the brachial artery is present, collateral circulation around the elbow is often sufficient to keep the hand warm and pink, perhaps even with a palpable radial pulse. However, swelling of the forearm muscles may occur from the partial ischemia and the edema from the injury. As these muscles are enclosed within a tight, strong fascial compartment, progressive swelling of the muscles increases the tissue pressure within this compartment, making it more difficult for capillary blood flow to enter the muscle and blocking the exit of venous blood flow in the muscle. When the intracompartmental muscle pressure is as high as the capillary blood pressure, blood flow into the muscle stops, leading to progressive muscle cell necrosis. This will occur even if the hand remains warm and pink, with good capillary fill in the fingertips and a palpable radial pulse.

The first symptoms of a developing compartment syndrome are increasing pain in the forearm and a loss of sensation in the hand. The pain may be aggravated by attempts at passive hyperextension of the fingers, as this maneuver stretches the swollen flexor muscles. If these findings are present, muscle compartment pressures must be measured by insertion of a needle directly into the muscles. If a compartment syndrome is confirmed by these measurements, emergency fasciotomy of the forearm is essential to relieve the abnormal muscle pressures and allow blood flow to be reestablished to these muscles. If the muscles have had no blood flow for more than a few hours, permanent muscle damage will be present and will lead to progressive contractures, a condition termed Volkmann's ischemic contracture, with impaired hand function.

Lateral Condyle Fracture of the Humerus

Fracture of the lateral condyle is the second most common fracture in the distal humerus. This fracture also usually occurs from a fall on the outstretched hand, in association with some rotational force. The displaced fracture fragment serves as the attachment for the forearm supinators and the wrist and finger extensors.

Examination will usually demonstrate swelling and tenderness localized to the lateral half of the elbow, but at times swelling may be present medially as well, a finding important to note. Neurovascular injury is rare in association with this fracture.

Radiographs of the elbow must be assessed carefully. The most common fracture type is analogous to a Salter-Harris type IV injury, with the fracture line beginning in the distal lateral metaphysis and extending across the physis into the elbow joint, through the cartilaginous epiphysis (Figs. 5.12 and 5.13). Care must be taken to correctly diagnose this fracture as a fracture of the entire lateral condyle, and not call this a lateral epicondyle avulsion. The lateral epicondyle is the last ossification center to appear and is generally not ossified in the age group in which lateral condyle fractures occur.

If soft tissue swelling is present medially as well as laterally, the fracture line may extend from the lateral metaphysis along the physis to exit medially, in the pattern of a Salter-Harris type II fracture. An intercondylar fracture that involves both the medial and lateral condyles is less common (Fig. 5.14).

If the fracture is nondisplaced, treatment is accomplished by use of a long arm cast for 3 to 4 weeks with the elbow flexed 90°. However, if there is displacement of 2 mm

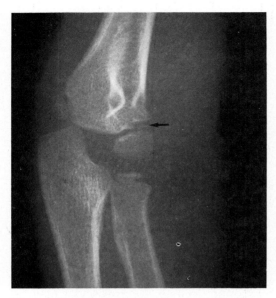

Figure 5.12. Fracture of the lateral condyle (capitellum). The *arrow* indicates the separated metaphyseal fragment. Surgical treatment is recommended for this fracture.

or more, operative reduction is needed to anatomically reduce the fracture, in this way restoring a congruent joint articular surface and realigning the physis to prevent later growth disturbance. A cast is used for 3 to 4 weeks postoperatively. Despite the fact that this fracture usually transects the physis, growth disturbance after open reduction is unusual. Angular deformity after this fracture is uncommon and the range of elbow motion is usually regained by several weeks after cast removal.

Medial Epicondyle Humeral Fracture and Posterior Elbow Dislocation

The medial collateral ligament of the elbow attaches proximally at the ossification center of the medial epicondyle of the distal humerus. If there is a fall on the extended arm, angular stress is placed on the medial part of the joint, with resulting avulsion of the medial epicondyle rather than a ligament tear. This may be associated with a posterior and lateral dislocation of the

elbow, although the elbow dislocation may be transient and may be reduced by the time the child presents for care.

If there is no elbow dislocation, examination will primarily show tenderness and swelling over the medial aspect of the distal humerus. Pain will be present on attempted elbow movement. If a dislocation is present, the ulna will usually be displaced laterally and posteriorly and the arm will be cradled in a flexed position to avoid painful movement. Distal function of the ulnar nerve should be carefully checked due to the anatomic proximity of the ulnar nerve to the medial epicondyle.

When the elbow is dislocated posterolaterally, the medial epicondyle may not only be fractured but may also be displaced into the elbow joint by the medial elbow ligaments. Reduction of such an elbow dislocation is generally accomplished readily with longitudinal traction followed by elbow flexion. While this reduction may be carried out on the athletic field or in the office, it is important to obtain elbow radiographs after reduction to assess the status of the medial epicondyle, which can remain incarcerated in the joint at the time of dislocation reduction.

Radiographs of the elbow need to be carefully evaluated for the position of the medial epicondyle if medial tenderness is present. Use of a comparison radiograph of the opposite elbow is recommended to determine the normal position of this ossification center. If displacement of the medial epicondyle is less than 5 mm and the elbow is stable, long arm cast immobilization is sufficient. The wrist should be placed in a flexed position and the forearm pronated to relax the pull of the forearm flexors and pronator teres on the medial epicondyle where they originate. If the medial epicondyle is displaced more than 5 mm (Fig. 5.15), elbow instability may be present and operative treatment may be necessary. If the medial epicondyle remains within the elbow joint

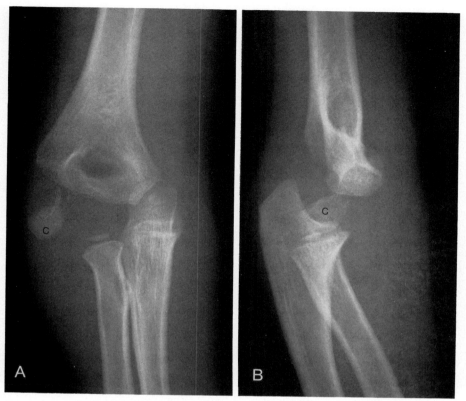

Figure 5.13. **A,** AP view of the humerus shows fracture through the lateral condyle with inferior and medial displacement of the capitellum (*C*) and its metaphyseal fragment and apparent dislocation of the radius and ulna. **B,** Lateral view with posterior displacement of the capitellum (*C*), radius, and ulna.

after reduction of an associated elbow dislocation, surgical reduction and internal fixation of the medial epicondyle are necessary to restore normal elbow movement.

Almost the only long-term complication associated with this fracture is the occasional development of a late ulnar nerve palsy several years after this injury. If the medial epicondyle remains markedly displaced, there is a tendency for the elbow to develop increased valgus deformity, in this way leading to a stretch of the ulnar nerve with resultant impairment of hand function.

Radial Neck Fracture

Although radial neck fractures are much less common than the fractures described above, if not treated properly they will result in limitation of forearm rotation secondary to a change in the position of the proximal radius against the capitellum. This fracture is also caused by a fall on the extended hand, in which the force is transmitted up the forearm to the elbow, resulting in a tilt of the proximal radius at the fracture site.

Physical examination will demonstrate tenderness at the lateral aspect of the elbow, though more distally than for a lateral humeral condyle fracture. Pain will be present on attempted forearm rotation and can be accentuated by longitudinal compression of the forearm.

Radiographs of the elbow will demon-

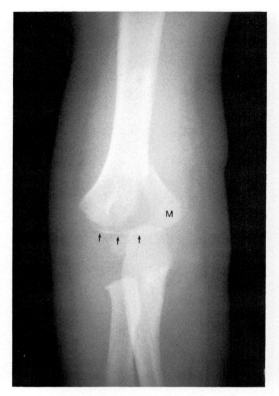

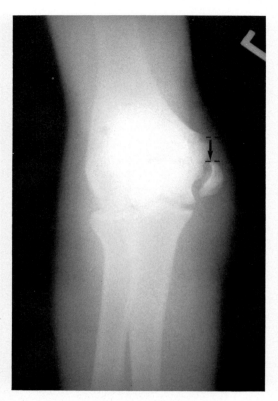

Figure 5.14.   Medial condyle fracture of the distal humerus (*arrows*) with a large metaphyseal fragment (*M*) and a small linear fragment of metaphysis laterally located. Medial displacement will lead to cubitus varus.

Figure 5.15.   Avulsion fracture of the medial epicondyle of the humerus. *Dashed lines* indicate the inferior displacement of the fragment.

strate a fracture through the radial neck with variable angulation, compression or displacement. In the normal elbow, the angle between the long axis of the radius and the horizontal line along the proximal aspect of the radial head is about 90°. These same lines should be drawn when a fracture is present. If this angle is still more than 60°, short-term long arm cast immobilization is adequate treatment, since remodeling will occur in the growing child. If this angle is less than 60°, either closed reduction or surgical reduction is needed to decrease the likelihood of later restriction in forearm rotation. If total displacement of the radial head and neck at the fracture site is seen, operative treatment is needed.

All children with this fracture, even when reduction is nearly anatomic, will have a tendency to have enlargement of the radial head over the few years following this fracture. While this radial head enlargement may lead to mild restriction of forearm pronation or supination, further treatment for this minor abnormality is not generally necessary.

Radial Head Subluxation

Subluxation of the radial head, commonly referred to as *"nursemaid's elbow,"* is generally found in children under the age of 6 years. Until the age of 5 or 6, the anatomical shape of the proximal radius and the annular ligament, which passes over the radial neck, allows the rather easy movement of the radius in the direction of the long axis of the arm (Fig. 5.16). In older children, progressive ossification of the radial head and tightening of the annular ligament are such that much more trauma is needed to lead to radial head subluxation.

In younger children, subluxation results from a longitudinal pull or traction being applied to the extremity. The most common mechanism of injury is the child being lifted by the hand over a curb or similar obstacle to initiate walking across a street. This injury may also result from the parent's swinging the child during play.

Whatever the mechanism of injury, the child will note sudden onset of pain and will be unwilling to use the affected arm. The arm is usually held in a flexed position. Hand function is normal. No swelling is generally seen and tenderness is hard to localize.

Radiographs of the elbow are almost always interpreted as normal. On occasion, a line drawn up the radius may pass into the lateral half of the capitellar ossification center, but no complete dislocation is present.

While the anteroposterior radiograph is being obtained by the technologist, the subluxation may reduce with forearm supination for positioning. In these cases, the child will often begin using the arm shortly after finishing the x-ray studies.

If the subluxation is not thus reduced, reduction is accomplished simply by supinating the forearm. At times, a small click may be felt or heard as the radial head slides back under the annular ligament, which is blocking reduction in the pronated position. The use of a sling for a day or two may be needed, but cast immobilization is not necessary. Return to full activity occurs rapidly when the symptoms subside.

Sometimes radial head subluxation is recurrent. If this injury is produced by the classic method of pulling on the arm, the same treatment of sling use for a short time should be sufficient. If this subluxation occurs more than three times, even with avoidance of pulling on the arm, consideration should be given to evaluating the child for a joint laxity syndrome (e.g., Ehlers-

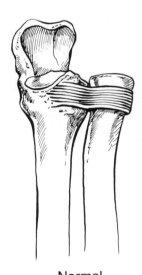
Normal

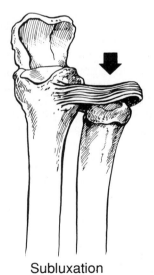
Subluxation

Figure 5.16. Radial head subluxation (nursemaid's elbow). In a child below the age of 6, the shape of the proximal radius is rather slender, allowing the radial head and neck to move distal to the annular ligament when the arm is pulled or the child is lifted by the arm. In the young child, this readily reduces with forearm rotation. As the child becomes older, the radial head enlarges, preventing this subluxation.

Danlos). If recurrent dislocation occurs following a more severe injury, surgical repair of the radiohumeral ligament complex may be needed.

The diagnosis of nursemaid's elbow should *not* be made in children over age 6. If recurrent dislocation or more subtle instability of the elbow in these children is present, a more thorough workup is needed, as surgical treatment will often be necessary. Imaging studies that can be helpful in this situation are radiographs to demonstrate bony alignment and magnetic resonance imaging to delineate cartilaginous and ligamentous abnormalities.

Medial Epicondylitis ("Little Leaguer's Elbow")

The bane of many a young pitcher, this condition arises from repetitive stress on the apophysis of the medial humeral epicondyle ossification center, generally from throwing a baseball.

In any overhand throwing motion, the elbow assumes a valgus position when the forearm and hand are brought forward, thus putting a great deal of stress on the medial ligaments of the elbow. Since the proximal attachment of the medial collateral ligament is onto the medial humeral epicondyle ossification center, the valgus stress is transferred to the cartilaginous attachment of this ossification center to the humerus. As in other conditions in the immature child, the cartilage is the weak link in the skeletal system, and the result is a microfracture through apophyseal cartilage, similar to the pathophysiology of Osgood-Schlatter "disease" of the knee. If throwing activity continues, further microfractures of this cartilage, with adjacent inflammation, will result.

The physical examination will demonstrate point tenderness over the medial humeral epicondyle. A mild limitation of full extension may result from the pain associated with this condition. Elbow swelling is not generally present. Because the medial humeral epicondyle also is the site of origin of the wrist flexors and the forearm pronator muscles, passive forearm supination and wrist extension may produce pain.

Radiographs of the elbow are almost always normal. However, if mild elbow pain suddenly becomes worse while throwing, displacement and fragmentation of the medial epicondyle may be seen on the radiographs (Fig. 5.17). Magnetic resonance imaging shows high signal in the cartilage between the medial epicondyle ossification center and the main part of the humerus on T1-weighted images.

Treatment consists primarily of rest, with avoidance of throwing. Injections of corti-

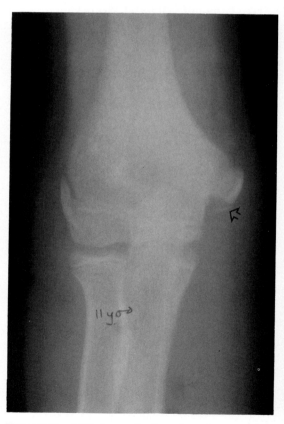

Figure 5.17. Little leaguer's elbow in an 11-year-old pitcher shows the result of repeated microfractures of the apophysis of the medial humeral epicondyle (*open arrow*).

costeroids or anesthetic agents into this area of the elbow should be avoided. Once the pain has resolved, strengthening exercises for the upper arm are appropriate, and stretching of the wrist flexors and forearm pronator should be accomplished prior to resuming throwing activities.

If medial epicondyle pain becomes recurrent, the child's throwing motion should be evaluated and modified to minimize valgus stress at the elbow. In some instances, the child should be switched to another position and avoid pitching altogether. Although some authors believe that throwing curve balls at a young age is the cause of this condition, by the sudden forearm supination needed at ball release, pain in the medial elbow may also result from throwing only fastballs.

Osteochondritis Dissecans of the Capitellum

This condition involves the lateral side of the elbow joint, and may occur alone or in conjunction with medial epicondylitis. Frequently associated with throwing sports, this capitellar lesion is thought to result from valgus stress at the elbow, in which the capitellum is compressed against the radial head as the throwing arm is brought forward from the cocked position.

Physical examination usually reveals a mild flexion contracture of the elbow and tenderness directly over the capitellum to palpation. Manual longitudinal compression of the radius against the distal humerus may reproduce or exacerbate the pain. An elbow effusion may be present.

Radiographs are often normal but may show a small radiolucency in the capitellum. At times a loose body of either bone or cartilage will be present within the joint. Tomograms of the distal humerus will define the extent of the lesion more clearly. A magnetic resonance image will allow visualization of the cartilaginous extent of the lesion.

If osteochondritis dissecans is diagnosed and no loose body is seen, the initial treatment consists of splinting the elbow and avoiding sports for several weeks. If, after rehabilitation of the arm strength and elbow movement, the pain recurs, surgical treatment is indicated. Arthroscopy of the elbow is difficult in this young age group, and open surgery is generally needed. The area of osteochondritis dissecans can be excised if it is relatively small and may be reattached if it involves a large portion of the capitellum. Return to sport is generally feasible after treatment is complete.

PHYSICAL THERAPY NOTE

Many of the conditions noted in this chapter may lead to rather prolonged periods of motion restriction in the elbow. Patience must be maintained by the physician and the family, as the large majority of these children will eventually regain full, or nearly full, elbow motion. If physical therapy is used, either in the office or at home, only active and active assisted exercises should be employed. Passive stretching by parents or therapists may lead to local hemorrhage or inflammation, which in turn usually leads to further loss of movement rather than to improved function. In the older child with an intra-articular injury, spring-loaded splints with variable tension adjustments may be used at night to facilitate return to full motion.

Suggested Readings

Abraham, E., Powers, T., Witt, P., et al.: Experimental hyperextension supracondylar fractures in monkeys. Clin. Orthop. 171:309-318, 1982.

Adams, J.E.: Injury to the throwing arm: A study of traumatic changes in the elbow joints of boy baseball players. Calif. Med. 102:127-132, 1965.

Brogdon, B.G. and Crow, N.E.: Little leaguer's elbow. Am. J. Roentgenol. 83:671-675, 1960.

Fowles, J.V. and Kassab, M.T.: Displaced fractures of the medial humeral condyle in children. J. Bone Joint Surg. 62A:1159-1163, 1980.

Haraldsson, S.: On osteochondrosis deformans juvenalis capituli humeri including investigation of intraosseous vasculature in distal humerus. Acta Orthop. Scand. 38(suppl):1-232, 1959.

Jakob, R., Fowles, J.V., Rang, M., et al.: Observations

concerning fractures of the lateral humeral condyle in children. J. Bone Joint Surg. 57B:430-436, 1975.

Mardam-Bey, T. and Ger, E.: Congenital radial head dislocation. J. Hand Surg. 4:316-320, 1979.

Murphy, W.A. and Siegel, M.J.: Elbow fat pads with new signs and extended differential diagnosis. Radiology 124:659-665, 1977.

Ogino, T. and Hikino, K.: Congenital radio-ulnar synostosis: Compensatory rotation around the wrist and rotation osteotomy. J. Hand Surg. 12B:173-178, 1987.

Pirone, A.M., Graham, H.K., and Krajbich, J.I.: Management of displaced extension-type supracondylar fractures of the humerus in children. J. Bone Joint Surg. 70A:641-650, 1988.

Rang, M.: Children's Fractures, 2nd edition. Philadelphia, J.B. Lippincott, 1983.

Rockwood, C.A., Jr., Wilkins, K.E., and King, R.E. (eds): Fractures in Children, volume 3. Philadelphia, J.B. Lippincott, 1984.

Salter, R.B. and Zaltz, C.: Anatomic investigations of the mechanism of injury and pathologic anatomy of "pulled elbow" in young children. Clin. Orthop. 77: 134-143, 1971.

Simmons, B.P. and Southmayd, W. W.: Congenital radioulnar synostosis. J. Hand Surg. 8:829-838, 1983.

6
Forearm and Wrist

The forearm and wrist region of the upper extremity is one of the most commonly injured areas in children. Any type of fall usually results in a child extending the arm to absorb the impact of landing. In so doing, a fracture may occur at the elbow but more often occurs in the mid-forearm or wrist area. It is important to remember the features of the child's skeletal system that make these injuries different than in the adult when evaluating injuries in the forearm and wrist.

Anatomy

The basic anatomy of this region consists of the radius and ulna, surrounded by the muscles, nerves, and blood vessels that allow for hand and wrist function. The ulna articulates with the trochlear portion of the distal humerus at the elbow and supports the medial or ulnar aspect of the carpal bones at the wrist. At the elbow, the ulna functions as a hinge joint, moving only in the flexion and extension planes.

The radius, on the other hand, moves in flexion and extension but also is responsible for allowing forearm rotation. The radius shaft has a bow of approximately 20° to facilitate rotation around the ulna, and normally 180° of rotation is possible at the proximal radioulnar joint. This rotation movement consists of 90° of supination (palm up) and 90° of pronation (palm facing down). The biceps tendon inserts into the

bicipital tubercle on the proximal metaphysis of the radius, thus acting as a major supinator of the forearm as well as the major elbow flexor. The distal radius articulates with the navicular and lunate bones in the wrist.

The wrist and finger flexor muscles lie on the volar or ventral aspect of the forearm, and the extensor muscles lie dorsally. The major neurovascular structures are mainly on the volar aspect of the forearm. The ulnar nerve runs with the ulnar artery on the medial surface and innervates multiple muscles of the hand as well as the muscles that flex the ulnar aspect of the wrist and the ring and little fingers. The median nerve accompanies the radial artery and innervates the majority of the flexor muscles of the wrist and fingers, in addition to some of the muscles controlling thumb motion. The radial nerve moves from a volar position to a dorsal position and is the primary source of innervation for the long extensors of the wrist and fingers of the hand.

There are eight bones that make up the carpus or wrist. The proximal row consists of, from radial side to ulnar side, the navicular or scaphoid, the lunate, the triquetrum, and the pisiform. The distal row is formed by the trapezoid, trapezium, capitate, and hamate. These carpal bones are connected to each other and to the distal radius and ulna by capsules and ligaments, the most recognized of which are the dorsal triangular cartilage complex and the conoid ligaments (see Figs. 7.1 and 7.2).

Examination

The physical examination in this region of the upper extremity consists primarily of evaluation of the region with the most tenderness, evaluation of rotation of the forearm, and evaluation of neurovascular function of the hand and fingers.

OBSERVATION

Is deformity present? Where is the swelling? What is the preferred resting position of the hand at the wrist? Is the hand well perfused or pale compared to the other arm? Are pulses present?

RANGE-OF-MOTION

Evaluation of the pronation and supination of the forearm should be performed with the elbow flexed 90° and the arm held at the side of the trunk. (To enhance the accuracy of measurement of motion with this examination, a pencil or other object of similar length can be held in the hand of the child being evaluated.) The child is then requested to pronate and supinate the forearm to the full extent possible with the arm held at the side. If the arm is not flexed and held at the side, it is difficult to eliminate the effect of shoulder rotation on forearm rotation.

NEUROVASCULAR EXAMINATION

The neurovascular function of the hand and fingers is similar to that noted for distal evaluation in the case of fractures around the elbow. Both radial and ulnar pulses can be readily checked. The autonomous area of sensory function for the median nerve is the volar tip of the index finger, for the radial nerve the dorsal web space between the thumb and index finger, and for the ulnar nerve the tip of the little finger on the ventral surface. Motor function of nerves in this area can be assessed quickly by evaluation of wrist extension (radial), flexion of the distal interphalangeal joint of the index finger (median), and flexion of the little finger (ulnar).

PALPATION

Unless dislocation is present, injury to the carpal bones generally results in only minimal swelling, so palpation is important to localizing the specific region of abnormality. The primary carpal bone that is injured is the carpal navicular or scaphoid. Palpation in the anatomical snuffbox (just dorsal to the thumb extensor at the radial aspect of the carpus) is the way to assess an injury to the navicular. If tenderness is present here, a navicular fracture is assumed to be present, even if the radiographs appear normal.

NORMAL RADIOGRAPHIC FINDINGS

As noted in Chapter 5, a line drawn up the long axis of the radius should intersect the midcapitellum at the elbow. This relationship should always be noted when a forearm fracture is present; both the elbow and wrist joints must be included in any radiograph of the forearm when a fracture is present. While the ulna is straight, the radius normally has a mild bow outward. At the wrist, the distal radius normally extends slightly farther distally than does the distal ulna. The distal radius ossification center is present early, appearing by the age of 1 year, whereas the distal ulnar ossification center does not appear until later.

Disorders of the Forearm and Wrist
CONGENITAL DISORDERS
Radioulnar Synostosis

Inherited as an autosomal-dominant condition, radioulnar synostosis may be present in the child's parent or sibling as well. During embryonic development, the radius and ulna fail to separate at the proximal end, leading to a cartilaginous bridge in this region followed by a bony bar connecting these two bones. This may affect one elbow or both.

The position of the radioulnar fusion determines the appearance of the forearm on visual examination. No significant arm deformity is seen in a young child unless the forearm has fused in an extreme position of rotation. The major finding on examination is complete loss of forearm rotation. The child will usually have some ability to rotate the hand, by rotating either the wrist or the shoulder, as a result of learning to cope with the rotation restriction.

The diagnosis is confirmed by anteroposterior and lateral radiographs of the elbow. A bony bar bridges the proximal ulna and radius, with angular change and bowing of the radial neck (see Fig. 5.6).

Treatment consists of appropriate diagnosis and explanation to the child and parents. Attempts at resection of this bar to restore forearm rotation have been unsuccessful, even with the placement of various interposition devices to prevent re-formation of this bar. No physical therapy is indicated. Surgical treatment is reserved for children whose synostosis has led to extreme positions of forearm rotation. In certain cases, osteotomy of the proximal radius and ulna to rotate the forearm to a preferred position is feasible. While this procedure does not lead to improved forearm rotation, the hand position is improved for better function.

Children with radioulnar synostosis generally adapt well to this abnormality. No restriction of activity or sports participation is usually needed.

TRAUMATIC DISORDERS

Midshaft Radius and Ulna Fracture

The primary traumatic disorder of the forearm in a child is a fracture of the radius and ulna, often termed a both-bones fracture. These fractures result from a fall on the arm. Fractures in this location are rarely associated with neurovascular injury or compartment syndrome unless there is marked displacement at the fracture site.

In the very young child, a fall on the arm may result in bowing of the radius and/or ulna rather than actual fracture. Because of the inherent elasticity of the bones of young children, plastic deformation of the bone occurs prior to the actual fracture. If the force dissipates before fracture occurs, the child may present with forearm pain and swelling

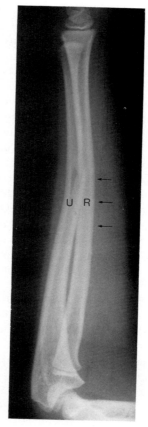

Figure 6.1. Lateral forearm radiograph shows midshaft ulnar (*U*) fracture with intact dorsal cortex, and acute plastic bowing fracture (*arrows*) of the radius.

and a radiograph showing bowing without fracture (Fig. 6.1). If a bone scan is performed in these cases, there is increased uptake of radionuclide, indicating that microfractures occurred. Treatment of a traumatically bowed bone is similar to that of a complete fracture, and reduction or straightening of the bone is followed by a few weeks of cast immobilization.

The more common result of a fall on the outstretched hand is a complete fracture of the radius and ulna, often with displacement. Swelling and deformity are obvious on examination, and radiographs confirm the fracture and degree of displacement. These fractures heal well and remodel with small degrees of malalignment, so the most important goal of reduction is to obtain realignment in such a way that forearm pronation and supination are not diminished. While these fractures in teenagers and adults usually require open reduction and internal fixation to preserve the best function and avoid limitation of rotation, in children below the age of 12, closed reduction and casting is almost always successful. When molding a cast for this fracture, it is important to try to prevent the ulna from being in contact with the radius at the fracture site to avoid bridging of these bones as the fracture unites. In addition, the normal bowing of the radius should be reestablished or else there is an increased risk of refracture. These fractures require cast immobilization of 6 to 8 weeks in a long arm cast.

Monteggia Fracture

Described first by Monteggia, this injury classically consists of an ulnar fracture associated with an anterior dislocation of the radial head. The ulnar fracture may occur anywhere along the shaft of the ulna, but most commonly is at the midshaft or slightly proximal to the midshaft (Fig. 6.2). The fracture of the ulna may appear only slightly angulated, so reduction is not needed in the young child. However, careful attention must be paid to the elbow joint, particularly the radiohumeral joint. For all children with forearm fractures the radiograph must include the elbow. (Remember, a line up the long axis of the radius should *always* intersect the capitellum of the distal humerus.)

The first step in treating this injury is to make the correct diagnosis. The second step is to manipulate the ulna, reducing the fracture to regain ulnar length and allow the radial head to reduce. If closed reduction is not feasible, operative treatment of the ulna fracture may be needed to regain the needed length to allow the radial head to slide back into place. Reduction of the radial head is

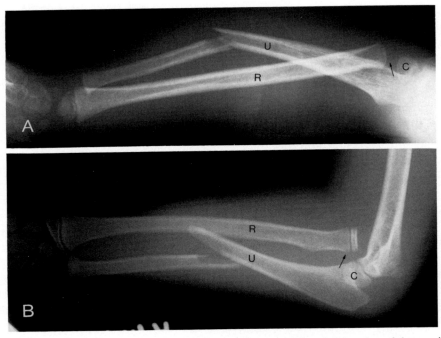

Figure 6.2. A, AP view of a Monteggia fracture with ulnar fracture (*U*) and dislocation of the proximal radius (*R*). The radius should articulate directly with the capitellum (*C*), and a line up the long axis of the radius should always pass through the capitellum. **B,** Lateral view of a Monteggia fracture with ulnar fracture (*U*) and anterior dislocation of the radial (*R*) head (*arrow*) from its usual articulation with the capitellum (*C*).

easiest in full forearm supination and elbow flexion, as this relaxes the biceps tendon pull on the proximal radius. Casting is used for approximately 6 weeks after injury.

Distal Radius and Ulna Shaft Fracture

A fracture of the distal radial and ulnar shafts is a very common injury in childhood. As a result of a fall onto the hand, the child may develop either a torus fracture or a complete displaced fracture at this location.

A torus or buckle fracture is seen in children or in adults with osteoporotic bone. Children have a more porous cortex in their long bones, so a bending deformity of the bone will lead to a cortical compression fracture on the concave side rather than on the convexity, where a fracture in a mature normal individual begins. Although a torus

fracture looks insignificant on the radiograph (Fig. 6.3) and may demonstrate only moderate tenderness on examination, one should remember that prior to the fracture, the elastic bone had deformed considerably more than can be seen in the radiograph. Unless a well-molded cast or splint is applied, with the normal resorption that occurs at a fracture site during healing, there may be further angulation at the fracture site in the 2 to 3 weeks following fracture. A short arm cast should be used for 4 to 5 weeks, and radiographs should be checked 7 to 10 days after cast application to see if the alignment has been adequately maintained.

When a fracture of the distal forearm is displaced, the distal fragment moves most often in a dorsal direction. Since the median

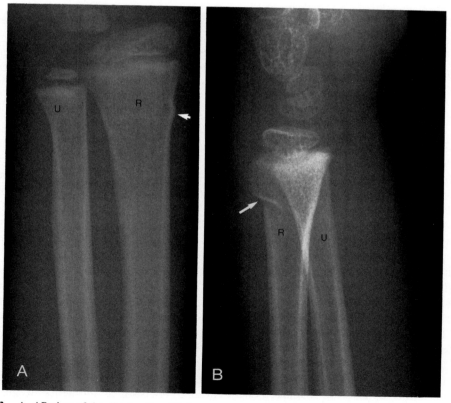

Figure 6.3. **A,** AP view of the distal radius (*R*) demonstrates a buckle fracture of the cortex (*arrow*) following a fall. **B,** Lateral radiograph of the wrist shows a buckle fracture of the dorsal cortex with impaction (*arrow*).

nerve may be stretched over the end of the proximal fracture fragment during injury, its function should be specifically checked prior to treatment. Before the teenage years, operative treatment of a distal forearm fracture is rarely needed, and closed reduction and casting for approximately 6 weeks will lead to very good results.

Distal Radial and Ulnar Physeal Fracture

With the same mechanism of injury that produces distal radial and ulnar shaft fractures, a fracture may occur through the open distal radial and ulnar growth plates or physes. Salter-Harris type I and II fractures occur most often. In many instances, the distal radius has a physeal fracture, while the distal ulna is fractured through the metaphysis or ulnar styloid.

Examination of the wrist after this fracture will show swelling and deformity on the dorsum of the wrist due to the usual dorsal angulation and displacement of the distal fracture fragments. If displacement is severe, median and ulnar nerve injury may coexist, so documentation of neurologic function in the fingers must be completed at initial evaluation prior to reduction attempts.

As with physeal fractures of other long bones, to minimize the risk of permanent injury to the growth plate, the number of attempts at reduction of this fracture should be limited. Adequate local or general anesthesia should be available to permit accurate, near-anatomic reduction to be completed with no more than two manipulations. It is preferable to accept a few millimeters of displacement at the fracture site than to repeatedly manipulate physeal fractures for perfect reduction of type I and II fractures here. After reduction has been accomplished, a well-molded cast is needed to maintain the reduction. Radiographs are checked within the first week following reduction, as fracture displacement can occur in the cast as the swelling diminishes. A distal radial and ulnar physeal frac-

ture should be nontender and healed 3 to 4 weeks after reduction. Growth arrests at this site are uncommon, but the family should still be counseled about this possibility as a result of this injury.

Other Wrist Fractures

A fall onto the hand may result in wrist pain without any deformity seen on examination and without any fractures apparent on radiographs. This tenderness must be carefully located by examination to reach an appropriate diagnosis. The differential diagnosis includes fractures to the carpal navicular and the hamate.

The more common of these is a fracture of the *carpal navicular*. Examination will elicit point tenderness to palpation at the anatomical snuffbox, an area on the radial aspect of the wrist between the extensor tendon and the abductor tendon of the thumb. While wrist radiographs are often normal, a special navicular series may show a fracture line (Fig. 6.4). Once diagnosed, the carpal navicular fracture requires casting in a thumb spica cast for 6 to 12 weeks.

Two main complications may result from this fracture: nonunion and avascular necrosis. If the diagnosis is not made and appropriately treated, scar tissue will form in the fracture site and wrist pain will continue to be present with activity. Navicular nonunions require either surgical treatment or, at times, prolonged cast treatment.

Since the blood supply to the carpal navicular enters the bone distally, a fracture through the middle or waist of the navicular may render the proximal pole of the navicular ischemic. This avascular necrosis may occur even in nondisplaced fractures and frequently requires surgical treatment to eliminate the wrist pain.

Pain and tenderness at the hypothenar eminence may result from a fracture of the hook of the *hamate*. This pain is exaggerated by twisting movements of the wrist, such as swinging a golf club or a bat. Since a regular wrist radiograph will not clearly

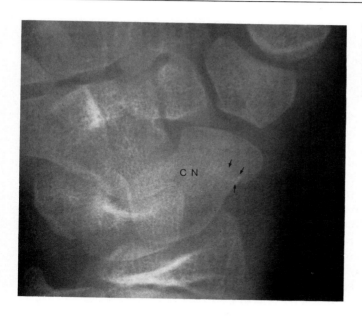

Figure 6.4. Fracture (*arrows*) of the carpal navicular (*CN*) is present after the patient fell on his hand. On examination, tenderness was present in the anatomical snuffbox, characteristic of a navicular fracture.

show this fracture, a special tunnel view of the wrist should be obtained if hypothenar tenderness is the key physical finding and the initial radiographs appear normal. Casting for 3 to 6 weeks will allow for fracture healing and pain resolution.

Sprains of the Wrist

Although physeal injuries should always be suspected if wrist area pain is present after a child falls, ligamentous injury can occur. To differentiate a ligament injury from a nondisplaced physeal fracture requires careful notation of the point of maximal tenderness. If the tenderness is mainly over the distal physis of the radius or ulna, casting is needed. If tenderness is maximal over the dorsal wrist between the distal ulna and the distal radius, a tear of the triangular cartilage complex may be present. If a sprain is diagnosed, a removable wrist splint will generally suffice to allow healing, though some of these fibrocartilage injuries become chronic, causing wrist pain with rotational movements and at times requiring surgical treatment for cure.

The author does not recommend cortico-

steroid injection in a child as a treatment for ongoing wrist pain. If initial splinting treatment is unsuccessful, magnetic resonance imaging may be useful in more clearly defining the soft tissue injury present. Surgical treatment may be needed in unusual circumstances, but most sprains will resolve with splinting and rest.

Wrist Pain in Gymnasts

A special problem may be seen in growing children who are very active in gymnastics. Highly competitive gymnasts often have wrist pain with tenderness at the distal radioulnar joint. Frequently the ulnar styloid appears to be longer than normal, and this finding can be confirmed by radiographs. Magnetic resonance imaging studies of the wrists of skeletally immature gymnasts have demonstrated growth plate abnormalities, accounting for the slower growth of the radius and the apparent overgrowth of the ulna. Evaluation of persistent wrist pain in a young gymnast who works out several times a week should often lead to a magnetic resonance study of this region. Treatment in this setting involves at least a temporary period of decreased gymnastics or complete rest until the wrist pain resolves.

Soft Tissue Injury in the Forearm

Contusions to the forearm musculature are common in sport activities. These contusions generally lead to localized hemorrhage within the muscles, with resultant tenderness and swelling that lasts for just a few days. The early initial treatment of contusions is the application of ice to slow the bleeding in the muscle. After the first 24 hours, heat on the bruised area increases comfort and may speed the resolution of the hematoma. Sports activity should not be begun again until pain is absent and the adjacent joint motion is normal. When athletic activity is started, stretching of the injured muscles prior to playing will assist in preventing a recurrent injury, at least for the first several weeks after the muscle contusion resolves.

Suggested Readings

Bailey, D.A., Wedge, J.H., McCulloch, R.G., et al.: Epidemiology of fractures of the distal end of the radius in children as associated with growth. J. Bone Joint Surg. 71A:1225-1231, 1989.

Davis, D.R. and Green, D.P.: Forearm fractures in children: Pitfalls and complications. Clin. Orthop. 120:172-183, 1976.

Larsen, E., Vittas, D., and Torrp-Pedersen, S.: Remodeling of angulated distal forearm fractures in children. Clin. Orthop. 237:190-195, 1988.

Mabrey, J.D. and Fitch, R.D.: Plastic deformation in pediatric fractures: Mechanism and treatment. J. Pediatr. Orthop. 9:310-314, 1989.

Mussbichler, H.: Injuries of the carpal scaphoid in children. Acta Radiol. 56:361-368, 1961.

Rang, M.: Children's Fractures, 2nd edition. Philadelphia, J.B. Lippincott, 1983.

Rockwood, C.A., Jr., Wilkins, K.E., and King, R.E. (eds): Fractures in Children, Volume 3. Philadelphia, J.B. Lippincott, 1984.

Tredwell, S.J., Van Peteghem, K., Clough, M.: Pattern of forearm fractures in children. J. Pediatr. Orthop. 4:604-608, 1984.

Vahvanen, V. and Westerlund, M.: Fracture of the carpal scaphoid in children: A clinical and roentgenologic study of 108 cases. Acta Orthop. Scand. 51:909-913, 1980.

7

Hand

Anatomy

The skeletal anatomy of the hand is relatively simple. Five metacarpals join the fingers to the carpal or wrist area. The thumb is composed of a proximal and a distal phalanx, while each of the other four fingers have three phalanges: proximal, middle, and distal (Figs. 7.1 and 7.2). The growth plate for the first metacarpal is located at the proximal end, while the growth plates for the other four metacarpals are located only at the distal ends. The physis for each of the phalanges is located only at the proximal end.

Normal movement at the carpometacarpal joints varies widely. The first metacarpal forms a saddle-type joint here and has a wide range of movement in several planes. The second metacarpal is nearly motionless at its articulation with the wrist. The third, fourth, and fifth metacarpals have progressively more dorsal and ventral mobility, a fact that needs to be considered to appropriately treat metacarpal fractures.

Each of the interphalangeal joints and the metacarpophalangeal joints move normally only in the flexion and extension plane, with 90° of motion present in this plane.

Movement of the fingers and thumb is provided by muscles of the forearm and of the hand itself. Interphalangeal joint flexion is provided mainly by the long flexors (flexor digitorum superficialis and flexor digitorum profundus), which pass through the palm in fascial sheaths to insert into the base of the middle (superficialis) and distal (profundus) phalanges (Fig. 7.3). The flexor pollicis longus is the long flexor of the thumb. In general, the major flexion power during grasping is provided largely by these forearm flexor muscles.

The intrinsic muscles of the hand include several interosseous and lumbrical muscles, originating from the metacarpals and inserting primarily on phalanges. Extension of the interphalangeal joints is provided by the long extensors of the forearm (extensor digitorum communis and extensor pollicis longus), as well as by the intrinsic muscles of the hand. The intrinsic muscles extend the interphalangeal joints only with the metacarpophalangeal joints flexed, while the long extensors extend the fingers even with these metacarpophalangeal joints extended.

Intrinsic muscles of the hand are also responsible for special hand movements. Opposition of the thumb to one of the other fingers allows one to pinch an object. Abducting or spreading the fingers is controlled by these intrinsic muscles, as is side-to-side pinching of the thumb against the index finger.

The arterial supply to the hand and fingers is provided by the radial and ulnar arteries, both palpable on the volar or ventral surface near the wrist. The radial pulse is just lateral to the palmaris longus tendon, while the ulnar artery is palpable adjacent to the flexor carpi ulnaris tendon just before its insertion. These arteries join to form the palmar arch, which distributes digital arteries to each of the fingers. In some cases, there is more vascular supply from either

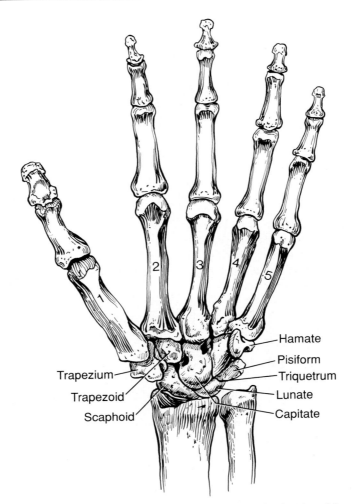

Trapezium

Trapezoid

Scaphoid

Hamate

Pisiform

Triquetrum

Lunate

Capitate

Figure 7.1. This diagram illustrates the skeletal anatomy of the hand and wrist viewed from the palmar aspect. The eight carpal bones are arranged in two rows of four bones each. As a result of the anatomic variation at the metacarpocarpal joint, the fifth metacarpal is the most mobile, while the second metacarpal is the least mobile.

the radial or the ulnar artery than from the other. Before radial artery catheterization is performed, it is important to make sure that the ulnar artery pulse is good and that the hand remains well perfused when the radial artery is temporarily manually occluded.

The primary nerve supply to the hand and fingers comes from the radial, median, and ulnar nerves. The radial nerve innervates the long extensor muscles of the wrist and fingers, while the median and ulnar nerves innervate the finger and wrist flexor muscles, the ulnar nerve serving the ring and little fingers and the median nerve the other fingers and thumb. The intrinsic muscles of the hand are supplied mainly by ulnar nerves, but some intrinsic muscles supplied by the median nerve are located in or near the thenar eminence and affect mainly thumb function.

The dorsum of the hand, thumb, and base of the fingers derives its sensation from the radial nerve. The palmar aspect of the thumb, the index and long fingers, and half of the ring finger is innervated by the median nerve, while the entire little finger and half the ring finger are supplied by the ulnar nerve. There may be some overlap in this sensory distribution, but certain autonomous areas for each of these nerves exist. The autonomous areas are the dorsal web space between the thumb and index finger for the radial nerve, the palmar tip of the index finger for the median nerve, and the palmar tip of the little finger for the ulnar nerve (Figs. 7.4 and 7.5).

The nail at the dorsal tip of each finger arises from a nail bed located just below the skin proximal to the visible fingernail. In some ways, this nail bed functions as a growth plate, pushing the nail distally as growth proceeds. Damage to this nail bed may lead to nail deformity or failure of further nail growth (Fig. 7.3).

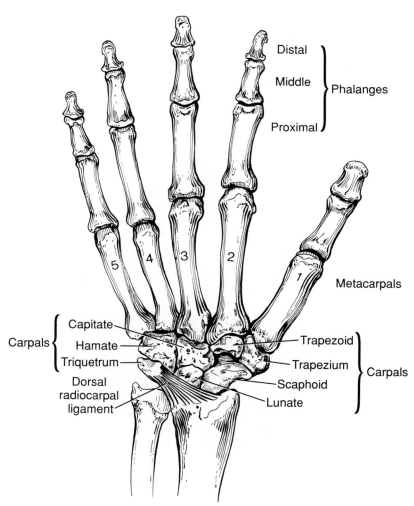

Figure 7.2. This dorsal view of the skeletal anatomy of the hand and wrist also includes the dorsal wrist ligament that is prone to injury with sports. Injury to the dorsal ligament complex at the distal radioulnar joint may lead to chronic pain with repetitive movements of the wrist.

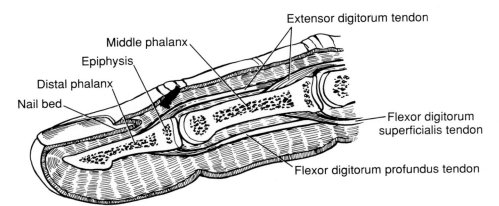

Figure 7.3. This sagittal section through a finger demonstrates several important anatomic features. Because of the position of the tendon insertions at or near the epiphyses of the middle and distal phalanges, avulsion fractures can readily occur with sudden forced flexion or extension of the finger during sports activity. Because of their anatomic proximity, injuries to the nail bed may occur with crush injury of the distal phalanx. Due to the honeycomb-like arrangement of the fingertip on the palmar aspect, an infection at this site (a felon) commonly requires surgical treatment.

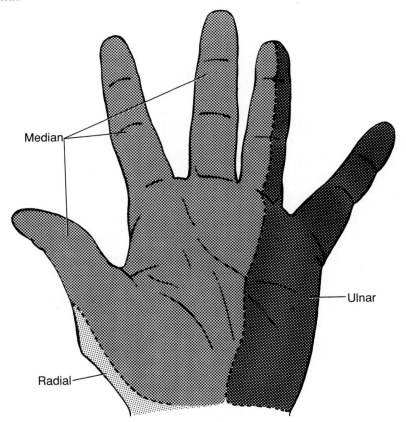

Figure 7.4. The skin innervation of the palmar aspect of the hand is generally constant for the radial, median, and ulnar nerves. The autonomous zone for the median nerve is the palmar tip of the index finger and the autonomous zone for the ulnar nerve the tip of the fifth finger.

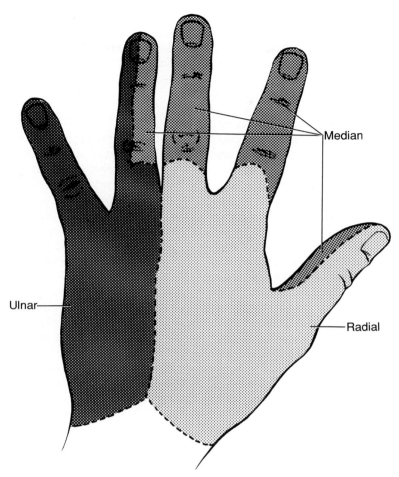

Figure 7.5. On the dorsum of the hand, the innervation of the skin is likewise relatively constant. The autonomous area of radial nerve sensation is on the skin web between the dorsal thumb and index finger.

Physical Examination

Simple observation of the hand will diagnose most of the congenital disorders and many of the traumatic injuries. If no deformity is present, it is useful simply to observe the young child trying to use the hand to assess for flexion and extension of the fingers and the wrist. Holding an object for the young child to grasp may enable the examiner to see active movements, even without the overt cooperation of the child. Does the thumb move out of the palm when an object is grasped? Do all fingers move together in flexion and extension or are some not moving? Will the child refuse to hold or reach for an object?

Areas of tenderness can be palpated easily in the older child, though exact localization of pain is more difficult in the toddler or young child. Swelling will lead to limitation of adjacent joint motion, as will pain from a recent injury. As a general rule, 90° of flexion from the straight or extended position is normal for all interphalangeal joints and metacarpophalangeal joints in the hand.

A careful neurologic examination of the hand is important, particularly in the case of associated trauma of the upper arm, forearm, or wrist region. If the anterior interosseous branch of the median nerve is injured in the upper forearm or elbow, as with a supracondylar fracture of the distal humerus, distal interphalangeal joint flexion of the index finger is absent. If the median nerve is injured in the upper arm, this flexion is absent, as is index finger sensation. If the median nerve is injured at the wrist level, sensation in the median distribution is absent and the thenar muscles will not move the thumb normally. Injury to the ulnar nerve at or above the elbow will lead to sensory loss and motor loss of the long flexors of the ring and little fingers as well as weakness in metacarpophalangeal flexion and interphalangeal extension, usually provided by the intrinsic muscles of the hand. If the ulnar nerve injury is at the wrist, the ring and little finger long flexors will still function, but the other sensory and motor findings will be the same as for the elbow region injury. In a radial nerve injury in the upper arm, wrist extension and long finger extensor function will be absent. If the radial nerve is injured at the wrist level, motor function will be essentially normal, while dorsal hand sensation will be impaired. It is clear that a careful motor and sensory examination of the hand will allow better localization of any injury throughout the entire upper extremity.

Lacerations in the finger or hand require careful examination for nerve or tendon injury. The digital nerves and arteries run along the lateral aspect of the finger. The position of the neurovascular bundle can be estimated by flexing the finger fully; the neurovascular bundle will usually be found at the dorsal edge of the crease formed at the interphalangeal joint in this flexed position. If a laceration has occurred in this region, distal sensation must be carefully checked, since most digital nerve lacerations are best repaired early. If the laceration is on the palmar or dorsal aspect of the finger or hand, the function of each tendon possibly injured should be carefully noted. Particularly in the case of the flexor tendons, primary repair at the time of laceration offers the best chance for an excellent later result.

Normal Radiographic Features

The skeletal anatomy is demonstrated by anteroposterior and lateral radiographs. Each of the phalanges and the first metacarpal have a proximal growth plate without a distal physis. The other four metacarpals have only a distal physis that provides the longitudinal growth for these bones.

Radiographs of the hand can be used to assess a child's skeletal maturity, based at first on the pattern of ossification center formation, then on the pattern of progressive epiphyseal maturation, then on physeal closure as growth and skeletal maturation proceed. By comparison with a text of standards (e.g., Greulich and Pyle), it is possible to estimate the bone age of the child. Full skeletal maturity is reached in a female at a bone age of 16 years and in a male at a bone age of 18 years. However, little growth occurs during the final year before skeletal maturation.

Traumatic and Sports Injuries
METACARPAL FRACTURE

Metacarpal fractures are common, and are usually caused either by the hand being struck or by the hand striking an object. Physical examination will reveal swelling and tenderness over the site of fracture. Inspection of the knuckles may reveal that one is not as prominent as usual when the fingers are flexed. Neurovascular injury is rarely associated with this fracture.

Radiographs of the hand will demonstrate the site of fracture and the amount of displacement present, two features that will determine the type of treatment recommended (Figs. 7.6 and 7.7). With a fifth metacarpal fracture, the so-called boxer's

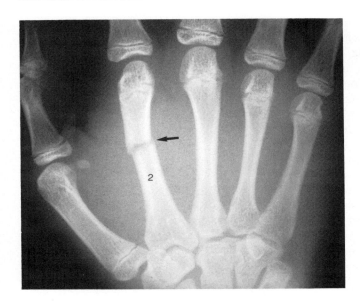

Figure 7.6. A transverse fracture (*arrow*) of the midshaft of the second metacarpal is present, sustained by the child being struck with a block. A fracture of the second metacarpal requires near-anatomic reduction.

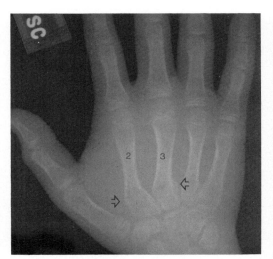

Figure 7.7. These fractures (*open arrows*) of the proximal second and third metacarpals were secondary to a crush injury.

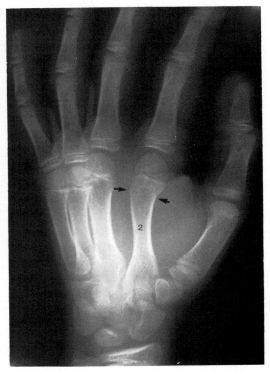

Figure 7.8. A boxer's fracture (*arrows*) of the second metacarpal, sustained by punching a friend in the face, shows volar angulation of the distal fragment and cortical impaction.

fracture usually sustained by hitting someone or something, up to 45° of palmar angulation of the distal fracture fragment is acceptable, because the base of this metacarpal moves about 45° at the articulation with the wrist bones. In the second metacarpal (Fig. 7.8), less than 10° of angulation can be accepted because little carpometacarpal motion is present to compensate for residual distal angulation. In the first metacarpal, exact anatomic reduction is not needed because of the multiplane motion present at its carpometacarpal joint.

Even though some angulation is acceptable in specific metacarpals, an attempt at closed reduction should be made, followed by casting using a short arm cast with an extension on at least the palmar aspect of the hand and affected finger. The metacarpophalangeal joint should be immobilized with a cast at a position of about 80° flexion, with the interphalangeal joints flexed about 20°, the so-called position of function. A cast should not be applied with the metacarpophalangeal joint and fingers fully extended. If, after closed reduction is attempted, the remaining angulation is not acceptable, open reduction and pinning are appropriate. These fractures generally are healed after 3 weeks of cast immobilization.

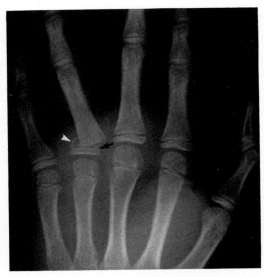

Figure 7.9. Salter-Harris type II fracture of the proximal phalanx of the ring finger shows displacement of the metaphysis (*arrowhead*) on the epiphysis (*arrow*).

PHALANGEAL FRACTURES

Four main types of phalangeal fractures occur: shaft fractures, physeal fractures (Fig. 7.9), intra-articular fractures, and avulsion fractures. (Avulsion fractures are usually associated with dislocations and are discussed under Interphalangeal Joint Dislocations below.)

Phalangeal shaft fractures tend to be oblique, though transverse fractures will result from a direct blow to the hand. Rotation and angulation at the fracture site commonly occur, as well as shortening of the finger due to the pull of the tendons that cross the fracture site. Radiographs will localize the anatomic position of the fracture, but rotation of the fracture fragments may be difficult to judge from the plain films. The fingers should be carefully inspected to assess any rotational deformity that may be present.

Normally, as the fingers are flexed toward the palm, the tips of all fingers tend to point toward the thenar eminence and the radial artery location. Rotational deformity

is difficult to judge with the fingers fully extended but can be demonstrated readily by careful active flexion of the fingers on the injured hand. Rotational deformity needs to be corrected if the injured finger tends to overlap an adjacent finger with this flexion maneuver.

Closed reduction with splint or cast immobilization is sufficient treatment for many phalangeal fractures. The joint above and below the fracture should be included in the immobilization. The interphalangeal joints should be held in a position of about 20° flexion; if the metacarpophalangeal joint needs to be immobilized, 80° of flexion is used for this joint. After reduction and splinting, the finger rotation is again assessed and postreduction radiographs are obtained to confirm the fracture reduction. If angulation, shortening, or rotation cannot be controlled by a splint, operative treatment is recommended. Phalangeal fractures take 2 to 3 weeks to heal. After healing is complete, taping the index and long fingers or the ring and little fingers together ("buddy-taping") is indicated for a few weeks during sports activity to prevent early re-injury.

If unrecognized rotational or angular deformity is present at the time of fracture healing, a corrective osteotomy may be needed to restore good hand function. Since the only phalangeal growth plate is present proximally, fractures in the more distal shaft have less remodeling capacity with growth than those in the proximal half.

Attempts to reduce physeal fractures should be limited to two manipulations. If reduction is not satisfactory, open reduction is needed. Open reduction is also needed if an intra-articular fracture involves more than 20% of the joint surface.

FINGERTIP CRUSH INJURY

A crush injury to the fingertip, such as a child getting a finger caught in a closing car door, can result in a variety of injuries. In the most mild case, a subungual hematoma forms, causing marked pain to the fingertip. Ice can be used to diminish the swelling, but pain relief is best provided by draining the subungual hematoma. The simplest way to do this is to heat a paper clip end over a flame, then apply the hot paper clip end to the base of the nail. The hot paper clip will readily burn a hole into the nail and the hematoma will exit, usually with immediate relief of some pain. Aftercare includes soaking this finger for a few days until the nail hole seals and the pain is absent.

In more severe cases, the distal phalanx sustains a comminuted fracture (Fig. 7.10), the palmar soft tissue is severely bruised, and the nail bed is lacerated. Ice is applied initially to decrease the swelling somewhat. The comminuted distal phalanx fracture requires immobilization only for comfort, as this will heal in 2 to 3 weeks. However, if the nail bed laceration has caused displacement of the nail bed, suture repair under aseptic conditions and local anesthesia should be performed to allow for later normal nail growth. A soft splint or bandage is used for 2 to 3 weeks.

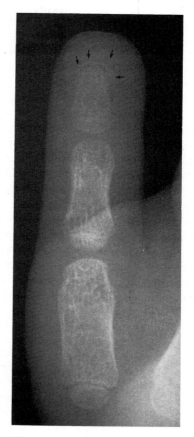

Figure 7.10. Radiograph after a crush fracture of the thumb shows avulsion of a crescent of bone (*arrows*) of the terminal tuft of the distal phalanx. A subungual hematoma is usually associated with this injury.

INTERPHALANGEAL JOINT DISLOCATIONS

A common athletic injury, particularly in ball sports, dislocation of the interphalangeal joint is immediately obvious when the injured hand is observed, because of the deformity present. Occasionally a coach or fellow player will have reduced the dislocation by applying traction to the injured finger before the injured player is seen by a physician. If the finger is still dislocated by the time the player seeks medical attention, reduction is usually readily obtained by longitudinal traction. After reduction has been achieved, an anteroposterior and lateral radiograph of the injured finger should be obtained to assess the injured joint for the position of reduction and for a possible associated avulsion fracture of the phalanx at the site of tendon or ligament attachment. If an avulsion fracture fragment consists of one-third of the joint surface or more, operative treatment is recommended to maintain good joint function. If no avulsion fracture is present, splinting the injured finger to the adjacent finger will immobilize it enough to allow healing. Active movement of the injured joint is begun within a few days of injury. Buddy-taping of the injured finger to the appropriate adjacent finger (index/long or ring/little) should continue for several weeks after the injury, but the teenager can resume sports when the pain has resolved. Localized nontender swelling of the injured interphalangeal joint will persist for months after pain has resolved and motion has returned.

MALLET FINGER

This injury to the distal interphalangeal joint occurs when the tip of an extended finger is struck on the end by a ball, forcing the fingertip into sudden flexion at the distal interphalangeal joint. This injury is common in baseball and football, but can also be found in other sports.

On examination, the teenager holds the distal phalanx of the injured finger in flexion, being unable to actively extend this phalanx. The joint is swollen and tender. Full passive extension is possible. Radiographs generally show a small avulsion fracture from the dorsal aspect of the base of the distal phalanx, where the long extensor tendon of the finger inserts.

Nonsurgical treatment is generally successful but requires patience by all concerned. A splint is applied with the distal interphalangeal joint in a hyperextended position, and this splint is left on for 6 to 8 weeks. In this position, the avulsion fracture fragment reattaches and active phalanx extension is regained. However, premature removal of this splint will result in a persistent extension lag at this joint. Surgical

treatment can also be used, but since the nonoperative treatment is so successful, the teenager should be urged to wear this splint religiously for the entire 6- to 8-week period.

SKIER'S THUMB

Also known as "gamekeeper's thumb," this condition consists of an injury to the ulnar collateral ligament of the thumb. Usually seen now in skiers using poles with wrist straps, this ligament injury results from a sudden forced abduction of the thumb, usually during a fall on the slopes. This injury is less common if ski poles with handles allowing the hand to slip out easily are used.

On examination, tenderness is present over the ulnar side of the thumb metacarpophalangeal joint. Pain is worsened by passive abduction of the thumb at this joint. Instability with abduction stress may be noted compared to the normal thumb. Radiographs may be normal or may demonstrate an avulsion fracture from the base of the proximal phalanx on the ulnar side, where this ligament inserts.

Treatment depends on the severity of the injury. If the joint is stable to abduction stress and no avulsion fracture is seen, a thumb spica cast or splint is used for 3 or 4 weeks. If joint instability is present or displacement of an avulsion fracture is obvious on the radiograph, surgical treatment is warranted, with splinting postoperatively. Although chronic instability at this joint can be treated later with ligament reconstruction, it is preferable to diagnose and treat this injury in the acute phase.

Congenital Disorders

POLYDACTYLY

Supernumerary digits generally form on the ulnar aspect of the hand, adjacent to the little finger. This digit may be only a nubbin of soft tissue or may contain phalanges. Usually there are only five metacarpals, despite the extra digit. Bilateral polydactyly is common, and polydactyly of the feet may also be present. A parent or siblings may have also had polydactyly, though in a slightly different form.

Voluntary control of the extra digit is generally not present. If only a small projection of soft tissue is noted at birth, a suture is commonly tied around this vestigial digit. The extra digit becomes necrotic and falls off. During the time the necrotic digit is still attached, the hand should be observed for possible superimposed infection.

If bony elements are included in the digit, as demonstrated by plain radiographs, formal elective surgical removal under operating room conditions is indicated. If there are supernumerary metacarpals to match the extra fingers, removal is not indicated since hand function is not impaired. One of the features of the Ellis-von Creveld syndrome is the presence of extra metacarpals and fingers.

SYNDACTYLY

Syndactyly is the failure of two or more fingers to separate into individual digits during intrauterine hand development. Diagnosed at birth, this condition may be unilateral or bilateral. Certain genetic disorders, such as Apert's syndrome, have syndactyly as a part of the classic syndrome.

Radiographs are useful for the classification of syndactyly. If all the phalanges are normally formed and the fingers are joined only by skin bridges, a simple syndactyly is present. A complex syndactyly consists of side-to-side fusion of the phalanges of adjacent fingers in addition to the skin bridges.

Surgical treatment is necessary to improve hand function with this condition, though this operative correction is not done in the infant. If surgical treatment is delayed too long, however, angular deformity of one or more fingers can occur. For example, if the little and ring fingers are joined, the ring finger will begin to curve toward the shorter and slower-growing little finger as the child becomes older. Surgical correction is indicated at a younger age to separate the syndactyly between fingers with different growth rates than for fingers with similar growth rates, such as the long and ring fingers. However, surgical correction should be completed by a few years of age in most cases to allow for the development of independent finger movement and to improve dexterity.

Syndactyly of the toes may exist in the same children with finger syndactyly. However, surgical separation of the toe syndactyly is rarely indicated or necessary, since independent toe movement is not essential in most people for normal foot function.

CAMPTODACTYLY

This congenital deformity consists of a flexion contracture at the proximal interphalangeal joint, likely related to anomalous intrinsic muscles. The little finger is most commonly involved. However, this can occur in any finger, and multiple fingers may be affected in the same hand.

Examination will show failure of active or passive full extension at the involved joint. The flexion contracture may be mild or nearly 90°. A lateral radiograph of the involved finger(s) will demonstrate the flexion deformity at the proximal interphalangeal joint, with palmar subluxation of the middle phalanx at this joint.

Splinting may improve extension somewhat, but care must be taken to not increase the joint subluxation. If treatment is thought to be necessary, surgical correction offers the best chance for improvement in both function and cosmetic appearance.

CLINODACTYLY

Clinodactyly is a congenital angulation of the distal phalanx of the fifth finger toward the ring finger. Commonly, both hands are involved. Mild limitation of full extension may also be present but flexion is usually full. Treatment is rarely recommended, though the teenager may have some concern about the cosmetic appearance of this finger.

RADIAL CLUB HAND

This congenital deformity occurs unilaterally or bilaterally. If a part of the thrombocytopenia-absent radius (TAR) syndrome, the condition is bilateral. Because of the congenital absence of the radius, the hand is deviated radially at birth. The thumb may be present or absent, but the other fingers are generally normal (Fig. 7.11).

The deformity is obvious on physical examination at birth. A key feature to note on examination is the active elbow flexion present, since this finding will aid in determining the treatment recommendations for the hand deformity. Abnormalities of the knees have also been associated with this syndrome, particularly various forms of knee instability.

The initial treatment consists of application of a splint to prevent further radial deviation of the hand at the wrist and to stretch the soft tissues on the radial side to allow easier surgical correction later. Thrombocytopenia may persist for several months or even years, and this low platelet level may delay surgical correction.

Surgical correction consists of centraliz-

ing the hand over the ulna to keep the hand at the end of the forearm. If elbow flexion is good, this procedure will improve hand function and stability well. However, if active elbow flexion is poor, the hand will function better in its radially deviated position, preserving active movement at the wrist and accepting the cosmetic deformity.

CONGENITAL CONSTRICTION BANDS

Though not congenital in the same sense as the other deformities described above, this condition is present at birth. The lower extremities may also be involved. No one clinical picture is characteristic of this disorder, which may include amputations (Fig. 7.12), hypoplastic digits, or a form of syndactyly.

The etiology of this condition is not completely clear. Premature membrane rupture is often associated with this condition. Some have reported that the constriction bands are amniotic tissue, but others have disputed this as the primary cause.

At birth, constriction bands may be present in any part of any extremity, though the fingers and toes are the most commonly affected. If the constricting band caused distal necrosis intrauterinely, a congenital amputation results. If the band is not tight enough

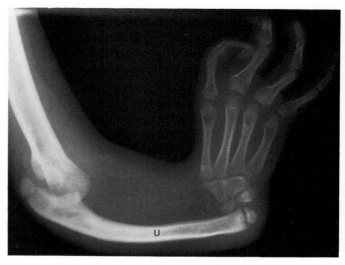

Figure 7.11. This child with a radial club hand has an ulna (*U*) that is present but short, thickened, and curved. The thumb is entirely absent and the wrist is displaced in a radial direction.

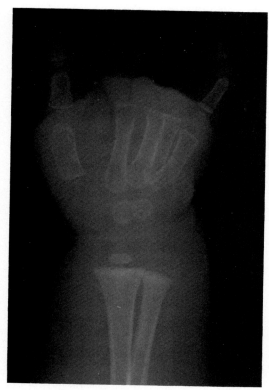

Figure 7.12. Secondary to constriction bands, there was an absence of the second, third, and fourth fingers and hypoplasia of the fifth finger at the time of birth. The thumb and metacarpals are normal.

to cause distal necrosis, edema of the digit or extremity distal to the band will result. Particularly in the lower extremity, a neuropathic club foot may result from this type of band. If the band caused only superficial constriction, a deep skin crease will be present but normal distal function will be present.

Urgent surgical treatment for release of the constriction band is indicated only in the infant with a markedly edematous, but viable, extremity or digit distal to the band, in which case release of the band may spare function of this distal part. If a digit or extremity has a deep skin crease but otherwise normal function, surgical excision of this crease with Z-plasty is performed when the child is a few months old. If several fingers

have had a congenital amputation from these bands, hand reconstructive procedures can be utilized when the child is larger and older, if hand function is severely compromised.

Infections

PARONYCHIA

This infection, based in the area of the nail bed, is characterized by increasing pain, swelling, redness, and tenderness on the dorsum of the distal phalanx. The palmar aspect of the fingertip is not tender nor swollen initially. Radiographs are generally not ordered, and if obtained show only soft tissue swelling.

If seen early, a broad-spectrum antibiotic, such as a cephalosporin, combined with warm soaks may control and eradicate this infection. Usually the infection is more advanced when medical attention is sought, in which case incision of the infected area adjacent to the nail bed is performed under local anesthesia in the office to drain the pus collection. Antibiotics and warm soaks are continued until the infection resolves. Inadequate drainage of this infection may damage the nail bed and affect subsequent nail growth.

FELON

This infection of the palmar aspect of the distal phalanx of the finger is potentially more serious than a paronychia and requires more aggressive surgical treatment. Pain, swelling, redness, and tenderness are present on the soft tissue of the fingertip. If inadequately treated, this infection can spread proximally along the flexor tendon sheath to involve more of the finger.

Surgical drainage, using lateral and medial incisions, is the initial treatment of choice. Care must be taken to avoid the digital nerve and artery in the distal phalanx. A drain may be used for a few days to prevent premature wound closure, depending on the extent of the infection. Appropriate antibiotics are administered and warm soaks are employed to facilitate wound drainage. As the infection heals, the wound heals secondarily.

PURULENT TENOSYNOVITIS

Infection within the flexor tendon sheath is a serious infection of the finger and hand. These infections track along the flexor sheath into the palm and can even go proximally into the forearm. Several distinct sheaths are present within the palmar aspect of the hand, and the infection may involve one or more of these.

Pain and swelling are present in the involved finger and/or in the palm. Active joint motion is limited, and attempts at passive movement are painful. An ascending lymphangitis may be present, as evidenced by a red streak up the forearm. Fever is common.

This infection requires urgent surgical incision and drainage in the operating room, leaving the wound open initially, together with parenteral antibiotics in an in-patient setting. The hand is elevated, and dressing changes with whirlpool treatment are employed until the infection is controlled. Failure to treat this condition adequately will lead to scarring within the tendon sheath with resultant stiffness of the involved finger(s).

Infection on the dorsal aspect of the hand or finger is less serious than on the palmar side, since the extensor tendons do not have tendon sheaths as do the flexor tendons. However, surgical drainage may be required dorsally as well if antibiotics alone are insufficient to control and eradicate the infection.

Suggested Readings

Barton, N.J.: Fractures of the phalanges of the hand in children. Hand 11:134-143, 1979.

Kleinman, W.B. and Bowers, W.H.: Fractures, Ligamentous Injuries to the Hand. In Bora, F.W., Jr.(ed): The Pediatric Upper Extremity: Diagnosis and Management. Philadelphia, W.B. Saunders, pp. 150-175, 1986.

Leddy, J.P.: Infections of the Upper Extremity. In Bora, F.W., Jr. (ed): The Pediatric Upper Extremity: Diagnosis and Management. Philadelphia, W.B. Saunders, pp. 361-371, 1986.

Leonard, M.H. and Dubravcik, P.: Management of fractured fingers in the child. Clin. Orthop. 73:160-168, 1970.

Moses, J.M., Flatt, A.E., and Cooper, R.R.: Annular constricting bands. J. Bone Joint Surg. 61A:562-565, 1979.

Smith, R.J. and Lipke, R.W.: Treatment of congenital deformities of the hand and forearm (first of two parts). N. Engl. J. Med. 300:344-349, 1979.

Smith, R.J. and Lipke, R.W.: Treatment of congenital deformities of the hand and forearm (second of two parts). N. Engl. J. Med. 300:402-407, 1979.

Tada, K., Yonenobu, K., and Swanson, A.B.: Congenital constriction band syndrome. J. Pediatr. Orthop. 4:726-730, 1984.

Wood, V.E.: Congenital thumb deformities. Clin. Orthop. 195:7-25, 1985.

8

Thoracolumbar Spine: General Features

The thoracic and lumbar portions of the spine present a variety of problems different than those associated with the cervical spine. From a functional standpoint the thoracic spine can be considered as providing trunk stability, providing attachments for the ribs of the thoracic cage, and allowing limited mobility, while the lumbar spine is the primary region allowing multiple-plane motion of the trunk.

Anatomy

The thoracic spine consists of 12 vertebrae, through the central canal of which passes the spinal cord. Adjacent vertebrae articulate by means of facet joints, anatomically positioned in a manner to allow gliding of the facets in flexion and extension but allowing little rotational movement. Each facet joint is surrounded by a joint capsule. A rib attaches by ligaments to the transverse process and lateral vertebral body on each side of every thoracic vertebra.

The lumbar spine is generally composed of five vertebrae, though a small percentage of normal individuals will have either four or six lumbar vertebrae. The vertebral body of a lumbar vertebra is larger than its thoracic counterpart both in height and width, enabling these vertebrae to better withstand the loads applied here by the erect position. The facet joints of the lumbar region are vertically oriented, an anatomic feature that al-

lows motion in more directions here than in the thoracic region. Forward flexion and extension occurs largely in the lumbar spine, with segmental motion being greatest in the lower lumbar spine. Lateral flexion and rotation occur to a greater degree in the lumbar area than in the thoracic region.

The interspinous ligament attaches one spinous process to another, providing a posterior tether against abnormal forward flexion. Specific names for muscles in this posterior trunk adjacent to the spine are rarely used clinically, with all the muscle groups being referred to as paraspinal muscles. These muscles are of three types, some joining only two vertebrae, some joining three or four vertebrae, and some running over multiple vertebral segments. On the anterolateral aspect of the lumbar spine lies the psoas muscle, with origins on the upper lumbar vertebrae. The psoas muscle courses distally, joining the iliacus in the pelvic region and inserting onto the lesser trochanter of the proximal femur.

Although the thoracic and lumbar vertebrae differ somewhat in height and width depending on their relative position in the spine, the basic anatomic configuration and growth mechanisms are the same. At the superior and inferior ends of each vertebral body lies a ring apophysis, which is analogous to the physis in long bones and produces vertebral body growth. Between the vertebral apophysis and the disc is a secondary ossification center (Fig. 8.1) that fuses with the vertebral body as growth is completed.

The intervertebral disc is composed of a central jelly-like region termed the nucleus pulposus, which is completely ringed by the strong, fibrous annulus fibrosus. The inherent stability resulting from the disc-vertebra construction is further enhanced by the anterior and posterior longitudinal ligaments spanning the entire length of the thoracolumbar spine.

Segmental arteries from the aorta and veins to the vena cava pass transversely over the anterior midsection of each thoracic vertebral body, carrying the blood supply to and from both the spinal cord and the vertebral bodies. Individual variability of these segmental arteries occurs, but, in general, the area of the spine with the most

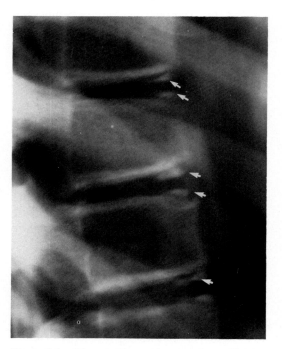

Figure 8.1. Ring apophyses (*arrows*) in an 11-year-old child represent the secondary ossification centers of the vertebra, analogous to the epiphysis of a long bone.

tenuous collateral circulation to the spinal cord is between the fifth and ninth thoracic vertebrae, making this level more prone to permanent spinal cord injury after regional trauma. In growing children, particularly at an early age, there is a greater vascular supply to the periphery of the disc than is seen in this area in the adult. The central 75% of the intervertebral disc itself is avascular.

Containing the essential neural elements for lower-extremity and trunk function, the spinal canal is completely surrounded by bone. The spinal canal gradually enlarges in diameter from the lower thoracic region to the lumbosacral area, helping to explain why lumbar region spinal injury is less often associated with permanent neurologic loss of function. The diameter of the spinal canal reaches its adult size by age 5 or 6 years.

The spinal cord lies within the spinal canal and tapers to form the conus medullaris at its distal end. From this the cauda equina originates with the lumbosacral nerve roots. The conus medullaris lies at the level of the second to third lumbar vertebra in an infant, but as spine growth progresses, the conus medullaris comes to lie at the level of the first lumbar vertebra, thus moving cephalad relative to the bony spine (Fig. 8.2). Failure of cephalad migration of the spinal cord relative to the vertebrae may be associated with a thickened filum terminale at the cauda equina of the cord, with this tethering of the spinal cord often leading to lumbosacral nerve root dysfunction and lower-extremity deformity.

Nerve roots exit from the spinal canal, passing out the neural foramina at each level. The nerve root number corresponds with the vertebral body superior to its exit point. In the thoracic area, the nerve joins the adjacent intercostal artery and vein to course along the inferior margin of the corresponding rib. In the lumbar area, the nerve root passes just inferior to the transverse process of the corresponding vertebra before joining adjacent nerve roots to form

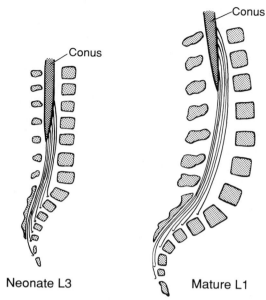

Neonate L3   Mature L1

Figure 8.2. There is a normal cephalad migration of the tip of the spinal cord or conus medullaris relative to the lumbar spine during early childhood. In the newborn, the conus medullaris lies adjacent to the second or third lumbar vertebra, but by early childhood the conus medullaris is properly at the level of the first lumbar vertebra. Failure of the spinal cord to ascend relative to the lumbar spine constitutes a "tethered cord," which usually leads to lower-extremity neurologic abnormalities.

the peripheral nerves of the pelvis and lower extremities. The sacral nerve roots provide some contribution to lower-extremity motor and sensory function and are the nerve roots responsible for maintaining bladder and bowel continence.

The sacrum and coccyx are formed by a coalescence of several vertebrae during fetal life. Five sacral vertebrae form a single bone, while the four lower vertebral segments form the coccyx, with these vestigial vertebrae held together by synchondroses or cartilaginous attachments. The sacrum acts as a keystone to anchor the spine to the pelvis, but the coccyx has little discernible functional role, except potential protection of the rectum, which lies directly anteriorly to the coccyx here.

Physical Examination

OBSERVATION

The first feature of the spine to observe is the position in which the child holds the trunk. The head should be centered over the sacral region in both frontal and sagittal planes. Is the trunk decompensated? Does this decompensation change when standing compared to sitting or lying (perhaps implicating leg length discrepancy and pelvic obliquity as the cause of the trunk shift)? When the child bends forward, is there asymmetry of the back surface, indicating a possible spinal deformity?

When the standing child is viewed from the side, there are normally a physiologic thoracic kyphosis (rounding) and cervical and lumbar lordosis (swaying) that allow the head to balance over the sacrum. Are these normal contours present? Are changes present with examination from the side with the child sitting or bending forward?

Abnormalities of the skin on the back may provide a tip-off as to an underlying condition affecting the spinal cord or spine in the thoracolumbar region. Most striking is a patch of hair in the lumbar area, virtually always indicating abnormalities in the development of the adjacent neural structures. The same is true of a deep lumbosacral dimple, which may communicate with the distal spinal cord dural sac. If this dimple is in the coccygeal area, associated abnormalities are uncommon. A hemangioma of the back is also a signal that underlying vertebral or neural abnormality may be present.

Observation of the ability of the child to move from one position to another and to walk will provide some information as to the amount of pain present and the most likely source. For example, if a child walks bending forward at the waist, this position may be due to pain being present with spine or hip extension that may be caused by inflammation or injury in the lumbar region, pelvis, or hips. In younger children, back pain may result in simple refusal of the child to stand or walk.

RANGE OF MOTION

Forward flexion should always be assessed when examining the back. Although goniometers or other measuring devices can be used, the simplest method to record the amount of forward spine flexion is to note the distance from the fingertips to the floor with the child bending forward with the knees kept straight. Lateral flexion of the spine can similarly be quantitated by noting the position of the fingertips relative to the knee as the hand is slid down the lateral aspect of the thigh while lateral trunk flexion takes place. Rotational movements are not generally quantified, but trunk rotation to both sides should be tested to determine if this motion causes pain. Hyperextension of the spine likewise should be evaluated with regard to the production of low back pain.

As a part of the examination of the range of motion of the lumbar spine, evaluation of flexion and extension of the hip needs to be assessed, since contractures in the hip will alter the lordosis of the lumbar spine. In a child with a hip flexion contracture, in order to place that leg on the ground to stand or walk, the child will arch the lumbar spine, increasing the lumbar lordosis with standing. The lumbar lordosis will flatten with the child in the sitting position, indicating that with hip flexion contractures the increased lumbar lordosis is a secondary or postural change that reverses with change in hip position. Hip flexion contractures are much more often the cause of excessive lumbar lordosis than is intrinsic spinal pathology.

PALPATION

Since the only part of the spine that can be palpated directly is the posterior tip of the spinous process, palpation for tenderness or masses in the back is less specific than in the extremities. The primary finding with palpation is either no tenderness or a diffuse discomfort to pressure on the paraspinal muscles. In an acute injury, muscle spasm may be felt, but this finding is less common in children than in adults.

If tenderness is present directly in the midline of the spine, over the spinous process, imaging evaluation for a possible tear of the interspinous ligament is needed, though this injury is more common in the cervical region than in the thoracic and lumbar spines. Tenderness in the sacroiliac joint region in an adolescent male may be an early sign of sacroiliac joint infection or arthritis.

LOWER-EXTREMITY EXAMINATION

There are two primary reasons to include a lower-extremity assessment in the routine back examination: spinal abnormalities may affect the nerves that supply the muscles of the lower extremity and lower-extremity disorders may affect the position of the trunk.

The essential elements of a brief neurologic assessment of the lower extremities include evaluation of gait, deep tendon reflexes, sensation to light touch, motor power of selected muscles, hamstring tightness, and the effect of a sciatic stretch maneuver. A more complete neurologic examination is conducted if any of these are abnormal.

Gait evaluation will allow the detection of asymmetrical muscle weakness and joint contractures. For example, a child with a foot drop secondary to a lumbar area neural deficit will lift the knee higher on the affected side when swinging that leg forward in walking. Or, a child with marked hamstring tightness from a spinal cause will be unable to take a long step when walking without obvious rotation of the pelvis.

Deep tendon reflexes at the knee and ankle should be symmetrically obtainable by tapping the patellar tendon and Achilles tendon, respectively. If reflexes are easily obtained by tapping the muscle itself, hyperreflexia is present and should be compared with both upper-extremity reflexes and other lower-extremity reflex responses. One or two beats of ankle clonus may be considered normal, but several beats or sustained clonus is pathologic.

Dermatomal sensory loss due to lumbar nerve root disorders are usually detectable by evaluation of light touch and pin prick in an older, cooperative child or teenager. More subtle sensory changes in proprioception, vibratory detection, and temperature are very difficult to detect in pre-adolescents and younger children.

The motor power corresponding to specific nerve roots is easier to assess than is sensory function, but in the young child even this examination may need to be incomplete. Foot dorsiflexion and plantar flexion muscle power are best assessed by having the child walk on the toes first, then on the heels; particularly with early weakness of the foot dorsiflexors, this test will detect weakness before that seen with manual muscle testing. If specific muscles cannot be evaluated in a young or uncooperative child, tape measurement of the calf and thigh circumferences will provide a clue to possible muscle atrophy from spinal cord or nerve root pathology.

The straight leg raising test is valuable in assessing the child for spinal abnormalities. With the child supine and the leg extended at the knee, the hip is gradually flexed to 90° or until pain is produced or no further hip flexion is possible without rotating the pelvis. One leg is tested at a time and the untested leg is kept lying on the examination table. If pain in the calf or foot of the leg being tested is produced by this straight leg raising test, this indicates that there is irritation or inflammation of the sciatic nerve or the lower lumbar nerve roots. If no pain or back pain only is produced, the straight leg raising test is deemed negative. However, even if no pain is produced by this maneuver, tightness of the hamstrings may be diagnosed if hip flexion is less than 60°. Particularly if this hamstring tightness is asymmetrical between the two legs, this finding should alert the examiner to possible spinal or spinal cord disorders.

Normal Imaging Studies

Imaging studies generally employed in the evaluation of spine disorders include radiography, bone scintigraphy, computed tomographic (CT) and magnetic resonance (MR) scans, myelography, tomography, and ultrasound examination.

RADIOGRAPHY

Anteroposterior and lateral radiographs of the thoracic and/or lumbar spine are the initial imaging studies to obtain before moving to the other studies. Particularly in young children when the specific area of spinal involvement is difficult to localize, both the thoracic and lumbar spine should be studied. If the radiographs are abnormal, the diagnosis will often have been made. If they are normal, particularly in the lumbar spine, oblique views may be indicated.

If radiographs are normal and physical examination is abnormal, suggesting some problem in the spine, the next imaging study is either a bone scan or an MR scan of the spine. If the neurologic examination of the lower extremities is normal and back pain is present, a bone scan of the spine and pelvis is the most productive test. However, if a neurologic abnormality of the lower extremities is seen with back stiffness or pain, an MR scan of the thoracic and lumbar spine is the study of choice.

OTHER IMAGING STUDIES

CT or MR scans are used in two primary instances in children: to assess in more detail a vertebral lesion found on radiographs or by bone scan and, in conjunction with a myelogram, to assess neural compression from bone or disc. In cases of spinal tumor or stress fracture, a bone scan will localize the area of pathology and the CT can anatomically define the exact site to expedite treatment. Used less often than MR at the present to evaluate neural compression, myelography with CT scanning can provide equivalent information, though general anesthesia is often needed for myelography in children. CT scanning should not be used for a screening test by scanning the entire spine looking for the site of pathology.

Tomography of the spine is only occasionally used for the evaluation of bony relationships in the spine. Tomography remains an excellent method to accurately define complex congenital scoliosis or kyphosis of the spine.

Ultrasound evaluation of the spine is most useful in the first 6 months of life, while many of the lumbar and sacral spinous processes are cartilaginous. In this age group, evaluation for a tethered cord, a lesion within the caudal spinal canal, or a sinus tract can be performed. This evaluation requires an MR scan as further vertebral and sacral ossification occurs.

Spinal Disorders: Pain versus Deformity

Numerous conditions may affect the spine in childhood and adolescence. Some are relatively age-specific, while others can occur at any time during the growing years. In general, each of these spinal problems presents as either back pain or back deformity. Although there is some overlapping between these two broad categories, Chapters 9 and 10 address childhood spinal problems under one of these two headings.

Suggested Readings

Bradford, D.S. and Hensinger, R.M. (eds): The Pediatric Spine. New York, Thieme, 1985.
Parke, W. W.: Development of the spine. In Rothman, R.H. and Simeone, F.A. (eds): The Spine. 3rd edition, Volume 1, pp. 3-33. Philadelphia, W.B. Saunders, 1992.
Parke, W. W.: Applied anatomy of the spine. In Rothman, R.H. and Simeone, F.A. (eds): The Spine. 3rd edition, Volume 1, pp. 35-87. Philadelphia, W.B. Saunders, 1992.
Verbout, A.J.: The development of the vertebral column. Adv. Anat. Embryol. Cell Biol. 90:1-122, 1985.

9
Spinal Deformity

Although most think of scoliosis as being the condition described when talking about spinal deformity, this category also includes the disorders associated with excessive kyphosis or lordosis of the spine. All these spinal deformities are three-dimensional in nature, with components of both frontal plane and sagittal plane deformity.

Scoliosis

Scoliosis is best described as a lateral curvature of the spine, when the child is viewed in the frontal plane from either the back or the front. This lateral curvature may result either intrinsically from disorders within the spine itself or from extrinsic factors that affect spine position and alignment. Although several categories of scoliosis exist, this discussion centers on postural, idiopathic, congenital, neuromuscular, and miscellaneous types of scoliosis. As a general rule, all the types of scoliosis presented in this chapter are pain-free.

POSTURAL SCOLIOSIS

Postural scoliosis is a lateral curvature of the spine that results from a leg length discrepancy. Since one leg is longer than the other, the pelvis is tilted when the child stands, thus placing the lumbosacral region at an angle. Because the brain stem postural centers strive to maintain the head centered over the midpelvis, the flexible lumbar spine will develop a two-dimensional lateral curvature to allow this head positioning. The larger the leg length difference, the larger will be the postural scoliosis.

With the child standing, the examiner viewing the child from behind will note trunk asymmetry. Palpation of the position of the iliac wings in this standing position will demonstrate the leg length inequality. A sufficient thickness of wood blocks or other material should be placed under the short leg to level the pelvis in the standing position. With the pelvis level, the trunk will no longer appear asymmetrical, since the postural scoliosis will have disappeared.

To further confirm this diagnosis, the child's back should be evaluated in the sitting position. Since the effect of leg length inequality is eliminated in this position, the back examination should be normal with a symmetrical appearance of the waistline and shoulders.

To confirm the diagnosis of postural scoliosis radiographically, one standing posteroanterior spine radiograph can be obtained with the child standing in his or her normal position and one standing radiograph can be obtained with a sufficient lift under the short leg to level the pelvis. Without the lift present, the radiograph will demonstrate pelvic obliquity and a lateral curvature *without* vertebral rotation. With the lift, the pelvis will be level and the scoliosis will virtually disappear.

Since this is not a problem within the spine itself, children with postural scoliosis alone do not require sequential radiographic evaluation of the spine to assess for progressive deformity. Here, attention should be focused on the lower-extremity length difference. As growth continues, ongoing assessment of progressive leg length inequality may be needed, and shoe lift or surgical treatment is indicated if the leg length difference is great enough.

IDIOPATHIC SCOLIOSIS

The most common of the types of scoliosis that require continued evaluation or treatment, idiopathic scoliosis accounts for about 80% of this group. As the name implies, the cause of idiopathic scoliosis remains unclear, though much research has addressed this issue in the past and present.

Etiology

Some of the major areas considered as prime possibilities in causing idiopathic scoliosis include muscular disorders, connective tissue abnormalities, disc pathology, and subclinical neurologic dysfunction. Type I muscle fibers have been found with a greater preponderance in paraspinal muscles in idiopathic scoliosis patients than in those with straight spines. Electron microscopic examination of the neuromuscular junction has demonstrated abnormalities in muscles of those with idiopathic scoliosis not found in normal persons or in children with congenital scoliosis. Fibroblasts in tissue culture have been reported to be both normal and abnormal, and some connective tissue disorders, such as Marfan syndrome, have an increased incidence of scoliosis, but fibroblast abnormalities are not found in all children with idiopathic scoliosis. The glycosaminoglycan content of the intervertebral discs in those with idiopathic scoliosis is decreased compared to normal controls, but this is probably a result of the scoliosis rather than the cause.

It is an observed fact that most children with idiopathic scoliosis think they are standing straight, even when they obviously have a curved spine and may be decompensated a few centimeters away from the midline of the body. Recent sophisticated neurophysiologic studies have demonstrated minor aberrations of the "postural center" in the brain stem in some (but not all) children with idiopathic scoliosis. Proprioception studies, balance tests, and response to vibratory stimuli have likewise been reported to be abnormal more often in children with idiopathic scoliosis.

An additional factor that plays a role is the genetic influence present. Parents with scoliosis are more likely to have children with idiopathic scoliosis than are parents with straight spines. However, among siblings born to scoliotic parents, not all develop scoliosis, and the size of the curvature in those that do may vary widely.

Despite all of the above findings that have resulted from the research into the cause of idiopathic scoliosis, the fact remains that the large majority of children and teenagers with idiopathic scoliosis appear clinically to be healthy, otherwise normal children who function in daily life the same as their unaffected peers. Probably the best description of the etiology of idiopathic scoliosis at this time is that it is a multifactorial condition with a genetic predisposition to developing a spinal curvature.

Patterns of Curvature

The terminology used to describe the type of curve pattern present in idiopathic scoliosis assumes that the examiner is viewing the child from behind. The direction of the curvature is described by the location of the convexity of the scoliosis, and the spine location is determined by the apical vertebra in the curve. If the curve apex is in the thoracic spine, the child has a thoracic curve; if the apex is between T11 and L1, a thoracolumbar curve is present; and if the apex is below L1, a lumbar curve is diagnosed.

The most common curve pattern overall is a right thoracic scoliosis, being a single curve. If there are two curves of approximately equal size but with the curve convexity in different directions, the most common type is a right thoracic, left lumbar curve pattern.

The curve pattern that should alert the examiner to the possibility of an underlying neurologic problem, despite a normal neurologic examination, is the left thoracic curve pattern, which has been reported to be caused by an underlying, and often subtle, neurologic abnormality up to 75% of the time. Children with a left thoracic curve pattern should have a magnetic resonance (MR) examination of the spinal cord prior to initiation of any treatment for the scoliosis.

Clinical Features

The clinical features of children with idiopathic scoliosis are different in various age groups. The three main categories of idiopathic scoliosis are infantile, juvenile, and adolescent.

Infantile idiopathic scoliosis is clearly the least common type. Although rare in the United States, this type of scoliosis has been noted to be seen more often in Great Britain. By definition, the infantile type is diagnosed when the child is 3 years of age or younger. It affects males more often than females. The classic curve pattern is a left thoracolumbar scoliosis. An unusual feature compared to idiopathic scoliosis at other ages is that many of these curvatures, even without treatment, progressively resolve as the child grows. In children in whom the scoliosis does not resolve, the curvatures become severe, requiring multiple surgical procedures in an attempt to control the progression.

Juvenile idiopathic scoliosis is found in children between the ages of 4 and 10 years at the time of diagnosis. In a sense, this group is a bridge between the infantile and adolescent groups, sharing characteristics of each. The juvenile type occurs equally in boys and girls, though the boys predominate in the younger end of this grouping and girls predominate in the older subgroup. A double curve pattern may be present, but many also present with a single right thoracic curve pattern. The scoliosis does not resolve in this group, but some may stop progressing without treatment. Although they are diagnosed with "idiopathic" scoliosis, about one-third to one-half of these children

will have some abnormality noted on an MR of the spinal cord, such as a small syringomyelia, with a normal standard neurologic examination. Worsening of these curvatures may be continuous with further growth, or some may appear stable for a few years, only to worsen further during the adolescent growth spurt.

The most common form of idiopathic scoliosis is the adolescent type, defined as occurring after the age of 11 years. While mild curvatures are approximately equal in incidence between males and females, the scoliosis is 8 to 10 times more likely to worsen and require treatment in females. The predominant curve pattern is a single right thoracic scoliosis, and a right thoracic, left lumbar double curve pattern is second in frequency. The risk of curve progression depends on the skeletal age of the child and the size of the scoliosis at the time of diagnosis. Approximately half of the curves between 10° and 30° do not continue to worsen without treatment. In those that do worsen, the increase in curvature is approximately 10° to 15° per year, or about 1° per month during active growing.

History

Several questions should be asked of the parents and the older child. A family history of scoliosis should be sought. If a parent has scoliosis, was treatment needed? The family should be asked about other familial conditions present, mainly to determine if the scoliosis is part of a more systemic syndrome.

A complete medical history may reveal information about associated birth abnormalities or developmental delays. The presence of pain or back stiffness should be sought, as well as functional limitations. A history of shortness of breath with activity may indicate pulmonary compromise in conjunction with thoracic scoliosis.

In the child with adolescent scoliosis, an important component of the history relates to determining the amount of remaining growth to be expected in the child. If the child is a girl, when was the onset of menses? If premenarchal, has breast development started? Since scoliosis is progressive primarily during periods of growth, these questions can help in providing advice to the child and the parents not only about the possible need for treatment but also about the length of time that treatment may be needed.

Physical Examination

No matter what the age of the child with a possible scoliosis, the examination should include at least an evaluation of the back, the chest wall, and the lower extremities.

For the examination of the back, the child should be standing, facing away from the examiner. Clothing, except for underwear, should be removed for direct visualization of the back. (If screening examinations for scoliosis are being performed, the child is best examined in a swimming suit to see the entire trunk well.)

Noting asymmetry of the trunk is the key to detection of spinal deformity. Symmetry of shoulder height and scapular position are first noted. Although about half of the children with unequal shoulder position on standing do not have scoliosis, this can be a marker for scoliosis and should lead the examiner to a more careful examination of the rest of the trunk. Symmetry of the waistline is noted next. If one side of the waistline is flattened and the other accentuated, there is likely a scoliosis toward the flattened side. Another way to assess symmetry in the waist area is to look at the "open space" between the lateral side of the trunk and the arms hanging at the side. If this space is not the same on each side, a scoliosis may be present. With the child standing, the level of the iliac wings on each side is noted to check for leg length inequality. While this examination is proceeding, the examiner should check for any abnormal cutaneous markings (such as a hemangioma, cafe-au-lait spots, or a hairy patch) that may be associated with spine and spinal cord congenital anomalies.

After the child has been assessed while standing erect, the examination should proceed to the forward-bending test, described by Adams in England in the 1850s. This test is easily performed, with the child bending forward with the legs straight at the knees and with the hands held together, as if trying to touch the toes (Fig. 9.1). If scoliosis is present, this test will confirm the diagnosis. The Adams or forward-bending test is based on the fact that scoliosis is a three-dimensional deformity, so there is rotation of the involved vertebrae at the same time there is lateral curvature. This vertebral rotation leads to a prominence on the posterior trunk that corresponds to the position of the convex side of the curvature (Fig. 9.2). In the thoracic area, vertebral rotation leads to a rotation of the entire thorax, since the ribs are directly attached to the vertebral body. Children who have a posterior right-sided rib hump or prominence will also usually have an anterior left-sided rib protrusion, which in a female with breast development may lead to the appearance of asymmetrical breast size. In the lumbar area, even without the ribs present, the vertebral rotation causes a posterior prominence, easily seen as the muscles on the convex side of the curve are pushed posteriorly.

The examiner should observe the back of the bent-over child from both the cephalic and caudal directions. Thoracic curve rib prominences are most easily seen when viewed from behind the child, while lumbar prominences are easier to see when looking down the back with the examiner standing at the head of the child.

Devices to measure the amount of rib hump or posterior rotational asymmetry are commercially available and can be used serially in mild curves to evaluate the angle of trunk rotation. The most commonly used device is conceptually based on a marine device used to measure the amount a sailboat is heeling or inclining to one side. If

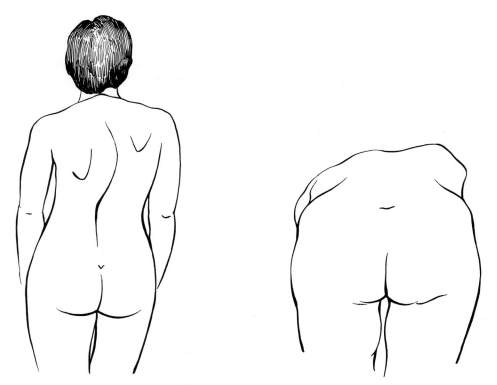

Figure 9.1. This diagram of a teenager with a right thoracic scoliosis demonstrates the primary physical findings noted. The right shoulder and scapula are higher than on the left side. The trunk is shifted slightly to the right and there is asymmetry in the waistline area. With the child bending forward, a posterior prominence is seen in the right thoracic region, corresponding to the convexity of the scoliotic curve.

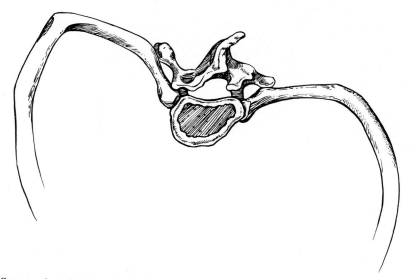

Figure 9.2. Structural scoliosis is a three-dimensional deformity, involving not only a lateral curvature but also a rotational component. This diagram is a superior view of the thoracic and vertebral changes noted in a right thoracic scoliosis. The spinous processes of the involved vertebrae rotate toward the midline. As the rib attaches to the vertebral body that has also rotated, the rib is pushed posteriorly on the convex side of the curve while the concave ribs move anteriorly. It is this thoracic cage deformity that is a valuable aid in the early detection of scoliosis.

the angle of trunk rotation is 5° or less, a significant scoliosis is generally not present. Because the amount of lordosis and kyphosis in the curved segment may vary, the correlation between the surface anatomy and the degree of scoliosis is not 1:1. Therefore, this inclinometer reading must be used somewhat cautiously, but it can be a good adjunct in following mild scoliosis over a period of growth, in this way avoiding the need for frequent radiographs.

Next, flexibility of the spine should be assessed by lateral bending and full forward flexion, noting if any of these movements cause pain. Examination by palpation does not generally locate areas of tenderness. If palpation of the spinous processes is used to try to estimate curve size, the scoliosis will always be underestimated because the spinous processes of the involved vertebrae rotate back toward the midline as the three-dimensional deformity progresses.

After the back examination is completed, the lower extremities are evaluated, particularly with regard to neurologic function. Thigh or calf atrophy is assessed, as is muscle strength. Deep tendon reflexes should be symmetrical and clonus should be absent. Hamstring tightness is noted by the straight leg raising test. The feet are checked for deformity or unequal foot size. The child's gait is observed in the examining room or the adjacent hallway.

The term idiopathic implies that there are no other abnormalities noted on physical examination that could be a cause of the scoliosis, so the examination is generally normal except for the spinal curvature. Nonetheless, this systematic examination should be completed whenever evaluating a child with scoliosis before the term "idiopathic" is applied to that particular curvature.

Radiographic Evaluation

If a child has physical examination findings to suspect a scoliosis, especially the presence of a posterior prominence on the forward bending test, a posteroanterior *standing* radiograph of the thoracolumbar spine should be obtained. Since all treatment and follow-up recommendations are based on the curvature measurement in the erect position, it is not recommended to obtain supine spine radiographs when evaluating a child for possible scoliosis. The so-called "scoliosis series" should not be ordered as the initial test, but simply one standing spine posteroanterior radiograph to avoid unnecessary radiation exposure to the child.

The magnitude of the scoliosis is measured on the radiograph by the Cobb method (Fig. 9.3). An angle of curvature is determined by drawing one line along the

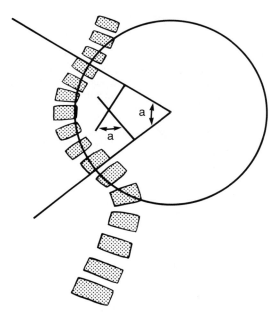

Figure 9.3.   The standard technique used to measure standing posteroanterior radiographs of the spine is the Cobb method. One line is drawn along the superior endplate of the vertebra tilted the most at the top of the curve and a similar line is drawn along the inferior endplate of the vertebra tilted the most at the bottom of the curve. If the scoliosis is large, these lines meet and form angle *a*. However, since most curves are not large enough to allow these lines to intersect on the radiograph, perpendicular lines can be drawn to each of the endplate lines to form angle *a*.

superior endplate of the vertebra at the upper end of the scoliosis and another line along the inferior endplate of the lowest vertebra in the curve (Fig. 9.4). Perpendicular lines are drawn to each of these vertebral lines and the angle of scoliosis is measured. The error of this measurement is ±3°, so sequential radiographic changes should be more than 5° to be considered significant. Although it is not needed to evaluate all idiopathic adolescent scoliosis, an MR study is valuable in assessing scoliosis with back pain or neurologic abnormalities (Fig. 9.5).

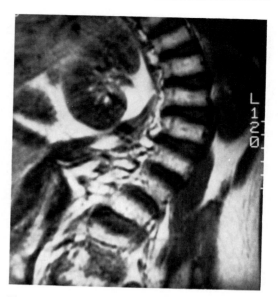

Figure 9.5. MR scan in this patient with idiopathic scoliosis shows wedging of the intervertebral discs, being narrow on the concave side.

Laboratory Studies

No serum studies are specifically useful in the evaluation of children with idiopathic scoliosis. The primary laboratory studies used at the authors' institution are for the evaluation of pulmonary function. If a thoracic scoliosis exceeds 50° or 60°, early abnormalities in pulmonary function studies appear. The most common abnormality is a decrease in vital capacity, probably related to the decrease in size of the hemithorax on the convex side of the scoliosis, a result of the rib deformity that occurs due to the vertebral rotation. If the scoliosis continues to worsen, hypoxemia may develop on room air, and with severe curves, carbon dioxide retention can occur.

Treatment

Treatment of idiopathic scoliosis falls into three categories: serial follow-up evaluation, bracing, and surgical treatment. The treatment method chosen depends on the age of the child and the magnitude of the scoliosis. The following guidelines for man-

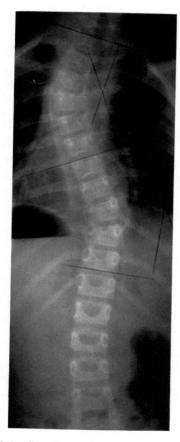

Figure 9.4. Standing posteroanterior radiograph of the spine in a 13-year-old demonstrates idiopathic scoliosis with a double thoracic curve pattern. Using the Cobb method, the upper curve measures 35 and the lower curve 25.

agement are for adolescent idiopathic scoliosis, since this is by far the most common form encountered in primary care.

As a rule of thumb, curves with a Cobb measurement of less than 25° require follow-up evaluation but no active treatment; progressive scoliosis of 25° to 40° is treated with a brace provided the child has growth remaining; and those with curves over 40° are generally surgical candidates.

The goal in early diagnosis and appropriate treatment of scoliosis is to keep the curvatures controlled during the period of rapid adolescent growth, when progressive curves increase at the rate of about 1° per month. Long-term follow-up studies have shown that if thoracic curves can be kept below 50° and lumbar curves below 40° by the completion of growth, the likelihood of the curve increasing during adult life is small. By diagnosing the scoliosis early and bracing progressive curves appropriately, the number of patients requiring surgical treatment should decrease.

If a young patient has a scoliosis of less than 25° at the time of diagnosis, no active treatment is needed at that time. If growth is nearly completed or finished, no further follow-up is needed for the scoliosis. However, if a few years of growth remain, a second radiograph of the spine should be obtained in several months. The time between radiographs can be estimated by the formula [25 − (present degree of curvature) = months until next radiograph]. If the scoliosis is less than 13°, a follow-up radiograph should be obtained in 1 year, but only if growth remains.

While a radiograph of the hand and wrist is needed to determine the bone age of a child, an estimate of growth remaining can be made clinically based on the menstrual history and the appearance of the iliac apophysis ossification center seen on the spine radiograph. In general, growth is largely completed within 18 months after the onset of menses. Between the initial appearance of breast development and the onset of menses, growth is quite rapid, tapering off after menses have begun.

The secondary ossification center of the iliac wing begins to appear just prior to the onset of menses. Risser classified the radiographic appearance of this apophysis into six grades, ranging from 0 in premenarcheal females to V in skeletally mature individuals

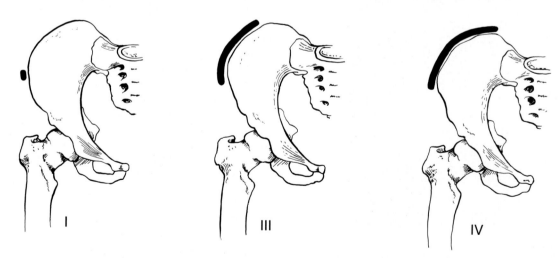

Figure 9.6.   Virtually always included on the standing posteroanterior radiograph used to evaluate spinal deformity, the iliac apophysis or secondary ossification center can be helpful in estimating skeletal age. Risser stage I, when lateral ossification has just begun, occurs between early breast development and the onset of menses, which typically appears between stages I and II. When Risser stage IV is reached, spinal growth is virtually complete. Risser stage V is achieved when the apophysis is fully fused to the rest of the iliac wing.

(Fig. 9.6). Since this iliac apophysis is seen on most spine radiographs, no further radiographs are necessary to determine the "Risser sign."

If growing children demonstrate an increase of the scoliosis to more than 25°, the use of a thoracolumbar sacral orthosis (TLSO) or brace is indicated to hold the curve in a straighter position until growth is completed. Since growth is slowed by an increase in pressure at the growth area, the concave side of a scoliosis grows more slowly than the convex side, leading to an increase in curve size, especially during the adolescent growth spurt. By holding the curve in a straighter position with the brace, spinal growth can take place more equally on both sides of the spine. The purpose of a spinal brace here is not to correct the scoliosis but to prevent further progression. When needed to control the scoliosis, this brace should be worn about 22 hours daily until growth ceases. If worn as prescribed, 80 to 85% of the treated patients will be able to avoid surgical treatment. During the period when the brace is worn, there is no need for restriction of activity and the child may participate in any sport desired.

If the scoliosis progresses past 40°, surgical treatment is generally needed. Current surgical techniques allow for correction of the scoliosis by 50 to 60% while maintaining the sagittal contours of the spine better than previously used techniques. Any area of the curved spine that requires spinal instrumentation also requires spinal fusion to maintain the correction for a lifetime. If children under the age of 10 or 11 years require spinal instrumentation and fusion, both anterior and posterior fusion may be needed to prevent progressive rotatory deformity as the child completes growth. Attempts are made to avoid fusion below the L4 vertebra, since fusion to lower levels may predispose the teenager to later back pain in early adulthood.

The results of surgical treatment are good. Fusion rates are approximately 99% in the teenage group. Current techniques allow for the avoidance of casting or bracing of the patient postoperatively. The fusion is healed by 6 months following surgery, at which time the patient can resume full activity, with the only restrictions being avoidance of collision-type sports like football. Once the fusion is healed, the instrumentation could be removed since the fusion is now holding the curve correction, but rod removal is rarely done. There is no evidence of long-term problems with leaving this hardware in the spine, and the surgical procedure for removing these segmental fixation devices is quite extensive.

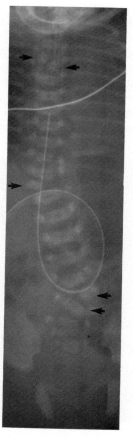

Figure 9.7. Anteroposterior projection of the full spine in a newborn with multiple anomalies shows multiple vertebral anomalies (*arrows*) with associated congenital scoliosis.

CONGENITAL SCOLIOSIS

Congenital scoliosis results from abnormal spinal formation during embryonic development. These congenital abnormalities may present in many different forms, but the most common is a hemivertebra, in which one lateral half of the vertebra fails to form (Figs. 9.7 and 9.8). Since the hemivertebra is a triangular-shaped piece of bone between the normal rectangular vertebrae, a lateral curvature results. The congenital anomaly that leads to the most rapidly progressive scoliosis is a unilateral unsegmented bar (Fig. 9.9), in which several vertebrae are joined on the concave side of the scoliosis while the convexity has had formation of discs and will continue to grow.

Congenital scoliosis can be associated with a number of congenital anomalies in other organ systems. About 30% of infants with congenital scoliosis have a congenital genitourinary abnormality, the most common being unilateral renal agenesis. Neural abnormalities may be present, and about one-third of children with congenital scoliosis also have a spinal cord anomaly seen

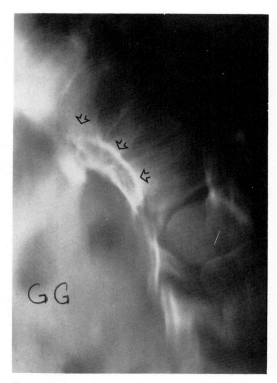

Figure 9.9.   A congenital bony bar (*open arrows*) is tethering the lateral masses of three vertebrae on the concave side, resulting in progressive scoliosis.

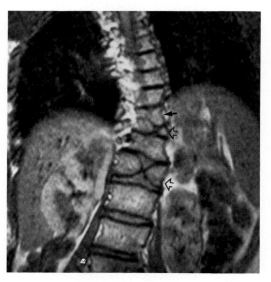

Figure 9.8.   MR scan of child with congenital scoliosis shows multiple butterfly vertebrae (*open arrows*) and a wedged vertebra (*solid arrow*).

on MR studies (Fig. 9.10). Congenital heart disease may be present. In children with VATER (vertebral defects, imperforate anus, tracheoesophageal fistula, radial and renal dysplasia) syndrome, the abnormalities mentioned above are present in addition to the scoliosis. As a general rule, the finding of congenital scoliosis should trigger a thorough search for associated anomalies elsewhere.

All children with any congenital vertebral anomaly should have a renal ultrasound to assess possible anomalies of the genitourinary system. While unilateral renal agenesis is compatible with a normal life expectancy, children with only one kidney should refrain from contact and collision sports as they grow up.

The treatment for congenital scoliosis varies according to the type of congenital

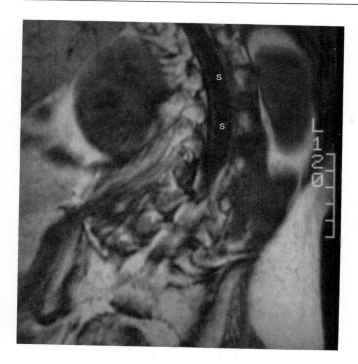

Figure 9.10. This child with congenital scoliosis has an associated syringomyelia (*s*), seen as fluid in the dilated central canal of the spinal cord. Congenital abnormalities of the spinal cord are present in about 30% of children with congenital vertebral anomalies.

defect present and the location of the deformity. The initial spinal radiograph is used as a baseline study, and serial standing spine radiographs are obtained as the child grows. If the congenital scoliosis segment increases by more than 10° on radiographs obtained with the same patient positioning, surgical treatment is warranted regardless of the young age of the patient. For the congenital scoliosis itself, bracing is rarely effective, though bracing can be used to control compensatory curves that may develop above or below the congenital scoliosis segment.

If surgical treatment is deemed necessary, an MR study should be obtained preoperatively to determine whether a neurosurgical procedure, such as the release of a tethered cord, is needed at the same time as the spinal fusion. In the cervical and thoracic area, fusion is primarily done to prevent progression, since hemivertebra resection or other surgical correction attempts have a high risk of iatrogenic neurologic injury in this location. In the lumbar spine, hemivertebra excision is more commonly

feasible and usually allows for substantial correction of trunk imbalance.

NEUROMUSCULAR SCOLIOSIS

Scoliosis is seen in a large number of neuromuscular diseases, the most common of which are cerebral palsy, muscular dystrophy, spina bifida, and spinal muscular atrophy. This same type of scoliosis is seen in children following spinal cord injury at an early age.

Scoliosis is relatively uncommon in children with neuromuscular disease who are able to walk. In cerebral palsy, scoliosis is primarily seen in the spastic quadriplegia patients who are unable to stand or walk. Scoliosis is rare in the spastic hemiplegic or spastic diplegic types in children who continue to walk. In Duchenne's muscular dystrophy, scoliosis is unusual until the child becomes wheelchair bound, at which point the majority develop scoliosis of varying degrees.

The curve pattern seen in neuromuscular scoliosis is relatively constant, being a long

C-shaped curve associated with pelvic obliquity. The scoliosis generally involves the entire lumbar spine and the lower half of the thoracic spine. Pulmonary function may not be compromised by this type of scoliosis unless the entire thoracic spine is involved or if the scoliosis has a large collapsing component, as seen in spinal muscular atrophy.

Accurate radiographic assessment of the magnitude of the scoliosis is difficult in this patient group, since standing radiographs cannot usually be obtained. While erect sitting spine radiographs can be used, the difficulty in obtaining the same positioning from one radiograph to the next can result in less reliable measurements.

In a child with the spastic quadriplegia form of cerebral palsy, a TLSO should be used at the first signs of a structural scoliosis. These children often have other health problems (e.g. seizures, need for gastrostomy tube, pulmonary disease) and seldom tolerate wearing the brace for several hours daily. Despite the fact that the brace is less effective in preventing progression of the scoliosis in these children, an alternate benefit is assistance with maintaining a good sitting position, which may in turn facilitate head control and promote improved use of the upper extremities. If the scoliosis continues to worsen despite bracing, surgical treatment is warranted to maintain sitting position, especially if some independent hand function is present.

In boys with Duchenne's muscular dystrophy, progressive scoliosis usually begins when they stop walking and become dependent on the wheelchair. Braces are relatively ineffective in these cases, and surgical treatment is indicated for curves greater than 30° on a sitting radiograph to preserve sitting ability and to delay increasing pulmonary compromise that occurs with worsening scoliosis.

Children with spina bifida who have no neurologic function below the thoracolumbar region have a high incidence of progressive scoliosis. Successful bracing is difficult in these children, in large part because of associated medical problems. Surgical treatment is often needed in these children, but MR evaluation prior to corrective surgery should be obtained and may detect a tethered cord or a lumbosacral lipoma that could complicate surgical correction.

If a young child becomes paraplegic following an accident at an early age, scoliosis frequently develops with growth. If the paraplegia occurs before the age of 5 years, virtually all children develop scoliosis that will require surgical fusion in later childhood. If the paraplegia develops near the end of growth, surgical treatment for scoliosis is often not necessary.

MISCELLANEOUS TYPES OF SCOLIOSIS

Scoliosis is a common feature of several syndromes or disease complexes, which are combined together under the miscellaneous group. Examples include connective tissue disorders such as Marfan syndrome and osteogenesis imperfecta and genetic conditions such as neurofibromatosis (Fig. 9.11) and dwarfism syndromes.

The evaluation of children with scoliosis as a part of a syndrome or genetic condition is essentially the same as for those with idiopathic curves, using standing spine radiographs. However, treatment has to be modified in many instances. For example, children with scoliosis associated with osteogenesis imperfecta cannot be well treated with a brace. Rather than controlling the scoliosis, pressure from the brace may lead to increased rib deformity. As a general rule, in this miscellaneous group, scoliosis more often requires surgical treatment than in the idiopathic scoliosis patient.

Kyphosis

A normal child has a physiologic amount of kyphosis or "rounding" in the thoracic spine, with cervical and lumbar lordosis or "swaying" that allows the head to balance

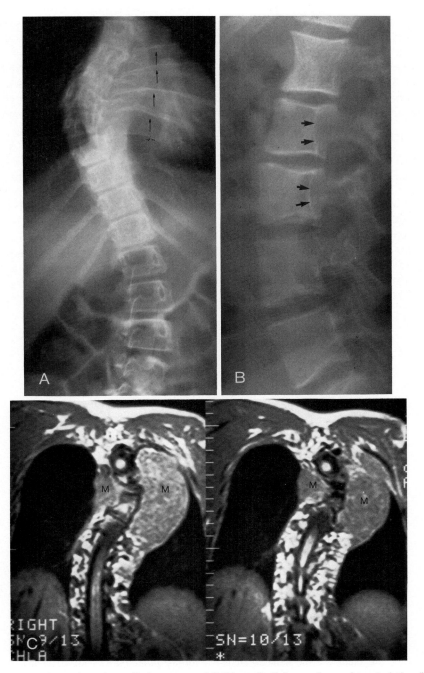

Figure 9.11. **A,** A sharp thoracic scoliotic curve and "ribbon ribs" (*arrows*) are characteristic of neurofibromatosis. **B,** Posterior vertebral body scalloping (*arrows*) in neurofibromatosis is caused by neurofibroma pressure and/or dural ectasia. **C,** A severe thoracic kyphoscoliosis and a posterior paravertebral neurofibroma (*M*) in a child with neurofibromatosis is demonstrated well by MR scan.

over the pelvis in the sagittal plane. When the term kyphosis is used clinically, it usually refers to an *increased* amount of rounding in the thoracic area or a reversal of the lordosis in the cervical and lumbar regions. The three most common conditions associated with an increase in kyphosis are postural roundback, Scheuermann's kyphosis, and congenital kyphosis.

POSTURAL ROUNDBACK

Postural roundback deformity is most common in the pre-adolescent or early adolescent child. Typically, the child has had a growth spurt earlier than his or her peers. In girls, a round-shouldered posture may be an attempt to de-emphasize breast development that has occurred earlier for her than for her friends. With boys or girls who are taller than their classmates, a roundback posture will serve to equalize their heights

more. In addition to the psychological reasons for this poor posture, there may be some trunk muscle weakness due to the muscle strength not keeping up with the rapid spine growth.

The child is usually brought reluctantly to the physician by parents who are concerned about this poor posture and who have been unsuccessful with parental discipline approaches in improving the child's standing position. Frequently the child is ahead of his or her classmates in development of secondary sexual characteristics and height. A history of pain is usually absent. The child is often relatively nonathletic, but weight lifters often seem to develop some excessive kyphosis.

Physical examination will demonstrate a child who stands with poor upper trunk posture at rest, with the shoulders positioned forward. The key finding here is that this

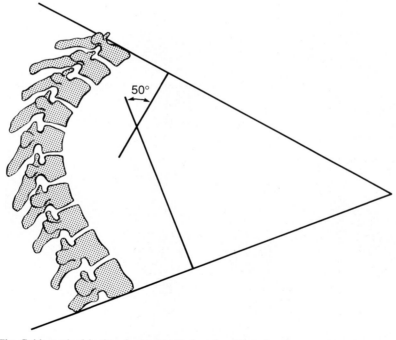

Figure 9.12. The Cobb method is the standard technique for measuring the amount of kyphosis present. On a standing lateral radiograph of the spine, one line is drawn along the superior part of the T3 vertebra and a similar line is drawn along the inferior portion of the T12 vertebra. Perpendicular lines to these reference lines intersect to form the angle of kyphosis, as shown in the diagram. The normal thoracic kyphosis by the Cobb method is between 20° and 40°.

increased thoracic kyphosis is passively correctable by the examiner applying an extension pressure on the shoulders. In fact, when specifically asked, the child can often actively correct this postural roundback. With the child in the forward-bending or Adams position, there is a normal smooth contour to the spine when viewed from the side. The remainder of the examination is normal in this condition.

A standing lateral radiograph of the spine is used to confirm this diagnosis. With postural roundback, there is no anterior wedging of the thoracic vertebrae as is seen in other kyphotic conditions. The angle of kyphosis is measured by the Cobb method (Fig. 9.12), with this angle formed by the intersection of a line drawn along the superior endplate of the T3 vertebra and a line drawn along the inferior endplate of the T12

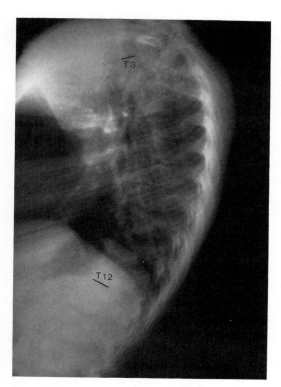

Figure 9.13. Postural roundback is seen in this lateral radiograph of a very tall young girl. Normal kyphosis from T3 to T12 is between 20° and 40°.

vertebra (Fig. 9.13). Normally, this angle of kyphosis is 20° to 40°. In postural roundback, this angle usually measures between 40° and 60°, rarely more.

Treatment for postural roundback is by exercises and posture modification. Hyperextension exercises of the posterior trunk muscles will strengthen weakness at this site that may be predisposing the child to this roundback position. Sit-ups are used to strengthen the abdominal muscles, which in turn will flatten the lumbar lordosis, leading to further compensatory straightening of the flexible thoracic kyphosis. In addition to these specific exercises, exercise to increase general fitness is recommended. No activity restrictions should be placed on a child with postural roundback. Visual hints are also provided to children to observe their own posture in mirrors or store windows on a day-to-day basis, with instructions to ''stand tall'' when they note this slumping posture.

Although children with postural roundback have a flexible spine in the region of the kyphosis, if this posture persists, permanent changes can occur in the vertebral bodies that cause progressive deformity and require bracing or surgical treatment. Subtle hints to the child of the possible progressive nature of postural roundback and the possible need for bracing may be useful in obtaining better compliance with the recommended exercise program.

SCHEUERMANN'S KYPHOSIS

More commonly seen in teenage boys than girls, Scheuermann's kyphosis is the condition that results when the kyphotic segment loses its flexibility and demonstrates vertebral wedging on the lateral spinal radiograph.

Etiology

The cause of Scheuermann's kyphosis remains unknown, though several theories have been advanced.

The presence of anterior vertebral body wedging and narrowing of the thoracic intervertebral disc spaces with invagination of disc material into the vertebral bodies has prompted the theory that repetitive trauma may cause this disorder. Scheuermann's kyphosis is seen in some weight lifters, but the exact link is not clear.

Juvenile osteoporosis of the thoracic vertebra has some support as the cause of this disorder. Biopsies of vertebral bone at the time of anterior spinal fusion for advanced kyphosis have demonstrated this osteoporosis, but it is not known if this change is primary or secondary. Using dual-photon absorptiometry, a decrease in bone density has been noted in teenagers with Scheuermann's kyphosis, but others have reported normal vertebral bone density demonstrated by quantitated computed tomographic (QCT) scans in teenage boys with the same disorder.

Although the influence is not as strong as in scoliosis, there does appear to be some genetic impact on the development of this kyphosis, as family groups have been reported with Scheuermann's kyphosis.

History

Teenagers with Scheuermann's kyphosis seek medical advice for two reasons: pain in the low thoracic area and an unsightly appearance. Teenage boys with this disorder often are involved with school athletics and may have back pain after playing their sport. Many will have a history of weight lifting as a part of their sport training. Although teenage boys are probably as concerned about their physical appearance as girls, some physicians may tend to play down complaints from males about the way they look. In some instances when pain is the presenting complaint, the principal reason for seeing the doctor is really the hunched-over appearance of the back.

If back pain is present, the pattern and location of pain should be elicited in the history. In thoracic Scheuermann's kyphosis, the pain usually follows activity and is in the lower thoracic region without radiation into the lower extremities. Scheuermann's kyphosis involving the thoracolumbar or lumbar regions produces pain at these respective locations, and the pain may radiate into the buttocks and posterior thighs.

In 30% to 50% of teenagers with Scheuermann's kyphosis, spondylolysis of the fifth lumbar vertebra is present. Since this stress fracture of the pars interarticularis may be the source of back pain, localization of the exact site of back pain becomes important in addressing treatment to the appropriate area.

Physical Examination

The evaluation of a child for excessive kyphosis is similar to the examination for scoliosis. Clothes should be removed from the back for a thorough evaluation.

With the teenager standing, the trunk is viewed from the dorsal aspect. Even if excessive kyphosis is the primary problem, a mild or moderate scoliosis may also be seen.

Next, the trunk is viewed from the lateral side, both in the standing and forward-bending positions. In the standing position, the amounts of thoracic kyphosis and lumbar lordosis are noted in a resting position and in a position when the teenager tries to actively stand as straight as he or she can. In the Adams or forwardbending position, a structural kyphosis, as seen in Scheuermann's kyphosis, will be readily seen by the appearance of a sharply angular kyphotic segment in the midthoracic region. By flattening the lumbar lordosis with forward bending, the nonflexible kyphosis becomes much more obvious. In the forward-bending position, the neck is then hyperextended actively as the patient attempts to actively correct the kyphosis, a test that may provide useful information about the flexibility of the kyphotic deformity. In true Scheuermann's kyphosis, this hyperextension will *not* reverse the kyphotic deformity.

Evaluation of the lower extremities, as

with scoliosis, is an important part of the examination for excessive kyphosis. Hamstring tightness is commonly present symmetrically in Scheuermann's kyphosis. Asymmetrical limitation of the straight leg raising test may be due to a lower lumbar problem instead. The remainder of the neurologic examination should be normal in this condition.

Radiographic Evaluation

The standing lateral radiograph of the spine is essential to confirm the diagnosis of Scheuermann's kyphosis (Fig. 9.14). Using the Cobb method described above, the thoracic kyphosis between T3 and T12 is normally 20° to 40°. In thoracic Scheuermann's kyphosis, this angle is greater than 60° and wedging of the apical vertebrae is noted. In

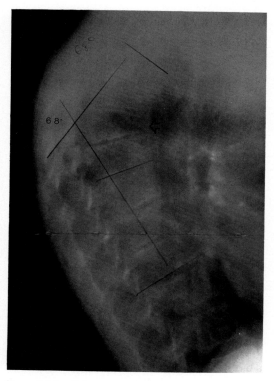

Figure 9.14. Scheuermann's disease with thoracic kyphosis of 68° is seen in this standing lateral radiograph. Note the anterior wedging of T4 and T5 (*open arrow*), producing this kyphosis.

fact, at least three of the apical vertebrae should have anterior wedging of 5° or more to make the diagnosis of thoracic Scheuermann's kyphosis. An additional radiographic finding is the presence of thoracic intervertebral disc narrowing and Schmorl's nodes from invagination of disc material into the vertebral bodies.

Treatment

The treatment recommended for Scheuermann's kyphosis depends on the magnitude of the kyphosis and the skeletal age of the teenager. The management options include no treatment, bracing, and surgical correction.

If a teenager has Scheuermann's kyphosis of 70° or less and has at least 1 year of growth remaining, brace treatment is generally recommended. The brace used is either a Milwaukee brace or, more often, a TLSO with anterior shoulder pads to extend the shoulders. If bracing is chosen, the brace needs to be worn for 22 hours daily for at least a year; thereafter, wearing the brace at nighttime is often needed until growth is complete. Unlike in scoliosis, where bracing infrequently will correct the curvature, the use of a brace in Scheuermann's kyphosis can usually improve the kyphosis significantly. As a general rule, a kyphosis of 60° can be improved to about 35° or 40° by the end of 1 year of brace wear, provided growth is still occurring.

If a marked kyphosis is present in a skeletally mature teenager, or if the brace is ineffective, surgical treatment can correct the kyphosis by 50% or more. Anterior and posterior spinal fusion with posterior spinal instrumentation is most commonly employed for the correction of Scheuermann's kyphosis.

The decision to undergo surgical treatment for Scheuermann's kyphosis is based mainly on the amount of pain present and the psychological impact of the spinal deformity. Pulmonary function is not impaired in marked kyphosis. Progression of the untreated deformity may occur in adult life, but mainly in females with later osteoporosis. Within 6 months of surgical treatment, the patient may resume normal activity, including sports, with the exception of collision or active contact sports.

CONGENITAL KYPHOSIS

Pure congenital kyphosis is less common than congenital scoliosis. As with congenital scoliosis, the presence of congenital kyphosis requires a close look for other congenital anomalies. The most common associated congenital anomalies are in the genitourinary system and the spinal cord, with about one-third of children with congenital kyphosis having one or both of these abnormalities.

The two types of congenital kyphosis generally seen are a single hemivertebra (Fig. 9.15) or failure of anterior segmenta-

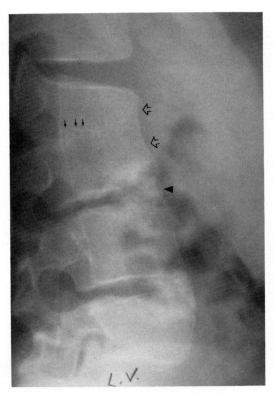

Figure 9.16.   Failure of anterior segmentation of two lumbar vertebrae is seen. The involved vertebral segments show a rudimentary disc posteriorly (*small arrows*), anterior fusion of two vertebral bodies (*open arrows*), and osteocartilaginous fusion at the lower margin (*arrowhead*).

tion, in which the intervertebral disc has not formed properly in its anterior aspect, producing a bony bar that bridges several vertebrae (Fig. 9.16). Because posterior vertebral growth exceeds the limited anterior growth, these kyphotic deformities are nearly always progressive.

Anterior spinal cord compression is the principal complication resulting from a progressive congenital kyphosis. Neurologic deficits are much more often seen in conjunction with congenital kyphosis than with congenital scoliosis. As the rigid kyphotic deformity progresses, the spinal cord is drawn anteriorly against the posterior aspect of the vertebra at the apex of the kyphosis.

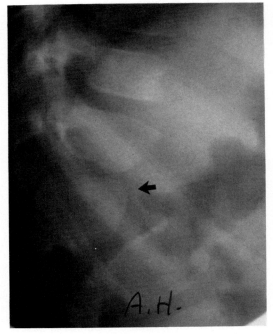

Figure 9.15.   A dorsal hemivertebra is present with anterior wedging (*arrow*) and resultant focal congenital kyphosis. Surgical treatment is indicated to prevent the progression of kyphosis and to avoid neurologic disorders in the lower extremities.

The initial step of treatment in a child with congenital kyphosis is a thorough baseline spine and neurologic evaluation. A renal sonogram and MR scan of the thoracic and lumbar spine should be obtained, as well as anteroposterior and lateral spine radiographs. If no neurologic deficit is present at the initial evaluation, re-examination is performed 4 to 6 months later to see if any progression of deformity has occurred by measuring the kyphosis by the Cobb method.

If the congenital kyphosis increases in size or if the initial congenital kyphosis exceeds 40°, surgical treatment is needed. Bracing as a primary treatment is ineffective in this condition. If no neurologic deficit is present, the surgical treatment consists of an *in situ* posterior fusion if the kyphosis is less than 50° and an anterior and posterior spinal fusion if the kyphotic segment is greater than 50°. If a neurologic deficit is present, anterior spinal cord decompression is completed at the same time as this anterior and posterior spinal fusion. Laminectomy alone does not provide sufficient decompression in this condition. Spinal instrumentation to obtain correction of the deformity is not commonly employed because of the risk of iatrogenic spinal cord injury with excessive correction and instrumentation.

Excessive Spinal Lordosis

Physiologic lordosis is present normally in the lumbar spine. In some clinical situations, this lumbar lordosis can be increased, but this change is usually secondary to other conditions rather than an intrinsic increase in the lumbar spine itself.

The two most common causes of lumbar hyperlordosis are the presence of hip flexion contractures and the existence of excessive thoracic kyphosis. In both of these instances, the flexible lumbar spine increases its lordosis to try to balance the trunk and head over the pelvis. Treatment may be deemed necessary for the hip or thoracic spine problem, but the flexible lumbar hyperlordosis itself needs no treatment and will resolve as the other abnormalities are improved.

Sometimes children in the 5- to 9-year-old age range will stand with exaggerated lumbar lordosis. This is painless, is passively correctable, and is not associated with hip or thoracic spine abnormalities. This condition virtually always resolves without active treatment, and bracing is not needed. If this flexible lordosis persists for a few years, a regimen of sit-up exercises may be helpful in strengthening the abdominal muscles and flattening the lumbar spine.

Relative or actual lordosis of the thoracic spine is at times associated with a progressive thoracic scoliosis. If present, this hypokyphosis or lordosis makes brace treatment less likely to succeed and leads to a larger decrease in vital capacity of the lungs than in patients with scoliosis and thoracic kyphosis. In some syndromes, such as Marfan syndrome, this thoracic lordosis is associated with the presence of a pectus excavatum deformity of the anterior chest wall.

Suggested Readings

Crawford, A.H.: Pitfalls of spinal deformities associated with neurofibromatosis in children. Clin. Orthop. 245:29-42, 1989.

Ferguson, R.L. and Allen, B.L., Jr.: Considerations in the treatment of cerebral palsy patients with spinal deformities. Orthop. Clin. North Am. 19:419-425, 1988.

Jacobs, R.R. (ed): Pathogenesis of Idiopathic Scoliosis: Proceedings of an International Conference. Scoliosis Research Society, Chicago, 1984.

Lonstein, J.E. and Carlson, J.M.: The prediction of curve progression in untreated idiopathic scoliosis during growth. J. Bone Joint Surg. 66A:1061-1071, 1984.

McMaster, M.J.: Occult intraspinal anomalies and congenital scoliosis. J. Bone Joint Surg. 66A:588-601, 1984.

McMaster, M.J. and Ohtsuka, K.: The natural history of congenital scoliosis: A study of two hundred and fifty-one patients. J. Bone Joint Surg. 64A:1128-1147, 1982.

Sachs, B., Bradford, D., Winter, R.B., et al.: Scheuermann kyphosis: Follow-up of Milwaukee-brace treatment. J. Bone Joint Surg. 69A:50-57, 1987.

Smith, A.D., Koreska, J., and Moseley, C.F.: Progression of scoliosis in Duchenne muscular dystrophy. J. Bone Joint Surg. 71A:1066-1074, 1989.

Tsou, P.M., Yau, A., and Hodgson, A.R.: Embryogenesis and prenatal development of congenital vertebral anomalies and their classification. Clin. Orthop. 152:211-231, 1980.

Weinstein, S.L.: Idiopathic scoliosis: Natural history. Spine 11:780-783, 1986.

Winter, R.B. (ed): Congenital Deformities of the Spine. New York, Thieme-Stratton, 1983.

Winter, R.B.(ed): Scoliosis. Orthop. Clin. North Am. 19:227-465, 1988.

Winter, R.B. and Lonstein, J.E.: Juvenile and Adolescent Scoliosis. In Rothman, R.H. and Simeone, F.A. (eds): The Spine. 3rd edition, Volume 1. Philadelphia, W.B. Saunders, pp. 373-430, 1992.

Winter, R.B., Lonstein, J.E., Drogt, J., et al.: The effectiveness of bracing in the nonoperative treatment of idiopathic scoliosis. Spine 11:790-791, 1986.

10
Back Pain

Back pain in children differs from that seen in adults, in whom degenerative disc disease is common. While about 40% of the adult population is bothered by intermittent back pain, back pain is unusual in children. In children, the complaint of pain in the back needs to be taken seriously, since medical—as well as psychological or emotional—causes of back pain occur uncommonly in this age group of patients. Even muscular causes of back pain are less common than in adults. In fact, 60 to 75% of children who have back pain for more than a few days can be found to have an underlying orthopaedic or neurologic reason for that pain. Thus, back pain in children should not be ignored.

The differential diagnosis in a child presenting with back pain includes muscular injury, spondylolysis, spondylolisthesis, disc infection or injury, spinal fracture, spinal deformity, tumors of the spine or spinal cord, and ankylosing spondylitis.

Muscular Injury

Although it is less commonly a cause of back pain in children than in adults, muscular injury can occur in the skeletally immature, particularly in pre-adolescents or teenagers engaged in sports. However, this should be a diagnosis of exclusion, with care being taken to rule out more serious causes of back pain.

Muscular injury may present as either acute or chronic back pain. If there is acute pain from an injury or accident, tenderness is present over the paraspinous muscles, usually on one side of the lumbar spine. The child is reluctant to shift position because of the pain. Neurologic examination is normal. Radiographs of the lumbar spine are normal. Treatment consists of rest until the pain resolves; in the teenager, muscle relaxants may be useful during the acute stage.

In teenagers with back pain that is intermittently present over a period of several weeks, particularly when sitting or standing for long periods, the cause may be a muscle injury or muscle fatigue in the back. A specific injury in the past is not generally recounted. Physical examination may be normal or may demonstrate mild low back discomfort with forward or lateral bending. Muscle spasm is generally absent, and the neurologic examination and lumbar spine radiographs are normal. In teenagers with this type of pain, muscle strengthening exercises for the paraspinous and abdominal muscles are often the most successful treatment. Temporary use of a lumbosacral corset during activities that produce delayed pain, such as a specific sport, is often useful to protect the teenager against moving the spine to the full extremes of motion. In this way, the pain with activity is diminished while strengthening exercises of the weakened muscles are continued. As the paraspinous and abdominal muscle strength improves, the corset can be eliminated, with concomitant return to full activity.

Muscle relaxants, nonsteroidal anti-inflammatory medications, and narcotic pain medication are seldom indicated for back pain in young children resulting from a muscular cause. If rest and an exercise program do not lead to resolution of the pain, further workup is needed to search for other, potentially more serious, causes of the back pain.

Spondylolysis

ETIOLOGY AND INCIDENCE

Consisting of a fracture through the pars interarticularis portion of the posterior elements of a vertebra, spondylolysis occurs in 5 to 6% of children and adolescents. This fracture may be due to an acute injury, but much more often it is a stress fracture that develops a fibrous union; it usually affects low lumbar vertebrae.

Infants are not born with a spondylolytic defect, but children develop the defect after walking begins. Although spondylolysis usually occurs by 6 or 7 years of age, a small percentage of spondylolysis occurs in the teenage years, often related to sports activity. Even though the pars interarticularis stress fracture occurs in the younger child, pain is usually not noted until the child is a pre-adolescent or a teenager, at which time increased sports activity and intensity may take place.

There is a higher incidence of spondylolysis in specific sports. In competitive young gymnasts the incidence may reach 20%, with this high rate of spondylolysis possibly due to the hyperextension of the lumbar spine needed in some gymnastic routines. As this lumbar hyperextension occurs, the thin pars interarticularis appears to have excessive force placed on it, with a resultant stress fracture. There is also a relatively high rate of spondylolysis in weight lifters, wrestlers, and interior linemen in football.

Genetic and ethnic factors also play a role in determining the incidence of spondylolysis. Eskimos have a very high rate, and a familial incidence of spondylolysis has been noted, though it is not clear whether this is a genetic predisposition or the result of shared family sports activities.

HISTORY

The primary fact to be learned in the history is when and how the pain began. Was there a sudden sharp pain or was the onset more gradual over a period of several weeks? Does the pain radiate into the buttocks or lower extremities? In what kind of sports has the child participated on a regular basis? The type and time of onset of the pain may help, as discussed below, to determine the type of treatment recommended.

PHYSICAL EXAMINATION

Physical findings with spondylolysis may be similar to those seen with muscular problems. Tenderness may be vaguely present to low lumbar palpation. Pain is usually produced by lumbar hyperextension more than by forward or lateral flexion. Straight leg raising may cause low back pain but does not usually produce pain radiating down the leg. The neurologic examination is normal in the lower extremities.

IMAGING STUDIES

The initial study to obtain is an anteroposterior and lateral radiograph of the lumbosacral spine. Spondylolysis is most common at the fifth lumbar level, with decreasing frequency from L4 to L1. If the spondylolysis is bilateral (as it usually is), a radiolucent line will be seen on the lateral radiograph extending through the pars interarticularis of the involved lumbar vertebra, most commonly L5. On the anteroposterior radiograph, sclerosis may be apparent adjacent to the pedicle region and the affected lower segment is rotated ventrally. In unilateral spondylolysis, the sclerosis is maximal on the side opposite the spondylolytic defect, and this radiodensity may denote an early stress fracture on the apparently intact side.

Although many spondylolyses can be diagnosed on the anteroposterior and lateral radiographs, further information is obtained with oblique radiographs. These radiographs, taken at an angle of 45° to the frontal plane, directly visualize the lamina better. In this view, the outline of a "Scotty dog" can be seen (Fig. 10.1), with the pars interarticularis being the neck of the dog. If a spondylolysis is present, it will appear as if the dog's neck has a collar, which is the radiolucency resulting from the stress fracture here.

In addition to noting the presence of a spondylolytic defect on the radiographs, it may be possible to judge the length of time the spondylolysis has been present. If a spondylolysis has been present for several months, the edges of this defect will be sclerotic, a finding that is absent if a spondylolysis is acute.

Another useful imaging study here is a technetium-99 pertechnetate bone scan. The bone scan in spondylolysis can be useful to estimate the age of the fracture, which has ramifications for the type of treatment to be recommended. If the bone scan shows no increased activity at this site, the fracture is old and will not heal with immobilization, while a "hot spot" at this location may be indicative of a fresh injury, which may heal with immobilization. Another use for a bone scan is to detect occult or early stress fractures here in athletes for whom the plain radiographs are normal.

A computed tomographic (CT) scan of the lumbar vertebra with spondylolysis will demonstrate the fracture well but is not necessary to guide management recommendations. Magnetic resonance (MR) studies are not used for imaging of spondylolysis except to evaluate the cauda equina in the rare instance of associated nerve root signs.

TREATMENT

Treatment recommendations are based in large part on the radiographic and bone scan findings. If the spondylolysis has sclerotic margins on the radiographs and shows no increased uptake on the bone scan, treatment is symptomatic. Rest from sports activity is prescribed until the pain is gone. A lumbosacral corset may speed the recovery from this pain; when the pain is better, sit-ups are used to strengthen the abdominal muscles, as gradual return to sports and other activity is implemented. If pain begins again with return to sport, a lumbosacral corset is often helpful in limiting this pain while sports participation continues.

If the area of spondylolysis shows increased uptake on the bone scan, an attempt to produce healing of this fracture is worthwhile. Either a thoracolumbar-sacral orthosis (body-jacket brace) or cast can be used for 3 months, with the child refraining from

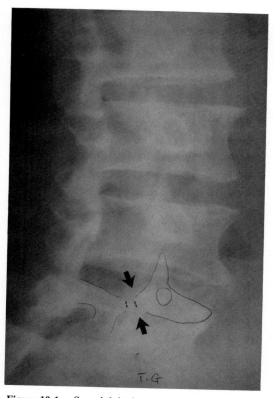

Figure 10.1. Spondylolysis at L5 shows the "Scotty dog" (drawing), which represents the lamina (body), superior articular facet (ear), pedicle (eye), and lateral mass (nose). The *arrows* and *dotted lines* indicate the defect in the pars interarticularis, which appears as a collar on the dog.

sports activity during this period. With this brace treatment less than half of the spondylolyses will heal, but even without healing, the brace is effective in the relief of the back pain. Following the brace treatment period, strengthening exercises and gradual return to sport are appropriate. All sports that do not produce back pain can be pursued, even with a persistent spondylolysis on radiographs.

Young adults with lumbar spondylolysis generally have occasional but not disabling episodes of back pain that last a few days, particularly with athletic activity. MR studies of lumbar spine discs in young adults with spondylolysis have demonstrated a higher rate of disc degeneration adjacent to the level of spondylolysis than in those without this fracture.

Spondylolisthesis

Spondylolisthesis is defined as a forward slip of one vertebral body relative to the vertebral body at the next caudal level. This most often is found at the lumbosacral level, with a slip at L4-L5 being next in frequency. While degenerative spondylolisthesis, secondary to lumbar disc degeneration, is common in adults, the dysplastic and isthmic types of spondylolisthesis are most often seen in children and adolescents (Fig. 10.2).

HISTORY

Back pain has frequently been present for some time but may not be severe. Difficulty in bending forward is often the main symptom noted, as well as increasing difficulty in running or walking quickly. The pain may radiate into the buttocks or posterior thigh. In some, a painful scoliosis will be the reason for seeking medical advice.

PHYSICAL EXAMINATION

In the most severe slips, inspection of the back will demonstrate a flattening of the mid and low lumbar area with an accentuation of the upper lumbar lordosis. Forward flexion will be limited and painful. Tightness of the

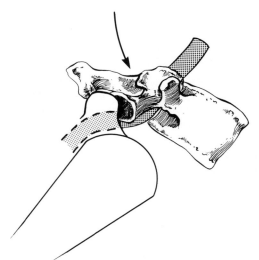

Dysplastic Spondylolisthesis

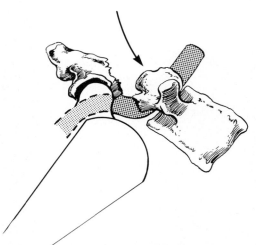

Isthmic Spondylolisthesis

Figure 10.2. The two most common forms of spondylolisthesis seen in children and adolescents are the isthmic and dysplastic types. The dysplastic type has attenuation or lengthening of the lamina, while the isthmic type follows a stress fracture at the pars interarticularis. The dysplastic type is more likely to cause compression of the cauda equina as the L5 vertebra moves forward on the sacrum.

hamstrings is often striking and frequently worse in one leg than in the other. While this hamstring tightness causes limitation of the straight leg raising test, the production of sciatica with this test is uncommon, though back pain may be produced with this maneuver. In long-standing cases, hypesthesia in the S1 dermatome on the dorsum of the foot can be noted, as well as mild weakness of the peroneal muscles that evert the foot.

In observing the gait of a child with hamstring spasm, the stride length will be shortened since the leg cannot be swung as far forward when taking the next step. If a long step is attempted, the pelvis needs to rotate. The result is a stiff-legged gait with relatively shorter steps than normal.

IMAGING STUDIES

A lateral lumbosacral spine radiograph will confirm the diagnosis of spondylolisthesis. To assess this film for a possible forward slip, the posterior margin of each lumbar vertebral body should be traced down the lumbar spine to the sacrum. Using the posterior margin as the reference point is more accurate than following the anterior vertebral margins (Fig. 10.3).

Once a slip is identified, the percentage of slip can be quantified by dividing the degree of displacement of the upper vertebral endplate by the width of the superior vertebral endplate of the vertebra immediately below the slipped vertebra. As the slip progresses, the sacrum is pushed dorsally, producing a localized lumbosacral kyphosis, which is measured by the angle of sagittal rotation or slip angle.

In addition to demonstrating the percentage of slip present, the lateral radiograph also will allow determination of the type of spondylolisthesis present. The *isthmic* type is the result of a slip at the site of a previous spondylolysis and will have a radiolucent gap at the spondylolysis approximately equal in width to the amount of forward vertebral body slip present (Fig. 10.3A). The *dysplastic* type has no spondylolysis initially but the laminae are elongated, like

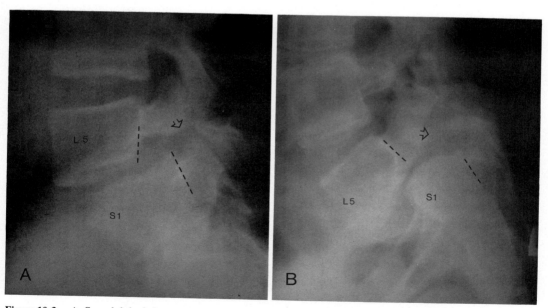

Figure 10.3. **A,** Spondylolysis is present at L5 (*open arrow*) with spondylolisthesis at L5-S1. *Dotted lines* indicate the degree of slip to be grade II, or between 25 and 50%. **B,** Spondylolysis (*open arrow*) with spondylolisthesis of the dysplastic type is present with a grade IV slip (greater than 75%) of L5 on S1 (*dotted lines*).

taffy being pulled. Spondylolysis may occur later as the slip increases. An additional finding in the dysplastic type is typically a rounded top of the sacrum on the lateral radiograph and a spina bifida occulta at S1 on the anteroposterior film (Fig. 10.3**B**).

Radiographs are usually the only imaging study used to diagnose and manage spondylolisthesis in children and adolescents. Bone scans are not helpful. CT and MR scans of the low lumbar area will demonstrate tenting of the dural sac over the posterior edge of the superior sacrum, with this indentation increasing as the slip percentage increases, but surgical decompression in this age group is not usually necessary. Unless a particular neurologic physical finding requires evaluation by an MR scan in this setting, these specialized imaging studies can be avoided.

PROGNOSIS

The majority of children with a mild spondylolisthesis will not worsen from the time of initial presentation, although periodic clinical and/or radiographic assessment should continue until growth is complete. If certain features of isthmic or dysplastic types of spondylolisthesis are present, worsening of the slip is more common.

The isthmic type is more common in boys, but progression is more common in girls. Those with recurrent pain and with initial presentation at an early age are at higher risk of progression. Slips that measure over 50% radiographically and that have more kyphosis at the lumbosacral level worsen more often.

The dysplastic type is more likely to worsen than is the isthmic type. Girls are at higher risk in this type as well. Recurrent pain, marked hamstring tightness, and painful scoliosis are more common in those that progress, as is a young age at first diagnosis. The presence of a spina bifida at both S1 and L5 together with a rounded superior sacrum tend to promote continued slip.

A genetic history is also of importance,

as several families have been reported with members of several generations involved, particularly with the isthmic type of spondylolisthesis.

TREATMENT

Three primary areas require assessment to tailor the proper treatment to the child with spondylolisthesis. First is the amount of back pain and hamstring tightness present. Second is the percentage of slip present on radiographs. Third is the amount of skeletal growth remaining in the particular child.

As a general rule, all children with over 50% slip require surgical fusion, because of the high likelihood of continued back pain and hamstring tightness unless stabilization of the slipped area is obtained. *In situ* posterolateral fusion of the affected 2 or 3 vertebrae is successful in over 90% at this age to relieve back pain, improve the hamstring spasm, and prevent further slipping. Although instrumentation to reduce these slips is often used in adults, there is seldom a need to risk iatrogenic neurologic injury by instrumental reduction in the skeletally immature.

If the slip percentage is under 50%, treatment depends on the severity of the symptoms present. A rigid body jacket brace will improve back pain symptoms, but this pain is often relieved as well by rest and transient restriction of activity. If pain and hamstring spasm persist with conservative treatment or if the slip increases as growth occurs, fusion is recommended.

Surgery is rarely needed for children with less than 25% slip. While these children need periodic assessment to detect a possible increase in the slip, most will have only occasional back pain that can be handled by exercise programs, periodic use of a lumbosacral corset, and rest as needed.

If the child or teenager desires, participation in all sports is allowed, provided the particular sport does not consistently lead to exacerbation of back pain. The sport itself will not lead to speedier progression of a spondylolisthesis, so the degree of symptomatology present with a particular sport becomes the main guide to which sports will be best pursued by an affected child. If lumbosacral fusion is needed, sports activity can generally be fully resumed after recovery from surgery.

A question often raised is how frequently radiographic reassessment is needed to detect the progression of spondylolisthesis in a growing child. While no exact answer covers all cases, the authors' approach is to obtain a second radiograph approximately 6 months after the first. If no change is seen, the next radiograph is obtained in 1 year, then a 2-year interval follows if no change is seen. If over this 3- to 4-year period of growth no increased slip has occurred, progression is unlikely, and patient management thereafter can consist of documentation of back pain and hamstring tightness. If either of these worsen on sequential examination, another radiograph is obtained. The authors limit these follow-up radiographs to a single standing spot lateral film of the lumbosacral region to facilitate the comparison of sequential measurements.

Discitis

Inflammation of the intervertebral disc may present in several clinical forms, depending largely on the age of the child. Included within the term "discitis" are relatively mild, transient episodes of back pain in the young, and bacterial infections that lead to systemic illness and the formation of vertebral abscesses. The child's age, the severity of systemic illness present, and the etiology must be assessed for each child with discitis to help guide recommendations for the most appropriate treatment.

GENERAL FEATURES

Discitis occurs primarily in the lumbar spine, with the lower lumbar spine more often involved. Two major age groups are present: birth to 4 years old and the preadolescent age range.

The cause of discitis is generally thought to be bacterial infection, especially due to *Staphylococcus aureus*, the organism most often seen when either the disc space or blood cultures are positive. However, a large number of children with discitis have negative bacterial cultures of the disc space and blood. Mild trauma has been suggested as a possible cause of discitis in such cases.

HISTORY

Older children may complain of back pain, but younger children usually present because the parents noted a limp or the child refused to stand or walk. In pre-walkers, refusal to move one leg may be seen.

There is no reported familial propensity for discitis. The child may have a history of a recent upper respiratory infection or a recent fall, but both are common in all children.

PHYSICAL EXAMINATION

The child is generally irritable. High or low-grade fever may be present. If a low thoracic disc is involved, abdominal tenderness and pain may be present. The child will hold the back straight and will resist attempts at spine flexion. Straight leg raising tests will show hamstring spasm. Flexion of the hips and cervical spine at the same time will cause an increase in pain or crying.

In children who refuse to walk, the hips and lower extremities need to be carefully examined. With discitis, the hip internal rotation is normal and symmetrical, while this rotation is routinely limited if there is an intra-articular hip infection or injury. Areas of swelling or tenderness should be excluded as causes of this change in walking. Neurologic examination of the lower extremities remains normal unless vertebral abscesses have formed.

LABORATORY STUDIES

No single serum test will make this diagnosis, but the most useful are the erythro-

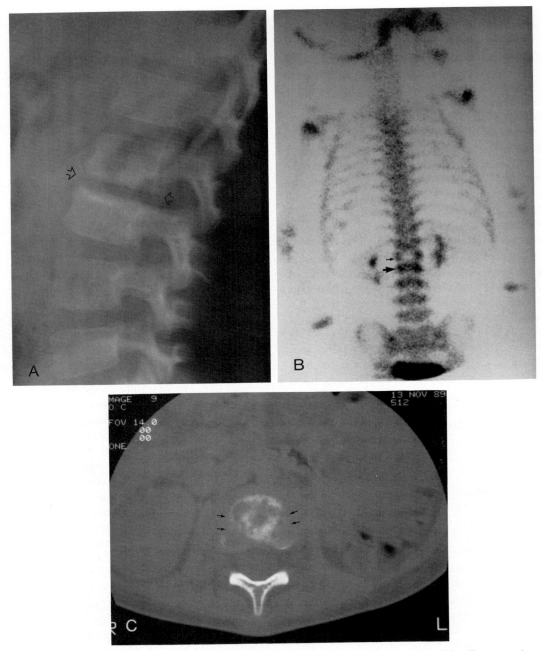

Figure 10.4. **A,** Lateral spine radiograph after 10 days of back pain shows narrowing of the disc space (*open arrows*) and irregularity of the adjacent vertebral endplates, secondary to discitis. **B,** Tc-99 MDP bone scan in a child with back pain for 10 days shows increased uptake at L2 (*large arrow*) and an area of destruction and lack of uptake at L1 (*small arrow*) consistent with discitis or early osteomyelitis. **C,** CT scan in the same child shows diffuse bone changes in the disc region (*arrows*) consistent with the diagnosis of discitis.

cyte sedimentation rate and the white blood cell count. The sedimentation rate is elevated, and the leukocyte count, while usually elevated, will be higher in sicker children. If abdominal pain is present as a result of the discitis, a serum chemistry panel will help assess the function of the gastrointestinal and renal systems.

IMAGING STUDIES

In children with a history of pain or problems walking for a few days to a week, anteroposterior and lateral spine radiographs are usually normal. In the young child, the entire thoracic and lumbar spine should be included in the study.

After discitis has been present for 1 to several weeks, the intervertebral disc space becomes narrower than the neighboring ones on the lateral radiograph (Fig. 10.4A). This decreased disc height persists even after resolution of the discitis. In more long-standing cases, especially in older children, abscess formation within the adjacent vertebral body can be seen as endplate irregularity, erosion, and loss of vertebral height.

In the early stages of discitis, a bone scan is extremely effective in confirming this diagnosis (Fig. 10.4B). Both blood flow sequences and static images will demonstrate increased isotope uptake in the affected disc space.

In the early stages, it is not necessary to obtain a CT or MR study unless a specific neurologic deficit can be demonstrated on physical examination. These studies will demonstrate changes of edema and disc irregularity at the affected level (Fig. 10.4C), but there is generally no change in clinical management as a result of this imaging information. If abscess formation and vertebral body destruction have occurred in untreated vertebral infection, these transverse imaging studies can be very helpful in defining the extent of this bone destruction and spinal cord compression, as well as the relationship of this spinal infection to the psoas muscle and to the ureters and kidneys (Fig. 10.5).

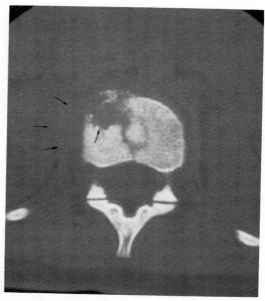

Figure 10.5. This CT scan of a 13-year-old child with back pain due to staphylococcal osteomyelitis shows focal vertebral body destruction (*arrow*) and focal soft tissue abscess (*three arrows*).

TREATMENT

The standard treatment for discitis consists of bed rest, body jacket cast immobilization, and, in most cases, the use of appropriate antibiotics.

No real controversy exists regarding the need for initial bed rest and later spine immobilization for discitis. The child is kept under bed rest until the above studies are performed and the child's illness is observed. Once the diagnosis of discitis is confirmed, a body jacket cast is applied and is usually worn for 3 to 6 weeks, depending on the length of time needed to achieve full resolution of symptoms. In the cast, the child is able to comfortably move and to begin walking again. The long-term sequelae of uncomplicated discitis are negligible. While radiographs may demonstrate spontaneous fusion of the two vertebral bodies at the site of this prior discitis, problems with later back pain and disability due to this cause have not been noted.

There continues to be some controversy, however, about the need for prolonged antibiotic treatment in certain forms of discitis in the younger child. All children with radiographic evidence of vertebral osteomyelitis require several weeks of appropriate intravenous antibiotics after surgical debridement is completed. Outside of this group, the need for extended antibiotic treatment is less clear.

In children below the age of 4 with negative blood cultures, the time until symptom resolution using cast immobilization has been shown to be the same whether or not antibiotics are added. Additionally, no higher incidence of later sequelae is apparent in those treated without antibiotics.

Antibiotics should be used in children with positive blood cultures and in those with signs of systemic sepsis. In younger children without systemic signs of sepsis and with negative cultures, it is the author's opinion that treatment with casting but without antibiotics can be safely recommended, although not all pediatric orthopaedists agree on this last point.

Tuberculosis of the Spine

Tuberculosis continues to be an important infection in the United States, particularly in large urban areas. When there is

Figure 10.6. **A,** A CT scan of a 15-year-old with sudden onset of back pain shows bilateral psoas muscle abscesses (*open arrows*). **B,** MR scan of the same teenager one vertebral segment lower shows bilateral paravertebral abscesses (*A*) and osteomyelitis of the body (*arrows*). The vertebral body is outlined by *dotted lines*. Note that the area of infection extends into the spinal canal (*open arrow*) and partially surrounds the spinal cord (*C*).

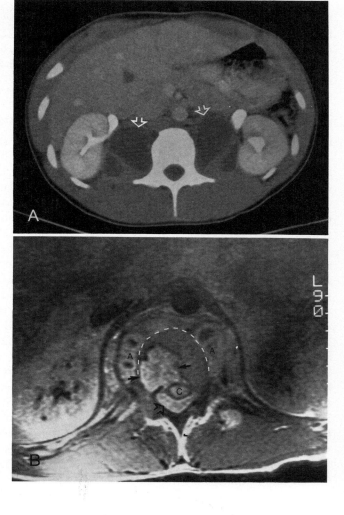

spine involvement tuberculosis has a predilection for the thoracolumbar region. Spinal infection in this region associated with vertebral body destruction should alert the physician to this possible cause. In longstanding cases of spinal tuberculosis, spinal cord compression from collapse or an extradural abscess with lower-extremity neurologic involvement is common. If the abscess tracks down the psoas muscle, it may localize to the medial groin, near the insertion of the psoas tendon.

Positive skin testing for tuberculosis may be the first clue to this diagnosis, which can be confirmed by needle or open biopsy of the affected vertebral region. If diagnosis is made early, medical treatment will be curative. If spinal cord compression is present or if an abscess is identified by CT or MR studies (Fig. 10.6), surgical treatment, followed by multiple drug therapy, is more appropriate.

Intervertebral Disc Trauma

In the skeletally immature child, there is rarely rupture of the nucleus pulposus through the posterior portion of the annulus fibrosus of the intervertebral disc, as is seen quite commonly in the adult with sciatica. Until skeletal maturity, the child has a cartilaginous apophysis at the superior and inferior aspects of each vertebral body, and it is this region that is most at risk for disc injury in the child (Fig. 10.7).

HISTORY

A specific history of trauma resulting in low back pain and leg pain on one side is almost always elicited with this condition. Generally, the mechanism of injury is from sudden compressive forces on a lumbar spine that is in a partially flexed position. A history of possible neurologic problems should be sought, particularly sensory or motor changes in the lower extremities, as well as urinary or bowel control problems.

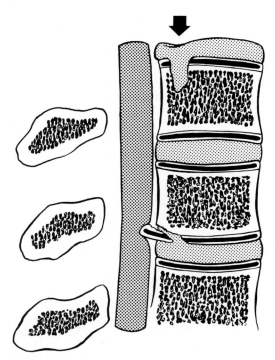

Figure 10.7. Compression-type injury to the immature spine most often results in a fracture through the vertebral apophysis, located at the top and bottom of each vertebral body. This may lead to invagination of disc material into the vertebral body (Schmorl's node on radiographs), anterior avulsion that appears as an ossification defect (Fig. 10.8), or posterior displacement of the apophyseal fragment into the spinal canal to cause lower-extremity neurologic signs and symptoms.

PHYSICAL EXAMINATION

Back pain is present with attempted movement. The child is unable or unwilling to bend forward very far. If the disc injury has led to displacement of a fragment against the cauda equina or a specific nerve root, the compressed area will demonstrate a neurologic abnormality in the legs and the straight leg raising test will cause pain radiating into one leg. If raising one leg causes pain down the other (contralateral straight leg raising test), this is very strong evidence of a low lumbar nerve root compression syndrome on the side of the leg pain.

For assessing motor function of the L4-

S1 region, it is better to have the child walk first on the toes and then on the heels than to attempt manual motor testing. Weakness of foot dorsiflexion with heel walking usually indicates L4 nerve root compression, while weakness with toe walking occurs with S1 nerve root compression.

IMAGING STUDIES

Anteroposterior and lateral radiographs should be the first study ordered. Since compression at the disc level often leads to disruption of the cartilaginous vertebral ring apophysis, intervertebral disc material may be displaced in a variety of directions, depending on the direction of forces involved. Accordingly, the radiographs may show a variety of changes in the vertebral body.

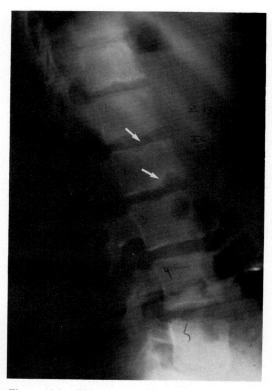

Figure 10.9. This 13-year-old runner shows several rounded defects (*arrows*) in the endplates of vertebral bodies, indicating herniation of disc material into the vertebral body. These defects are also called Schmorl's nodes. Disc spaces are narrowed.

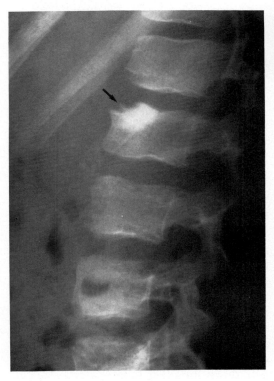

Figure 10.8. Anterior avulsion of the vertebral apophysis has resulted in a well-defined, sclerotic defect (*arrow*) of the anterosuperior margin of L2. Note the disc height at L1-L2 is less than at the other lumbar levels as a result of this injury.

If the anterior ring apophysis has failed, the anterior lip of the superior vertebral body will be displaced anteriorly with extrusion of disc material into this gap (Fig. 10.8). If the forces have been less, disc material may have been "injected" into the vertebral body, being seen on the lateral radiograph as a radiolucency or Schmorl's node (Fig. 10.9). If the displaced fragment is posterior, a small bony fragment may be visible in the spinal canal. Disc herniation is detected by myelography (Fig. 10.10) or MR. In all these instances, the affected disc will have lost height when compared to the adjacent levels.

If the neurologic examination is normal, radiographs are sometimes sufficient to establish the diagnosis and guide the manage-

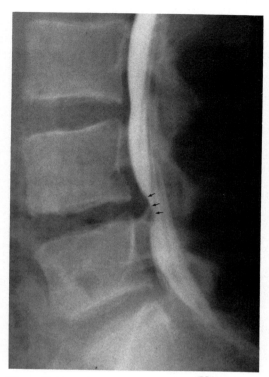

Figure 10.10. This myelogram in an athlete with pain in his legs shows the defect in the column of contrast material (*arrows*). This may be due to posterior displacement of an apophyseal fragment or disc.

ment. The primary role for a bone scan is to detect an occult fracture or to differentiate between a possible anterior compression fracture and a normal variation of vertebral body ossification. The MR study is useful to locate a posteriorly displaced fragment of apophyseal cartilage or disc material not visible on radiographs, a condition that is associated with neurologic abnormality in the lower extremity.

TREATMENT

If no neurologic deficit is present, as with anterior disc protrusion, the treatment is largely symptomatic. With an acute injury, bed rest is usually needed for a few days, followed by relative activity restriction until pain is absent. A lumbosacral corset or a body jacket brace may be needed for a few weeks to a few months, depending on the severity of the vertebral bony injury. Unless there is an associated spondylolisthesis, fusion is generally unnecessary. Permanent radiographic abnormality may persist in the area of ring apophyseal injury, but clinically the majority of patients will be able to resume full activity, including sports, within a few months of the injury.

If neurologic signs and symptoms are present in the lower extremity, surgical removal of the posteriorly displaced fragment is necessary for pain relief and return of neurologic function. After postoperative rehabilitation has been completed, return to full function can be anticipated.

Bone Tumors

Benign bone tumors of the spine include osteoid osteoma, histiocytosis X, aneurysmal bone cyst, osteochondroma, hemangioma, and assorted other unusual lesions. Primary malignant tumors of the spine are rare.

OSTEOID OSTEOMA

Osteoid osteoma may occur in any bone, but the spine is one of the most common locations. Histologically, this lesion consists of a nidus of inflammatory-appearing tissue surrounded by a substantial amount of new bone formation that appears to form under the stimulus of this nidus.

The child generally has intermittent back pain near the site of this lesion. Classically this pain is present more at night than during the day, when pain may be completely absent. Pain is relieved by salicylates and may not be improved by narcotic analgesics. Painful scoliosis is often present at the first examination, but other positive physical findings may be absent. The neurologic examination is normal.

Radiographs of the spine are often normal, though local scoliosis without pedicle rotation may be present. If the lesion has been present for several months, sclerosis

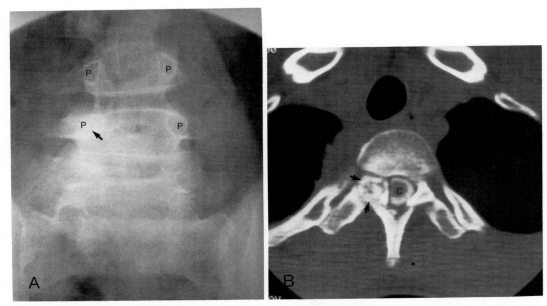

Figure 10.11.   A, This child had persistent back pain at rest. The lumbar spine radiograph shows sclerosis of the right L5 pedicle (*arrow*) secondary to an osteoid osteoma (*P,* pedicle). **B,** This CT scan of a thoracic vertebra of a patient with upper back pain shows a sclerotic and expanding pedicle lesion (*arrows*) with displacement of the cord (*C*) by the mass. Osteoid osteoma was confirmed by excisional biopsy.

of a part of the posterior elements may be seen (Fig. 10.11**A**).

A bone scan is useful to localize the site of the cause of the back pain. In osteoid osteoma, there is a marked increase in isotope uptake in the lesion. Once the bone scan has localized this lesion, a CT scan of the affected vertebra will demonstrate a lucent nidus surrounded by sclerotic bone (Fig. 10.11**B**).

If the diagnosis of osteoid osteoma is made on clinical and imaging grounds, treatment is surgical excision of the nidus and some of the surrounding sclerotic bone. It is not necessary to remove all the new bone that formed, since removal of the nidus will prevent further excess bone formation at the resection site and allow remodeling to occur.

Immediately postoperatively, the pain is improved, and the scoliosis secondary to osteoid osteoma usually gradually straightens after the surgical removal of this lesion.

If the nidus has been removed, there should be no recurrence.

HISTIOCYTOSIS X

One or more bones, including vertebrae, may be involved in this condition, which may present with pain in the back. If only one long bone or vertebra is involved, the term *eosinophilic granuloma* is used to describe the condition. If multiple bones and other organs are involved, the child is diagnosed with either Hand-Schüller-Christian disease or Letterer-Siwe disease.

Eosinophilic granuloma of the spine has a characteristic radiographic appearance called "vertebra plana," which is a wafer-like, sclerotic appearance of the compressed vertebral body involved (Fig. 10.12). This radiographic appearance is enough to make the diagnosis of eosinophilic granuloma of the spine, and surgical treatment or biopsy is usually not needed

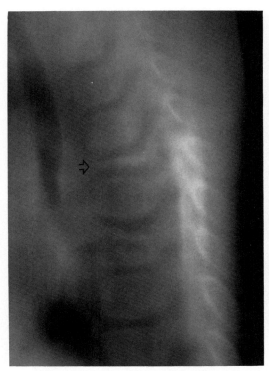

Figure 10.12. Lateral tomogram of a child with histiocytosis X shows typical sclerotic "wafer vertebra" (*arrow*) or vertebra plana secondary to collapse. Adjoining vertebrae are normal, except for the vertebra two levels below the flattened one.

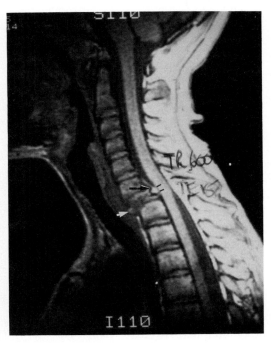

Figure 10.13. MR study of a patient with neck pain and arm numbness has collapse of a single vertebra (*white arrow*) with hemorrhage posteriorly (*black arrow*) and impression on the spinal canal (*lines*). Histiocytosis X was confirmed at the time of surgery.

except in the unusual circumstance of spinal cord compression (Fig. 10.13).

If a single vertebral lesion is present, evaluation of the entire skeletal system with a bone scan and skeletal survey is indicated to detect other occult lesions. In some instances, a liver and spleen scan is also needed to determine the extent of visceral involvement.

If a solitary lesion is present, treatment is usually observation with serial radiographic evaluation or low-dose local radiation therapy if spinal cord compression is present. If other lesions are also present, chemotherapy is used. Once the vertebral body lesion is cured, growth again proceeds, and the height of the affected vertebral body will increase with age. If there is no recurrence

of disease, no long-term sequelae are apparent.

ANEURYSMAL BONE CYST

Back pain and extremity neurologic dysfunction are the predominant presenting problems with an aneurysmal bone cyst of the spine. Though benign, this tumor may be locally recurrent if incompletely treated.

An aneurysmal bone cyst is one of the few tumors that can involve adjacent vertebrae, often spreading from one level to the next around the disc. If sufficient vertebral destruction occurs, spinal cord compression may result.

Radiographs will demonstrate an expansile, lucent area of well-defined bone destruction. The vertebral body or posterior elements are involved. Soft tissue or bony compression of the spinal canal is assessed with MR.

Treatment is surgical. The tumor must be completely excised and, if sufficient bone destruction has occurred to lead to spinal instability, fusion of the affected segments is needed. Radiation therapy is reserved for those with recurrent disease for whom further surgery is not safely possible.

OTHER BENIGN LESIONS

A wide variety of other lesions may be diagnosed radiographically in children with back pain; two are worthy of mention.

Osteochondromas may involve the vertebrae as a part of multiple hereditary exostoses. If these osteochondromata grow toward the spinal canal, neurologic signs and symptoms may result. Treatment is surgical excision of the osteochondroma.

Hemangioma may involve a vertebral body and lead to back pain. The radiographic appearance is relatively characteristic, with the vertebra appearing large and showing a striated lucency (Fig. 10.14). No treatment may be needed, although a biopsy may be necessary to confirm the diagnosis. When treatment is indicated, surgical or embolization therapy may be used.

MALIGNANT BONE TUMORS

Osteogenic sarcoma and Ewing's sarcoma (Fig. 10.15) are the two primary malignant bone tumors of the spine seen in children and adolescents. Ewing's sarcoma is most common in the sacral region, while osteosarcoma can affect any area of the spine. Survival rates of these disorders have historically been below 10%.

OTHER MALIGNANT TUMORS

The most common malignancies that involve several sites, including the vertebrae, are leukemia and lymphoma. Local surgical

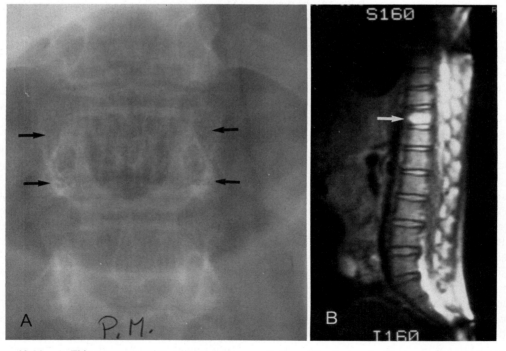

Figure 10.14. **A,** This anteroposterior radiograph shows a single vertebra (*arrows*) with coarse, linear trabeculae, typical of a vertebral hemangioma. **B,** MR study of a vertebra with a hemangioma (*arrow*) shows increased signal in the area of hemangioma on a proton-density series.

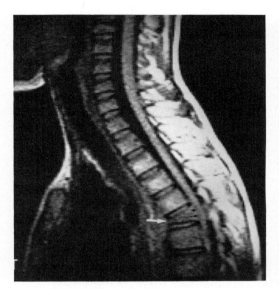

Figure 10.15. MR study of the cervicothoracic region shows a Ewing's sarcoma of the upper thoracic spine with collapse of an upper thoracic vertebra (*white arrow*). Low signal indicates destruction of the marrow. There is posterior extrusion of the body (*black arrows*) into the spinal cord. The patient had back and shoulder pain.

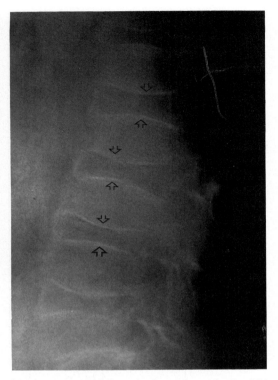

Figure 10.16. This lateral spine radiograph of a child with leukemia shows universal collapse of the vertebrae secondary to marrow and trabecular destruction. Collapse is indicated by *arrows*. Disc spaces are larger than vertebrae, and marked osteoporosis is present.

treatment is not undertaken unless biopsy is utilized for diagnosis and treatment is by chemotherapy. Children with leukemia often develop diffuse, severe compression fractures of all the vertebral bodies, which obtain a biconcave appearance and may require bracing to prevent progressive kyphosis while the underlying disease is being treated (Fig. 10.16).

Spinal Cord Tumors

About 25 to 30% of children with spinal cord tumors present with painful scoliosis as the initial finding. The common physical findings in this condition are pain in the back, associated with limitation of spine movement, particularly in the forward-flexed position.

Radiographs of the spine are normal. However, an MR scan of the spinal cord will demonstrate the spinal cord tumor, which most commonly is either an ependymoma or an astrocytoma (Fig. 10.17). The neurosurgical treatment depends on the type of tumor and the extent of involvement. If laminectomy in the thoracic area is used to treat the spinal cord tumor, particularly if radiation therapy is also needed, close follow-up is indicated to assess for progressive kyphotic deformity with growth (Fig. 10.18). If the thoracic kyphosis does become progressive, surgical fusion of the affected area is needed.

Congenital Scoliosis

In congenital scoliosis of the lumbar spine, especially if multiple vertebrae are involved, pain may result from the abnormal spinal mechanics resulting from the de-

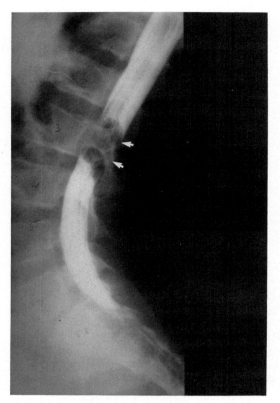

Figure 10.17. This myelogram demonstrates an intraspinal defect (*arrows*) from an ependymoma of the spinal cord presenting with back pain on forward flexion of the spine.

formity itself, even if the magnitude of the deformity is insufficient to warrant surgical treatment. If back pain in this setting is not controlled by conservative means, surgical fusion should relieve this pain.

Associated with congenital scoliosis may be a lipoma in the lumbar area with tethered cord (Fig. 10.19), or diastematomyelia (Fig. 10.20), all of which may cause back pain and lower-extremity neurologic abnormalities. Children with back pain associated with a congenital scoliosis should be studied with an MR scan to assess for any associated congenital neurologic anomaly. Approximately 30% of children with congenital scoliosis, even without pain, will have an abnormal spinal MR study. Neurosurgical

treatment is indicated if progressive pain or neurologic deficit is present.

Sacroiliac Joint Arthritis

Ankylosing spondylitis is the most common form of arthritis seen affecting the sacroiliac joint. This condition is frequently familial and affects primarily male teenagers. A history of pain in the low back is noted, and tenderness over the sacroiliac joints is present on physical examination. Limitation of lumbar flexion may be noted. Hyperextension of the hips may elicit sacroiliac area pain. Although later restriction of chest expansion and hip stiffness are pres-

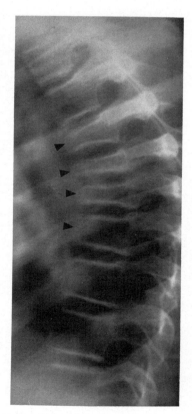

Figure 10.18. This child had previously received local radiation therapy for a tumor. The lateral spine radiograph shows regional flattened vertebrae (*arrowheads*), reflecting growth arrest of the ring apophyses and the effect of radiation necrosis with vertebral compression.

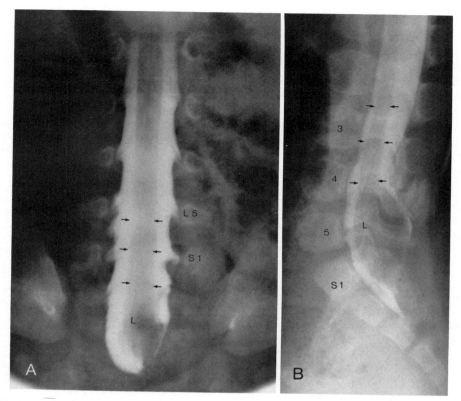

Figure 10.19. **A,** This anteroposterior myelogram view shows a tethered cord (outlined by *arrows*) with a lipoma (*L*) at the base of the cord. The conus medullaris or spinal cord tip normally ends at L2, but here extends to the S2 level. **B,** Lateral myelogram view of the same patient shows the tethered cord (*arrows*) and lumbosacral lipoma (*L*).

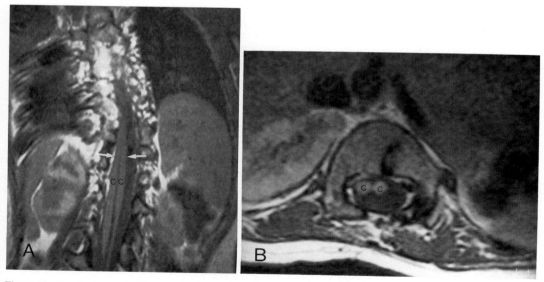

Figure 10.20. **A,** Coronal MR scan of a child with a diastematomyelia shows where the single spinal cord (*arrows*) splits into two (*C, C*) in the lower thoracic region. **B,** Axial MR scan shows the double spinal cord of diastematomyelia.

ent, these findings are not common at the time of initial presentation in the teenager.

Radiographs of the pelvis and lumbar spine may demonstrate narrowing and adjacent sclerosis of the sacroiliac joints. Later, ossification of the anterior longitudinal ligament will occur. If the serum demonstrates the presence of the HLA-B27 antigen in conjunction with the symptoms and radiographs described above, the diagnosis is confirmed. Initial treatment is by nonsteroidal anti-inflammatory medication. Spine surgery is not generally needed, but hip arthroplasty may be needed in advanced cases.

Sacroiliac arthritis may present occasionally in association with *inflammatory gastrointestinal conditions*, such as ulcerative colitis, though this is uncommon in this age group. Medical treatment of both conditions will control the back pain in most cases.

Juvenile rheumatoid arthritis is seldom a cause of low back pain in children. The primary spinal changes seen in this condition are in the cervical spine, where involvement of the facet joints will lead to spontaneous fusion of adjacent vertebrae in this region.

Suggested Readings

Azouz, E.M., Kozlowski, K., Marton, D., et al.: Osteoid osteoma and osteoblastoma of the spine in children: Report of 22 cases with brief literature review. Pediatr. Radiol. 16:25-31, 1986.

DeOrio, J.K. and Bianco, A.J., Jr.: Lumbar disc excision in children and adolescents. J. Bone Joint Surg. 64A:991-996, 1982.

Dillin, W.H. and Watkins, R.G.: Back pain in children and adolescents. In Rothman, R.H. and Simeone, F.A. (eds.): The Spine, 3rd edition, Volume 1. Philadelphia, W.B. Saunders, pp. 231-259, 1992.

Fredrickson, B.E., Baker, D., McHolick, W.J., et al.: The natural history of spondylolysis and spondylolisthesis. J. Bone Joint Surg. 66A:699-707, 1984.

Hay, M.C., Paterson, D., and Taylor, T.K.: Aneurysmal bone cysts of the spine. J. Bone Joint Surg. 60B:406-411, 1978.

Hensinger, R.M.: Current concepts review: Spondylolysis and spondylolisthesis in children and adolescents. J. Bone Joint Surg. 71A:1098-1107, 1989.

Ker, N.B. and Jones, C.B.: Tumors of the cauda equina: The problem of differential diagnosis. J. Bone Joint Surg. 67B:358-362, 1985.

King, H.: Evaluating the child with back pain. Pediatr. Clin. North Am. 33:1489-1493, 1986.

Peterson, H.A.: Musculoskeletal infections in children: Part VII. Disk space infection in children. In Evarts, C.M. (ed.): American Academy of Orthopaedic Instructional Course Lectures, XXXII. St. Louis, C.V. Mosby, pp. 50-60, 1983.

Pizzutillo, P.D. and Hummer, C.D.: Non-operative treatment for painful adolescent spondylolysis or spondylolisthesis. J. Pediatr. Orthop. 9:538-540, 1989.

Reilly, J.P., Gross, R.H., and Emans, J.B.: Disorders of the sacroiliac joint in children. J. Bone Joint Surg. 70A:31-40, 1988.

Seimon, L.P.: Eosinophilic granuloma of the spine. J. Pediatr. Orthop. 1:371-376, 1981.

Wenger, D.R., Bobechko, W.P., and Gilday, D.L.: The spectrum of intervertebral disc-space infection in children. J. Bone Joint Surg. 60A:100-108, 1978.

11
Pelvis

Anatomy

The pelvis provides stability as its primary function, anchoring the end of the spine and providing proximal support for weight bearing in the lower extremities. The pelvis is formed by two hemipelves, identical in shape and size to each other. The skeletal anatomy of each hemipelvis consists of the ilium, ischium, and pubis, joined together at the medial aspect of the acetabulum through a synchondrosis called the triradiate cartilage. Anteriorly the hemipelves join at the pubic symphysis through a cartilaginous and ligamentous attachment, and posteriorly the hemipelvis joins the lateral sacrum to form the sacroiliac joint. Although the pubic symphysis and sacroiliac joints normally have only slight motion, if hip or spine mobility is impaired these joints may become more mobile.

Growth of the pelvis in a child occurs in two primary ways. The triradiate cartilage acts as a growth plate for all three bones, seemingly growing in three directions at the same time as the pelvis and acetabulum develop. Injury to the triradiate cartilage will lead to a more shallow acetabulum and a smaller hemipelvis than on the normal side. In addition, appositional bone growth from the outer aspects of each pelvic bone provides further increases in size over time.

Besides providing a stable base for standing and walking, the pelvis serves as the attachment site for multiple muscles. In the retroperitoneal area, the iliacus muscle originates from the inner iliac wall, joining with the psoas from the lumbar region to form the iliopsoas muscle with a common tendon attachment to the lesser trochanter of the proximal femur, providing strong hip flexion (Fig. 11.1).

The other muscles that help to control hip and knee movement originate from the outer surface of the bony pelvis. Medially, the hip adductors (adductor longus, adductor brevis, and adductor magnus) begin on the pubis and attach distally on the medial femoral shaft (Fig. 11.2). Anteriorly, the sartorius originates from the anterior superior iliac spine, while the rectus femoris starts at the anterior inferior iliac spine; both of these muscles insert onto the proximal tibia, so they have an effect on both hip and knee movement (Fig. 11.1). Laterally, the tensor fascia femoris has a broad origin from the iliac wing, running distally to become the iliotibial band that inserts onto the proximal tibia and fibula. Adjacent to the tensor fascia femoris are the gluteus medius and gluteus minimus, which insert onto the greater trochanter of the proximal femur, providing hip abduction and stability for standing (Fig. 11.3). Weakness of the gluteus medius produces the well-recognized Trendelenburg gait indicative of hip disorders.

The gluteus maximus and hamstrings originate posteriorly, as do the hip external rotators. The gluteus maximus, the primary hip extensor muscle, begins on the posterior iliac wing and inserts onto the posterolateral femoral shaft just below the level of the

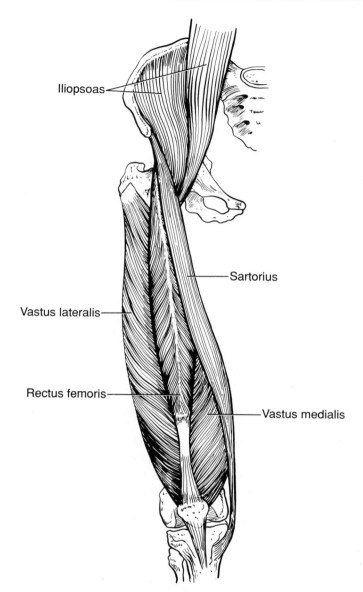

Iliopsoas

Sartorius

Vastus lateralis

Rectus femoris

Vastus medialis

Figure 11.1.   The primary muscles that flex the hip originate either on or near the pelvis. The iliopsoas is formed by the psoas and the iliacus muscles, coursing to insert onto the lesser trochanter of the proximal femur. The sartorius arises from the anterior superior iliac spine, and the rectus femoris, a part of the quadriceps, originates from the anterior inferior iliac spine.

lesser trochanter. The external rotators originate at the posterior lip of the acetabulum and ischium and attach onto the posterior greater trochanter. The hamstrings originate from the inferior pubis and the entire ischium, inserting onto the proximal tibia to provide strong knee flexion as well as some hip extension power. Medial hamstrings consist of the semimembranosus, semitendinosus, and gracilis muscles, while the lateral hamstring muscle is the biceps femoris. Because the hamstring muscles cross both the hip and the knee, tightness or contracture of the hamstrings will limit hip flexion when the knee is straight, being a common cause of a child's inability to touch the toes when bending forward from a standing position.

As with tendinous attachments in other bones, the origins of several of these muscles are on apophyses, or secondary centers of ossification. As these cartilaginous attachments are somewhat weak, avulsion may occur as a result of sports activities. Particularly at risk for this injury are the pelvic apophyses that provide the origins for the sartorius and rectus femoris muscles, as well as the hamstrings.

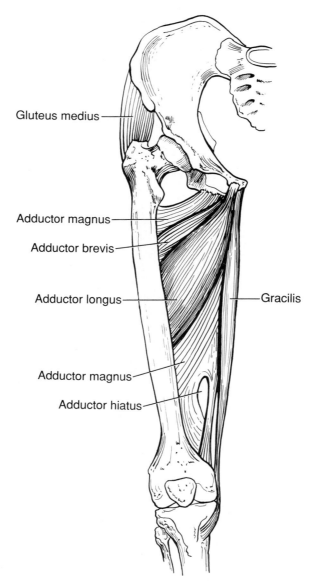

Figure 11.2. The primary adductors of the hip originate from the pubic and ischial rami of the pelvis, passing to insert onto the entire medial aspect of the femoral shaft.

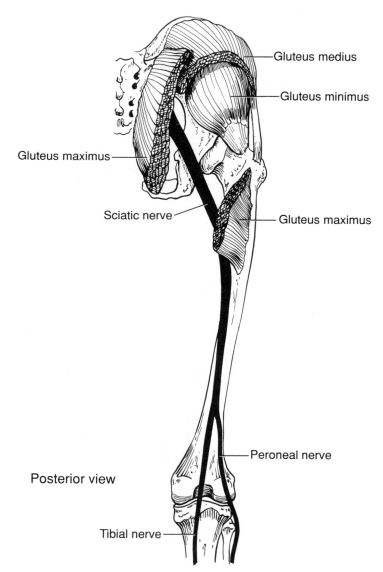

Gluteus medius

Gluteus minimus

Gluteus maximus

Sciatic nerve

Gluteus maximus

Peroneal nerve

Posterior view

Tibial nerve

Figure 11.3. The gluteus medius and gluteus minimus are the major abductors of the hip, running from the side of the iliac wing to the greater trochanter of the femur. The gluteus maximus is the principal hip extensor muscle. The sciatic nerve passes out of the pelvis through the greater sciatic notch, runs posterior to the hip joint, and extends distally to form the posterior tibial and common peroneal nerves to the lower leg.

The major arterial structures in the pelvic region are the external and internal iliac arteries and their branches. The superior gluteal artery, a branch of the internal iliac artery, passes through the sciatic notch with the sciatic nerve and may be a source of bleeding from pelvic fractures in this region.

The obturator artery passes through the obturator foramen with the obturator nerve. The external iliac artery continues into the proximal thigh as the femoral artery.

The femoral and sciatic nerves pass through the pelvic region on the way to the lower extremity. The femoral nerve, formed by the nerve roots of the second, third, and fourth lumbar levels, runs with the femoral artery to supply primarily the quadriceps muscle. The obturator nerve, also formed primarily by the second and third lumbar nerve roots, runs through the obturator fo- ramen of the pelvis to innervate the adductors and gracilis muscles (Fig. 11.4). The sciatic nerve, formed by the fourth and fifth lumbar nerve roots as well as the nerve roots from the first two sacral levels, courses through the greater sciatic notch,

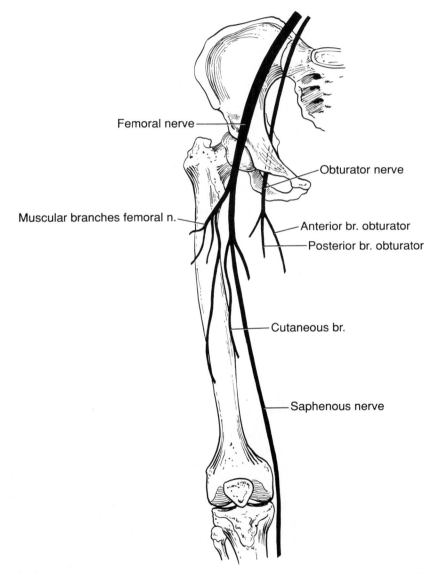

Femoral nerve

Obturator nerve

Muscular branches femoral n.

Anterior br. obturator

Posterior br. obturator

Cutaneous br.

Saphenous nerve

Figure 11.4. The femoral nerve is formed by the midlumbar nerve roots and passes over the hip joint anteriorly with the femoral artery and vein. Its primary muscle innervation is to the quadriceps muscle, but it provides distal leg and foot sensation through the saphenous nerve. The obturator nerve innervates primarily the adductor muscles of the hip.

passing posterior to the hip joint on its way to the posterior thigh. Besides providing the innervation for essentially all the muscles below the knee, the sciatic nerve also innervates the hip abductors and extensors (Fig. 11.3).

The hip joint itself is innervated by branches from the sciatic, femoral, and obturator nerves. Therefore, hip disorders, particularly those with a hip effusion and inflammation, may lead to pain in the groin, buttock, or anterior thigh. The obturator nerve will refer pain down the medial thigh to the knee level. The femoral nerve will refer pain down the anterior thigh, often causing pain just above the patella, the location of the autonomous zone of the femoral nerve. Irritation of the sciatic nerve, on the other hand, will lead to pain in the buttock and posterior thigh. Consideration of referred pain from an irritated hip should always be present when leg pain or a limp is being evaluated.

Physical Examination

OBSERVATION

Is symmetry present? Are the iliac wings at the same height when standing or are they uneven, indicating a leg length difference?

PALPATION

Where are the areas of maximal tenderness? Is there tenderness over specific tendon origins? Is the sacroiliac joint tender?

Hyperextension of the hip with the child lying prone will place stress on the sacroiliac joint, eliciting pain in conditions affecting this area. If pelvic area pain is produced by external rotation of the hip, infection of the sacroiliac or iliac areas should be considered as a possible diagnosis. Spine motion needs to be examined when tenderness is noted at the sacroiliac joint, a finding associated with ankylosing spondylitis.

Imaging Studies

An anteroposterior radiograph of the pelvis is the primary initial imaging study for the evaluation of possible pelvic disorders. Care must be taken to obtain this radiograph with the pelvis in a neutral position (Fig. 11.5), in which the obturator foramina are symmetrical. If pelvic rotation is present, noted by the obturator foramina being asymmetric, accurate evaluation is more difficult. The normal synchondrosis in a young child between the pubis and ischium in the inferomedial region of the pubic rami may simulate a fracture; in the absence of

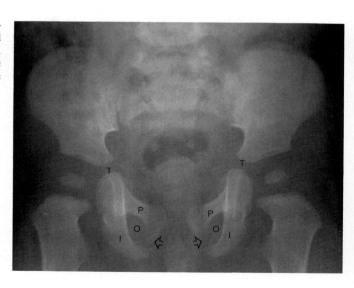

Figure 11.5.   This is a normal anteroposterior pelvis radiograph in a 7-month-old child. (*T*, triradiate cartilage; *P*, pubis; *I*, ischium; *O*, obturator foramen) The *open arrows* indicate the normal ischiopubic synchondrosis.

tenderness at this site, no fracture should be diagnosed.

Several apophyses can be noted in the pelvis as a child matures, though the major apophyses are in the iliac and ischial regions. The iliac apophysis starts to ossify laterally, and ossification proceeds toward the sacrum. The iliac apophysis begins to ossify just before the onset of menses and can be used as a guide to how much growth remains, particularly in the spine. When the iliac apophysis has ossified completely, spinal growth is essentially complete.

In the evaluation of traumatic injury to the pelvis, the physician should recall that the pelvis is a ring structure. Because of this, if a fracture is found at one site, a careful search for a second fracture needs to be made, since the ring usually breaks at two points. For example, if a pubic ramus fracture is noted on the anteroposterior radiograph, the sacroiliac joint or posterior sacrum on the same side is commonly injured.

Computed tomographic (CT) and magnetic resonance (MR) scans are extremely useful in the evaluation of orthopaedic problems in the pelvis (Fig. 11.6). Children with pubic or ischial rami fractures with tender-

ness at the sacroiliac area should have a CT scan to evaluate possible injury posteriorly that cannot be seen on the plain radiograph. CT or MR scans may also be the only way to definitively diagnose a bone tumor involving the iliac wings or sacral region (Fig. 11.7).

Nuclear medicine studies can be helpful in diagnosing an infection in the pelvis or adjacent region. Usually a technetium-99 bone scan will detect tumors and most infections, but in some cases of pelvic osteomyelitis, a gallium scan is needed to more clearly visualize the affected region of the pelvis.

Traumatic Disorders

PELVIC FRACTURES

Fractures of the pelvis range from the mild to the severe. The more displacement of the fracture the more likely the adjacent genitourinary or neurovascular structures are injured as well. Careful neurovascular examination of the distal extremity involved needs to be documented when a pelvic fracture is noted.

Isolated unilateral pubic or ischial rami

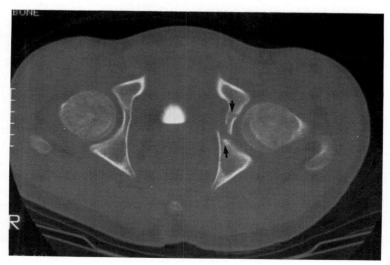

Figure 11.6. Although the radiograph was normal, this CT scan of the pelvis shows two fractures (*arrows*) and displacement of the ilium at the acetabulum.

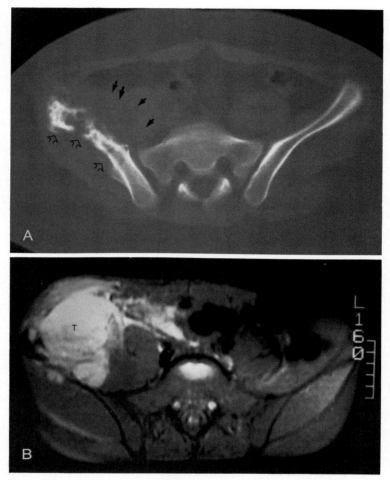

Figure 11.7.   A, A CT scan of the right ilium shows the destruction of the iliac wing (*open arrows*) and the tumor mass in the pelvis (*arrows*) of this child with Ewing's sarcoma. **B,** An MR T2-weighted scan of the same child with Ewing's sarcoma shows a high-signal tumor mass (*T*).

fractures require little treatment. This portion of the pelvis is not essential for weight bearing, the forces of which pass through the hip joint, so stability of the pelvis is not an issue. Pain and tenderness are present at the fracture site, so bed rest is initially used to relieve this discomfort. However, within a day or two crutch walking can usually be started and the child can be discharged home, provided oral intake is adequate. Pelvic fractures frequently lead to retroperitoneal bleeding, which in turn causes an ileus. When oral intake is good and bowel sounds

have returned, home discharge on crutches is appropriate. Crutches are used for a few weeks until pain with weight bearing is absent.

Bilateral fractures through the pubic and ischial rami, termed a Malgaigne-type fracture, can present a more serious problem. Because of the site of this fracture, a tear of the membranous urethra may occur at the time of this injury, and genitourinary evaluation is essential. If no urinary injury is present, walking with crutches is started once pain relief is sufficient to allow weight bearing. Fracture healing is complete when tenderness to palpation and pain with weight bearing are absent.

If a ramus fracture is diagnosed, careful palpation of the posterior pelvic region, especially at the sacroiliac joint, is needed. If tenderness is present posteriorly, a CT scan can help diagnose fractures not easily appreciated on the radiograph. If a fracture of the posterior iliac wing or the sacroiliac joint is discovered, weight bearing on the injured extremity is avoided for 6 weeks. Hospitalization and bed rest, often with traction, are needed for initial management, and avoidance of weight bearing is continued for 6 weeks. Walking on the injured leg too early may lead to further cephalad displacement of the iliac area at the fracture site, with a resultant leg length discrepancy.

A markedly displaced fracture of the pelvis can cause a severe loss of neurologic function and life-threatening hemorrhage. Injury to the sciatic nerve or avulsion of the lumbosacral nerve roots may accompany a vertical shear fracture through the posterior iliac wing. Bleeding from the iliac artery branches can lead to substantial blood loss that may require use of the G-suit to control bleeding while replacement is begun. Such displaced fractures may require internal or external fixation of the fractures to permit satisfactory reduction and healing, particularly in the teenage group.

APOPHYSEAL FRACTURES

The apophyses in the pelvic region are secondary ossification centers that serve as origins for muscles of the thigh or trunk. Fractures involving the apophyses generally result from sudden or excessive contraction of one of the muscles of the thigh (Fig. 11.8).

Fracture of the ischial tuberosity apophysis is often found in track athletes who run in the hurdle events. The hamstrings originate from the ischium and insert onto the proximal tibia. When the hurdler's leg is suddenly thrust forward (with the knee fully extended

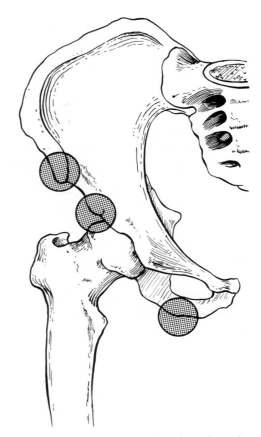

Figure 11.8. The three primary sites of apophyseal injury during sports activity are illustrated here. The sartorius arises from the anterior superior iliac spine. The rectus femoris originates from the anterior inferior iliac spine; an apophyseal avulsion occurs here with sudden hip extension with the knee flexed. The hamstrings begin on the ischial apophysis; sudden knee extension with the hip flexed, such as in hurdling, can cause an avulsion fracture at this location.

and the hip flexed) to clear a hurdle, the hamstrings may pull off the ischial apophysis (Fig. 11.9), resulting in sudden pain in the buttock. Though displacement of the ischial apophysis often occurs, operative treatment is rarely needed, as the apophysis will usually reunite with the ischial bone over a period of several weeks as new bone is formed by the periosteum. Crutches with limited weight bearing are used initially and until pain relief is complete. Generally 6 to

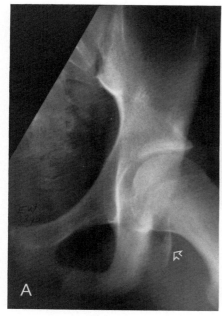

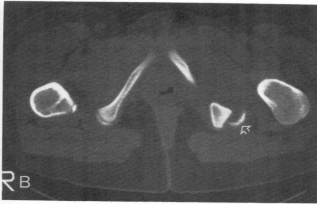

Figure 11.9.   A, Anteroposterior radiograph of the hip shows an ischial apophysis avulsion fracture (*open arrow*) in a hurdler at the origin of the hamstrings. **B,** A CT scan of the same teenage athlete demonstrates the avulsion fracture of the left ischium. Note the normal ischial apophysis on the right side.

8 weeks of limited activity is needed before return to sports is allowed. Adequate stretching before track participation is essential to lower the risk of sustaining this injury.

An avulsion fracture of the anterior inferior iliac spine apophysis (Fig. 11.10) can result from sudden contraction of the rectus femoris. This muscle originates here and inserts onto the tibial tubercle with the rest of the patellar tendon. Sudden hip extension with the knee somewhat flexed can provide sufficient force to cause this injury. As with other apophyseal injuries, nonoperative

Figure 11.10.   An anteroposterior radiograph of the pelvis shows an avulsion fracture of the anterior inferior iliac spine apophysis (*arrowheads*) that occurred in a runner at the start of a race. The rectus femoris muscle originates here.

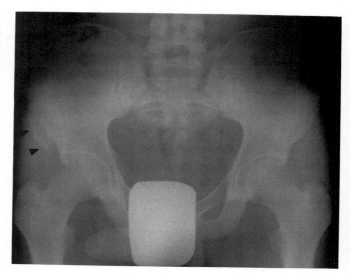

treatment will usually suffice, though use of crutches and avoidance of sports are needed until healing is complete.

The sartorius, which originates at the anterior superior iliac spine, inserts onto the medial proximal tibia. An avulsion fracture of this anterior superior iliac apophysis may result from sudden contraction of this muscle; treatment is conservative. Sports participation may be allowed when pain and tenderness are absent.

Each of these avulsion fractures of pelvic apophyses can be diagnosed by physical examination and a pelvis radiograph. Long-term disability from these fractures is rare, and sports activity can be resumed when signs and symptoms have disappeared. Upon return to sports activity, a muscle stretching program must be established to prevent re-injury.

"HIP POINTER"

A commonly occurring injury in contact sports, especially in football, is the condition known as a "hip pointer." When the side of the pelvis is struck by an opposing player, such as with the helmet in football, sudden pain may result. In the more mild cases, the pain will resolve quickly and the player can return to the game. However, in other cases, a hematoma can form, in which case tenderness and pain with leg movement may last for several days, making sports participation painful and unwise.

Physical findings of a hip pointer are primarily the localization of tenderness and perhaps hematoma swelling over the lateral side of the iliac wing of the pelvis. Pain with leg or hip movement can be produced by adjacent muscle injury.

Radiographs of the pelvis are normal. No fracture of either the primary bony pelvis or the apophyses is present.

Treatment consists of initial application of cold packs to the bruised area to prevent or slow local bleeding. Early return to sports activity is generally possible once the pain has resolved.

ORTHOPAEDIC INFECTION OF THE PELVIS

The two most common infections in this area are a psoas abscess and an osteomyelitis of the pelvic bones.

A *psoas abscess* generally begins with infection in the lumbar spine region. Since the psoas muscles originate from the anterior aspect of the upper lumbar spine, infections in this area can spread along the course of the muscle to appear in the pelvis or the upper medial thigh as an abscess. Pain is present with hip movement and the hip is held flexed, as stretching of the psoas by hip extension will aggravate the pain.

Prior to the days of antimicrobial therapy, psoas abscesses were classically associated with the presence of tuberculosis of the thoracolumbar spine. In urban areas the diagnosis of tuberculosis still needs to be considered as a likely cause of psoas abscess. *Staphylococcus aureus* is the most common bacterial cause of a psoas abscess, which generally will have resulted from a disc space infection or vertebral body osteomyelitis. Gram-negative organisms produce a psoas abscess secondary to gastrointestinal tract problems such as a ruptured appendix or Crohn's disease.

If a psoas abscess is present, the white blood cell count will be elevated, as will the erythrocyte sedimentation rate. Radiographs may demonstrate disc space narrowing or vertebral bone destruction in the lumbar spine if the process has been present for more than a few weeks. An MR or CT scan will clearly demonstrate the presence of an abscess within the psoas muscle and pelvic region. If the diagnosis has been delayed, the abscess may lead to ureteral obstruction, producing an enlarged proximal ureter.

The initial treatment of a psoas abscess is surgical drainage, with Gram stain and culture of the drained abscess contents. A skin test for tuberculosis should be done. If a staphylococcal infection is confirmed by Gram stain and culture, appropriate parenteral antibiotics should be administered for at least 6 weeks. Since cultures for tuberculous bacilli take a longer period of time, drug coverage for tuberculosis should also be given until it is clear that tuberculosis is absent. If tuberculosis is confirmed by culture, treatment for at least 1 year is indicated with the appropriate chemotherapeutic agents.

Osteomyelitis of the pelvis is uncommon but affects the ilium more often than the pubis or ischium. Diagnosis of this condition is often delayed because hip septic arthritis or proximal femoral osteomyelitis, which produce similar signs and symptoms, are much more common.

Pain is present with hip movement and the hip is held flexed, though not generally externally rotated as with septic arthritis of the hip. In fact, external rotation of the hip will usually aggravate the child's pain more than internal rotation maneuvers, a good sign that the infection is outside the hip joint.

Elevation of the white blood cell count and the erythrocyte sedimentation rate will be present as with infections of the hip, but imaging studies should allow differentiation of these conditions. Ultrasonography of the hip will show either no effusion or a small sympathetic effusion, which if aspirated will have a low white blood cell count. A technetium bone scan will generally allow proper localization of the infection, but in some cases a gallium bone scan will be needed to confirm the diagnosis. Magnetic resonance imaging has been proposed as a means to detect early infection by changes in the signal of the bone marrow, but other studies are still performed first at the present time.

Treatment of pelvic osteomyelitis is the same as for bone infection in long bones. If the diagnosis is made early, parenteral antibiotic treatment for 3 to 6 weeks should be curative. If an intrapelvic abscess has formed, surgical drainage is needed, followed by appropriate parenteral antibiotics for 3 to 6 weeks. Unless the diagnosis is markedly delayed, long-term effects are few.

Congenital Pelvic Disorders

PUBIC SYMPHYSIS DIASTASIS

Diastasis of the pubic symphysis does not occur as an isolated congenital defect but is associated with bladder or cloacal exstrophy, with failure of anterior closure of the genitourinary structures in this location.

As a part of this deformity, the pubic symphyses are widely spread. Because of this lateral movement of both sides of the pelvis, the acetabula are directed more laterally and the legs appear to have excessive external rotation at the hips. Even though a child will walk with the feet turned out, lower-extremity function is not otherwise affected.

From a functional standpoint, it is not necessary to surgically repair this pubic symphysis diastasis. However, closure of the exstrophy will not be successful in most cases unless bilateral iliac osteotomy is performed at the same time to allow bone reapproximation at the pubic symphysis. If iliac osteotomy is done as a part of an exstrophy closure, the child will walk with the feet turned out less than before the surgical correction.

Suggested Readings

Fernbach, S.K. and Wilkinson, R.H.: Avulsion injuries of the pelvis and proximal femur. A.J.R. 137: 581-584, 1981.

Martin, T.A., and Pipkin, G.: Treatment of avulsion of the ischial tuberosity. Clin. Orthop. 10:108-118, 1957.

McDonald, G.A.: Pelvic disruptions in children. Clin. Orthop. 151:130-134, 1980.

Quinby, W.C., Jr.: Fractures of the pelvis and associated injuries in children. J. Pediatr. Surg. 1:353-364, 1966.

Rang, M.: Children's Fractures, 2nd edition. Philadelphia, J.B. LIppincott, 1983.

Reichard, S.A., Helikson, M.A., Shorter, N., et al.: Pelvic fractures in children: review of 120 patients with a new look at general management. J. Pediatr. Surg. 15:727-734, 1980.

Rockwood, C.A., Jr., Wilkins, K.E., and King, R.E. (eds.): Fractures in Children. Philadephia, J.B. Lippincott, volume 3, 1984.

12
Hip and Thigh

Multiple problems may occur around the hip in children. Probably more so than in other parts of the body, abnormalities in the hip region are frequently age-specific, a fact that makes diagnosis of the appropriate condition easier.

Anatomy

The hip joint is a universal-type joint, able to move in multiple planes. The basic elements of the hip are the acetabulum, the femoral head, neurovascular structures, and adjacent muscles that control and position the leg in the desired location.

The acetabulum is formed by portions of the iliac, pubic, and ischial bones of the pelvis. These three bones are joined at the triradiate cartilage, positioned in the center of the acetabulum and responsible for appropriate enlargement of the acetabulum with growth. The acetabulum does not face directly laterally but is inclined slightly forward. The ligamentum teres originates from the central acetabulum and attaches to the center of the femoral head while carrying a small percentage of the femoral head blood supply. Acting as the socket for the hip joint, the acetabulum must be accurately fit with the femoral head for development of the acetabulum to progress normally.

The femoral head develops from a portion of the proximal femoral epiphysis and fits closely with the shape of the acetabulum. The only attachment onto the articular surface is the ligamentum teres. Because of a small amount of normal femoral antever-sion, with the leg in a neutral position the femoral head protrudes anteriorly from the acetabulum, a fact that helps allow for the great deal of motion in the hip joint, particularly in flexion. A tube-like capsule surrounds the hip joint, running from the acetabulum to the base of the femoral neck near the trochanters and providing much of the stability of the hip.

The femoral head forms from the medial portion of the proximal end of the femur. In the developing fetus, there is longitudinal growth potential along the entire proximal physeal region. However, with further development, the central portion of the physis evolves to provide appositional bone growth for the femoral neck, while the lateral portion develops into the greater trochanter, with its own physis. This medial part, however, is the primary source of proximal femoral longitudinal growth, accounting for approximately 10% of the length of the lower extremity.

The circulation to the femoral head is unique and is important in aiding the understanding of many of the childhood hip disorders. For the first 12 to 18 months of age, the primary circulation to the femoral head is directly through the physis, from the metaphysis to the epiphysis. A small amount of vascular supply passes through the ligamentum teres, but this is probably insignificant. By 18 months of age, the only significant blood supply to the proximal femoral epiphysis comes from the lateral and medial femoral circumflex arteries, which pierce the femoral epiphysis after passing proximally toward the hip in the hip capsule. Because these arteries pass from distal to proximal in the hip capsule, any injury to the hip capsule or femoral neck has the potential of obliterating the blood supply to the femoral head (Fig. 12.1).

Familiarity with the innervation of the hip joint, likewise, helps in understanding the signs and symptoms present with hip disorders. The hip joint itself is innervated by branches from the femoral, obturator, and sciatic nerves. Inflammation or irritation within the hip joint or capsule can refer pain along any of these nerves. Thus a child with a hip disorder may complain of pain in the anterior thigh or knee (femoral), medial thigh (obturator), or buttock and posterior thigh (sciatic).

The muscles around the hip are responsible for providing some hip stability and for positioning the hip appropriately for the lower portions of the leg to function normally (see Figs. 11.1, 11.2, and 11.3). Flex-

ion is provided mainly by the iliopsoas muscle, which originates from the lumbar spine and inner iliac wing and inserts onto the lesser trochanter. The rectus femoris muscle (a part of the quadriceps) and the sartorius are lesser hip flexors. Hip extension is primarily the role of the gluteus maximus, originating from the outer iliac wing and inserting on the proximal posterior femoral shaft just below the greater trochanter level, although the hamstrings of the thigh also help in hip extension control. The gluteus medius and gluteus minimus course from the iliac wing to the greater trochanter and are the prime hip abductors and lateral hip stabilizers. Hip adduction is provided by the adductors (longus, brevis, and magnus) and the gracilis muscles. While external rotation of the hip primarily results from the short external rotator muscles (gemelli, quadratus femoris, piriformis), whether internal or external rotation results from a specific muscle action may depend on the position of the

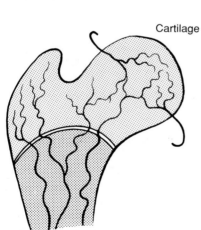

Cartilage

Ossification center

Neonate—Communicating   After 1 Year—Noncommunicating

Figure 12.1.   The vascular supply to the epiphysis of the proximal femur changes over the first 12 to 18 months of life. In the neonate, there is communication between the metaphyseal circulation and that of the epiphysis, through both blood vessels and cartilage canals. After 12 to 18 months of age, the epiphyseal circulation is solely from the medial and lateral femoral circumflex arteries, which run in the hip capsule to penetrate the epiphysis. The metaphyseal arteries after this age are blocked at the physis and form vessel loops in the metaphysis adjacent to the growth plate. Understanding this vascular anatomy at different ages is useful in the assessment of hip trauma or infection.

hip at the time of the muscle contraction (e.g., the iliopsoas may either internally or externally rotate the hip, depending on the amount of flexion present).

Physical Examination

A thorough examination of the hip area must include the evaluation of six planes of motion (flexion/extension, abduction/adduction, and internal/external rotation), observation of walking, and palpation for points of tenderness.

OBSERVATION

Is the leg held in a position of external rotation, flexion, and abduction? Is the foot externally rotated compared to the other side when walking? If a limp is present, is the time spent on each foot about equal (indicating gluteus medius weakness or a short leg) or unequal (indicating an antalgic gait with pain occurring on each attempt at weight bearing)? Is the back straight when sitting but has marked lordosis when standing, indicating a flexion contraction of the hip? Is the pelvis level with standing? In the infant or neonate, are the thigh folds symmetrical and do the leg lengths appear equal?

RANGE OF MOTION

Hip range of motion can be impaired by either an abnormality of the articular cartilage or the presence of fluid (pus, blood, effusion) within the joint capsule. Because of the oblique anatomical arrangements of the capsular fibers, the largest capacity for fluid within the capsule occurs when the hip is flexed, abducted, and externally rotated, while the smallest capacity is in the extended, adducted, and internally rotated position. Passive and active range of motion of the hips should be evaluated with the child lying down on a firm examination table. The supine position is used for flexion, abduction, and adduction, while the child is prone for evaluating internal and external rotation as well as hip extension.

Flexion is easily tested in an obvious manner. However, evaluation for a possible hip flexion contracture can be misleading. The lumbar spine may arch (increased lumbar lordosis) when a child with a hip flexion contracture lies supine, thereby making it appear that the child has no flexion contracture of the hip. The child should lie on a firm examining surface. To lock the pelvis adequately to assess for hip flexion contractures, it is necessary to fully flex the opposite hip so that the thigh is near the abdomen. By this maneuver, which flattens the lumbar spine and locks the pelvis, the presence of a flexion contracture of the opposite hip becomes obvious.

Abduction is evaluated with the hips both flexed and extended. The smaller the child, the more important it is to be certain the pelvis is level when testing hip abduction with the hips flexed. Particularly in the neonate and infant, the hip abduction examination should be performed with the perineum and pelvic area exposed so the examiner can directly visualize the pelvic and hip position with attempted abduction of both hips at the same time. Abduction and adduction testing with the hip extended is most useful in the ambulatory child to detect contractures that affect walking and apparent leg length differences.

Qualitative assessment of hip rotation can be obtained by the "roll test," in which the legs of the supine child are gently rolled into internal and external rotation. If limitation of hip motion exists, there will be increased resistance to this rolling action compared to the normal side. To quantitate hip rotation better, the child should be placed in a prone position and the knees flexed to 90°. The foot and lower leg are rotated laterally to assess hip internal rotation, and with the child in this position, minor differences of internal rotation between the two hips is readily apparent (Fig. 12.2). External rotation is assessed by medial movement of the leg in this position, taking care to hold the buttocks and pelvis

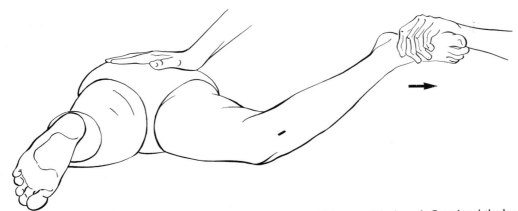

Figure 12.2.   Internal rotation of the hip is best assessed with the child prone. The knee is flexed and the leg is rotated in the direction of the *arrow*. The amount of rotation from the midline is the hip internal rotation.

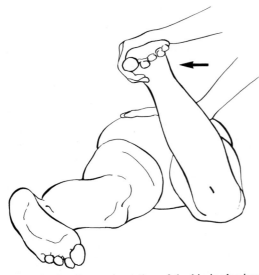

Figure 12.3.   External rotation of the hip is also best evaluated in the prone position. The pelvis is stabilized with the examiner's hand to prevent rocking of the pelvis. The amount of rotation in the direction of the *arrow* is the external rotation of the hip.

flat on the examining table (Fig. 12.3). Active extension is tested prone to assess gluteus maximus strength. Passive hyperextension puts stress on the sacroiliac joint and, when pain is present from this maneuver, may help to differentiate hip pain from sacroiliac joint pain.

Although all six planes of motion should be assessed for a complete hip examination,

internal rotation with the hip extended (prone examination position) is the most sensitive single motion test. If internal rotation in this position is equal to the unaffected leg, one can generally rule out intra-articular hip pathology as the cause of the leg pain or limp. Flexion may remain nearly fully normal despite advanced intra-articular hip pathology, and intact flexion is the least sensitive indicator of hip disorders.

PALPATION

The greater trochanter is the major hip structure that can be directly palpated. Tenderness may be present here after injury or with trochanteric bursitis. The position of the greater trochanter relative to the opposite side may help in the diagnosis of hip dysplasia. While the hip joint itself cannot be directly palpated, adjacent soft tissue tenderness and swelling should alert the examiner to a hip problem, particularly infection. Point tenderness will be present over a strained muscle in this area, with the most commonly injured being the adductor and proximal hamstring muscles.

STANDING EVALUATION

The child should be viewed from both the front and the back, although more useful information is usually obtained from the posterior examination. The height of the iliac crest is noted and compared with the opposite side to detect leg length differences. If a difference is present, blocks of varying heights should be placed under the short foot until the pelvis becomes level; in this way the the leg length difference can be assessed.

An important component of the hip examination is the evaluation of the strength of the gluteus medius, the principal hip abductor, by the use of the Trendelenburg test. This test is positive in all children with hip pain or problems for more than a few weeks. The test evaluates the position of the pelvis with the child standing on one leg and the examiner viewing the pelvis from behind. Normally, when a child stands on the right foot, the left side of the pelvis moves cephalad as the right-sided gluteus medius contracts and prevents the left side of the pelvis from dropping down, making the Trendelenburg test negative (Fig. 12.4). However, if the gluteus medius muscle is weak, it cannot hold up the opposite side of the pelvis, and as the opposite side drops caudally, a positive Trendelenburg test is observed (Fig. 12.5).

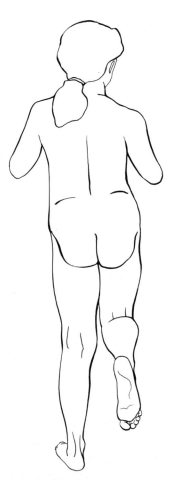

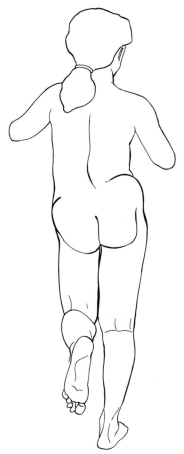

Figure 12.4. If a child stands on one leg and the pelvis on the opposite side remains as shown, the Trendelenburg test is negative or normal, indicating normal gluteus medius strength.

Figure 12.5. If the gluteus medius muscle is weak, as is commonly the case with hip disorders, when a child stands on one leg, the Trendelenburg test will be positive, as illustrated. In this illustration, the right hip gluteus medius is too weak to support the weight of the elevated leg, and the pelvis drops inferiorly on the opposite side.

GAIT EVALUATION

The most common gait abnormality with hip disorders is the Trendelenburg gait or gluteal lurch. Because in children with gluteus medius weakness the contralateral side of the pelvis drops down during the time the leg on that side is off the ground, the child will lean the trunk over the leg with a weak gluteus medius. This accomplishes two things: first, by centering the body weight over the weak hip joint, stability in standing is possible even without good muscle strength and second, by leaning to this side, the opposite leg can be more easily swung forward for the next step. Although they are not specific for any exact hip disorder, the presence of a positive Trendelenburg test and gait should point the examiner to a much more careful examination of the hip.

A Trendelenburg gait is usually painless, and the time the child spends on each foot during walking is approximately equal. If a painless limp is present and equal time is spent on each foot with the Trendelenburg test negative, the legs are probably of unequal length. If the child stands on one foot more than the other, the gait is termed antalgic, indicating pain somewhere in the extremity that bears weight less of the time.

Soft tissue contractures around the hip may cause significant gait disturbances. If an abduction contracture is present, the affected limb will appear to be longer than the opposite side, because the child will have to adduct the normal leg and tilt the pelvis to keep both feet centered under the trunk. If a fixed hip adduction contracture is present, the affected leg will appear much shorter for the same reasons. If hip flexion contractures are present, the child will compensate when standing by arching the back and increasing lumbar lordosis, at the same time the contralateral knee is flexed.

Imaging Studies

A variety of imaging studies are commonly applied to evaluation of the hip region, among them radiography, ultrasound, computed tomography (CT), magnetic resonance (MR) imaging, bone scintigraphy, and arthrography.

RADIOGRAPHY

The most commonly used of the imaging modalities, frontal and lateral radiography remains the initial method of evaluation for hip problems, especially after the neonatal period. A frontal radiograph of the pelvis provides a view of the hip in question and a comparison with the normal side (Fig. 12.6).

Figure 12.6. A normal frontal radiograph of an 8-month-old child with hips in neutral position is illustrated. Sacrum (*S*), ilium (*IL*), sacroiliac joint (*SI*), pubis (*P*), ischium (*I*), femoral head (*F*), lesser trochanter (*L*), and greater trochanter (*G*) are marked.

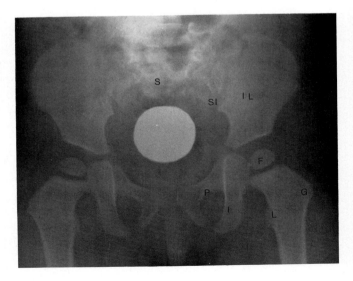

The initial pelvic radiograph should be obtained without a gonadal shield to allow visualization of the bony anatomy of the entire pelvis. For most hip conditions, anteroposterior radiographs with the hips in the neutral and frog-leg positions should be the initial radiographic studies. If radiographs are utilized for follow-up evaluation of a specific area of the hip, shielding of the gonads should be done routinely.

The ossification center in the proximal femoral epiphysis should appear between 4 and 6 months of age and continues to enlarge until growth is completed. The size of the proximal femoral ossification center in one hip should be equivalent to that in the other hip, though minor variations in ossification may occur.

In the neonate or infant, even without a femoral head ossification center, specific lines drawn on the anteroposterior radiograph can assist in hip evaluation (Fig. 12.7). These lines include the following:

1. Hilgengreiner's line: drawn horizontally through the triradiate cartilage of each acetabulum, this line serves as a reference line;
2. Perkins' line: a vertical line at a right angle to Hilgengreiner's line, beginning at the lateral edge of the ossified acetabulum;
3. Shenton's line: drawn up the medial cortex of the femoral neck, continuing as a crescent along the inferior cortex of the superior pubic ramus;
4. Acetabular index: an angle formed by Hilgengreiner's line and a line drawn along the ossified superior acetabulum;
5. Metaphyseal-teardrop distance: measurement of the distance between the medial proximal femoral metaphysis and the inner acetabular wall.

On radiography, the normal proximal femoral neck-shaft angle is approximately 135° to 145°. In pathologic conditions affecting the growth of portions of the proximal femur, this angle may be less or more. Since the child is usually positioned for this examination with the knees extended and the feet pointing straight ahead, in children with excessive femoral internal rotation, the neck-shaft angle will often appear to be 150° to 160°, though this apparent coxa valga is due to positioning rather than a true increase in neck-shaft angle; in such an instance, the true angle can be ascertained by an anteroposterior radiograph with the leg internally rotated.

With a normal neck-shaft angle in the proximal femur, the superior margin of the greater trochanter will be a centimeter or two caudal to the superior margin of the ossified femoral head. If a radiograph of the hip demonstrates the tip of the greater trochanter to be at the same level as the femoral head, the gluteus medius is functionally lengthened and a Trendelenburg gait would be expected.

Although radiography demonstrates the osseous structures well, the soft tissues should also be evaluated when interpreting a pelvic and hip radiograph. Hip or proximal femoral infection will cause local edema, which is apparent on radiographs as a widening of the soft tissues around the bone, especially in the infant.

ULTRASOUND

Two primary roles for hip sonography are in evaluating neonates for hip dislocation and in assessing infants and children for the presence of a hip joint effusion. In neonates and infants, ultrasound evaluation can accurately locate the cartilaginous femoral head in the cartilaginous acetabulum. This technique also allows the dynamic evaluation of the hip to assess stability as motion takes place. In evaluating for progress in the treatment of hip dysplasia, ultrasound evaluation can be performed with the child in a hip abduction brace.

Two potential drawbacks to ultrasound examination are the possibilities of inaccurate interpretation and overdiagnosis of hip

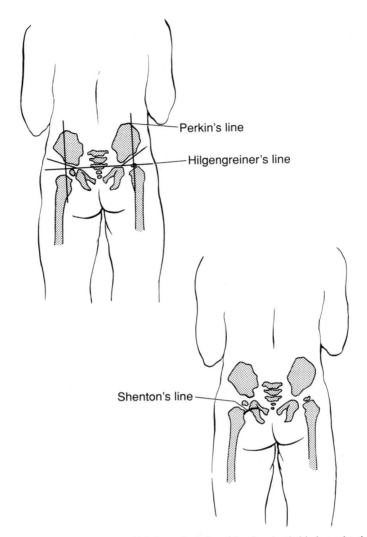

Perkin's line

Hilgengreiner's line

Shenton's line

Figure 12.7.   In these illustrations, the normal hip is on the left and the dysplastic hip is on the right. Hilgengreiner's line is a reference line drawn horizontally through the triradiate cartilage of the acetabula. Perkins' line is a vertical line beginning at the ossified lateral edge of the acetabulum and passing perpendicular to Hilgengreiner's line. Normally, the ossific nucleus of the femoral head should be in the lower inner quadrant formed by these intersecting lines. Shenton's line passes along the inferior edge of the superior pubic ramus and continues along the femoral neck in the normal hip. A disruption of Shenton's line generally implies lateral subluxation or dislocation of the hip.

instability. These studies are operator dependent and must be performed by one skilled in the interpretation of sonography to avoid misdiagnosis. In the newborn, laxity of the hips for the first 2 to 4 weeks of life may be incorrectly diagnosed as being unstable when stress is applied. Ultrasound examinations after 2 to 4 weeks of age are more representative of the presence or absence of pathologic hip instability.

Ultrasound is useful in the evaluation of effusion in a hip, prior to attempted aspiration. If the sonogram does not demonstrate fluid in the hip, aspiration attempts are probably not warranted.

COMPUTER-ASSISTED TOMOGRAPHY

CT scans of the hip are used primarily to add anatomic or pathologic information to that obtained by radiography. These studies should not be used as the initial diagnostic study in the assessment of the hip.

Acetabular structure or pathology is evaluated well with this modality. The relationship of the femoral head to the acetabulum can be well studied prior to hip surgery or following reduction of a developmental hip dislocation. The extent of tumors in the femoral head and neck or acetabulum is also readily determined.

CT scans can quantitate the amount of femoral rotation or anteversion. To accomplish this, a single cross-sectional image through the femoral head and neck is obtained, and an axial scan through the distal femoral condyle is performed without moving the extremity. Using the transverse axis through the condyles as the reference line, a line drawn up the femoral neck will form an angle that corresponds to the degree of femoral anteversion or internal femoral torsion.

MAGNETIC RESONANCE

Used as an adjunct to radiography for diagnostic purposes, magnetic resonance imaging assesses soft tissues, growth and articular cartilage, bone, and bone marrow.

Marrow and cartilage changes resulting from infection, infarction, and tumor are visualized prior to any bone changes on radiographs. Soft tissue masses or muscle injury may be identified in areas not easily palpated by physical examination. Articular cartilage lesions are readily seen, and disturbances in physeal growth after injury may be diagnosed with MR. MR is extremely useful in evaluation of the long-standing dislocated hip, demonstrating subtle abnormalities of cartilage, acetabular de-

velopment, as well as hip capsule and psoas tendon anatomy.

BONE SCAN

This scintigraphic imaging technique is useful in the hip to differentiate between inflammatory and infectious conditions and to evaluate the vascularity of the femoral head.

Skeletal scintigraphy provides a functional skeletal image with particular attention to blood flow and regions of growth or skeletal abnormality with repair (see Chapter 2).

HIP ARTHROGRAPHY

Not generally used by primary care physicians, arthrography is useful in the dynamic evaluation of the relationship between the cartilaginous femoral head and the cartilaginous acetabulum in the treatment of developmental hip dysplasia. A secondary use is in conjunction with nonproductive hip aspiration to show that the needle has been placed in the hip joint correctly.

Developmental Dysplasia of the Hip

Developmental dysplasia (or displacement) of the hip (DDH) is currently the preferred term for a variety of hip disorders, which include the condition previously called congenital dislocation of the hip. As used at this time, DDH includes hip subluxation, hip dislocation, and acetabular dysplasia, all of which imply potential or actual instability of the hip in the neonate or young child. Hip dislocation or subluxation is generally diagnosed at birth or shortly thereafter, whereas a child with hip displacement secondary to acetabular dysplasia may have a normal examination at birth, only to develop hip dysplasia sometime in the first several months of life. Terming this condition developmental dysplasia rather than congenital dysplasia takes into account the fact that this dislocation can occur during infancy despite being normally reduced at the time of delivery.

Hip dislocation occurs in approximately one infant out of each 1000 births. It more commonly is seen in babies with breech presentation and is more common in females than males. If the mother has a history of having a dislocated hip as a child, the risk that her female baby will have hip dysplasia is 1:25 for nonbreech presentation and 1:15 if the child is in the breech position. If an older female sibling has had hip dysplasia, the risk in subsequent siblings for a dislocated hip is increased.

All newborn children require a careful evaluation of the hips for potential or real instability. In children with a positive family history, more than one examination in the first few weeks of life is recommended. Children with coincident metatarsus adductus or torticollis at birth have a slightly higher incidence of hip dysplasia and should be examined extra carefully.

For an adequate hip examination in the newborn, the baby must not be crying. A crying child can generate enough muscle power in the legs to prevent the detection of hip instability. The thighs and buttocks are first observed for any asymmetry of soft tissue and skin folds in these regions (Fig. 12.8). While children with normal hips may demonstrate asymmetry of skin folds here, this can also be a sign of extremity shortening due to hip displacement.

Hip abduction with the hip flexed is tested first, with normal abduction being 70° or more (Fig. 12.9). The amount of abduction should be symmetrical, so if one hip abducts more than the other, carefully assess the hip that abducts the least for possible instability (Fig. 12.10). If abduction is less than 70° and yet the hip appears stable, the infant must be followed for later hip subluxation until the abduction increases, since infants with limited hip abduction are more prone to later instability due to acetabular dysplasia. Hip abduction should be estimated and recorded in degrees at each examination.

The next step in hip evaluation in the in-

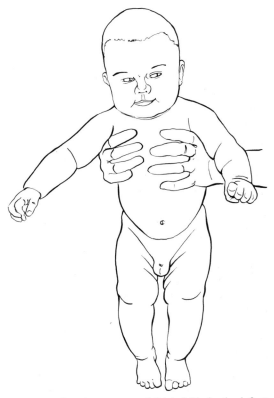

Figure 12.8. Asymmetry of thigh folds in the infant may be an indication of developmental dysplasia of the hip. In this illustration, the left thigh has more thigh folds than the right thigh. If this finding is combined with limited hip abduction, a hip subluxation or dislocation is likely to be present.

fant is to assess for possible instability. The Galeazzi or Allis test is accomplished by flexing both hips and knees with the feet on the examining table (Fig. 12.11). The height of the knees should be the same. If the knee height is unequal, the most common problem is hip dislocation, though this same finding occurs if a congenitally short femur is present.

The principal tests for instability of the hip itself are the Barlow and the Ortolani tests. The *Barlow test* is a provocative test, meant to detect latent instability. With the infant's hip and knee flexed, the examiner's hand is placed on the proximal thigh with the thumb medially over the adductors and

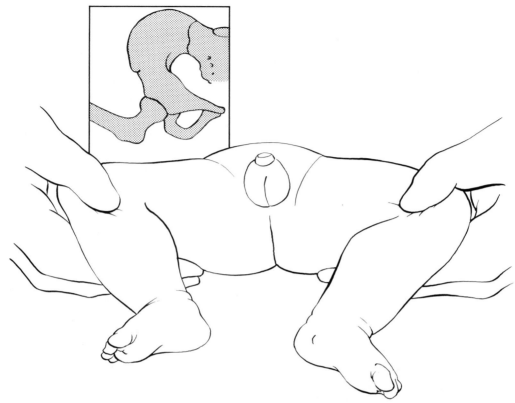

Figure 12.9. Normal hip abduction in the newborn should be symmetrical and generally ranges between 70° and 90° in each hip. As noted in the inset, the femoral head is reduced in the acetabulum if symmetrical and wide abduction is present as shown.

the long finger over the greater trochanter laterally (Figs. 12.12 and 12.13). The hip begins in a neutral position of abduction and adduction. The thumb then attempts to push the proximal femur laterally and displace the femoral head out of the acetabulum (Fig. 12.14). If outward movement of the proximal femur is produced, the hip is then abducted and medial pressure on the greater trochanter allows the palpable feel of reduction of the femoral head into the acetabulum. The *Ortolani test* produces reduction of a dislocated femoral head into the acetabulum. The hand is positioned as for the Barlow test (Fig. 12.15). As the hip is abducted, the long finger over the greater trochanter pushes medially and lifts the trochanter (Fig. 12.16). A positive Ortolani test is pro-

duced when the examiner feels the "clunk" of the femoral head reducing into the acetabulum. The palpation of a slight "click" when the hip is in 80° or 90° of abduction is not a positive Ortolani test and is usually of no consequence, being due to the tensor fascia femoris muscle and fascia snapping over the greater trochanter.

If the Barlow test is positive and the Ortolani test is negative in a neonate, no specific treatment is needed except a re-examination in 2 to 3 weeks. If the hips remain dislocatable at that time, treatment should be provided. Since well over 50% of hips with a positive Barlow test at birth will stabilize without treatment in 2 to 3 weeks, much unnecessary treatment is avoided if treatment for dislocatable hips is withheld

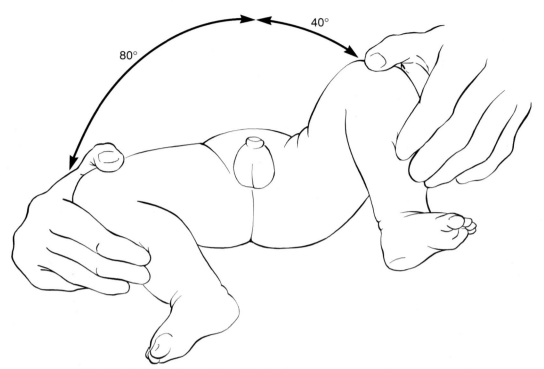

Figure 12.10.   If hip abduction is asymmetrical and limited to less than 60° on one side, developmental dysplasia of the hip (DDH) is likely. In the newborn with this limited abduction, ultrasound evaluation is helpful, while radiographs are used after 6 months of age.

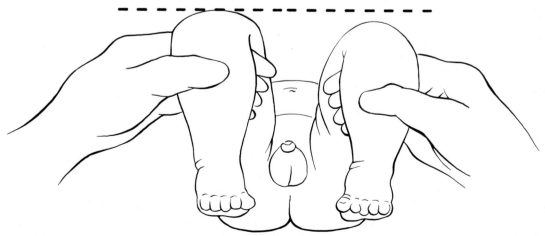

Figure 12.11.   The Galeazzi or Allis test is easily done by flexing the knee and hip bilaterally and looking at the level of the knees. In this diagram, the level of the left knee is obviously lower, which usually indicates that hip dysplasia is present in this leg. A congenital short femur should give the same sign but is much less common.

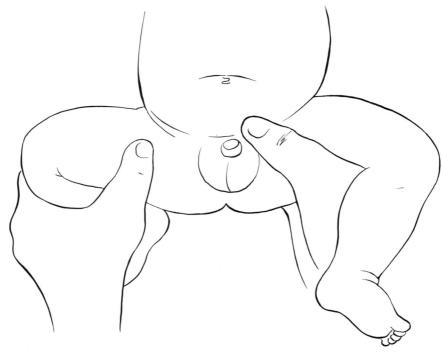

Figure 12.12. When assessing the infant with the Barlow and Ortolani tests, hand position is important. As shown in the diagram, the thumb on the right thigh controls hip movement while the left thumb is used to stabilize the pelvis.

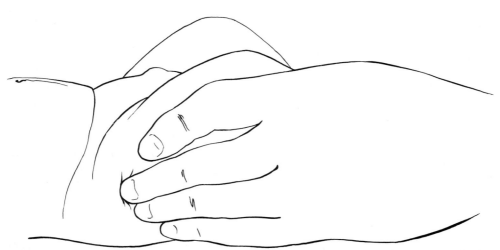

Figure 12.13. On the lateral side of the hip, the long finger is placed directly over the greater trochanter of the proximal femur to help control hip movement and to detect any hip instability present. The infant must not be crying during these tests or else subtle instability will not be detected.

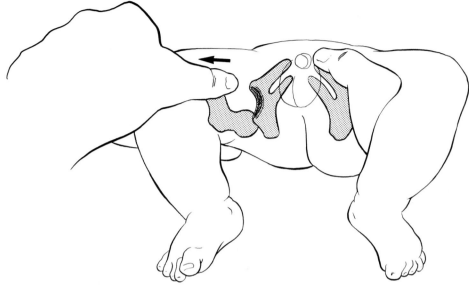

Figure 12.14. The Barlow test is a provocative test to detect any tendency of the hip to dislocate. At rest, the hip is reduced and abduction is near-normal or normal. With the leg in a flexed and adducted position, the examiner pushes laterally with the thumb. If the hip dislocates, as shown in the illustration, the Barlow test is positive. Reduction usually readily occurs with hip abduction after a positive Barlow test is found. See text for treatment guidelines.

for a few weeks. This is not true for hips that are dislocated at rest and are reducible; these require active treatment from the time of diagnosis.

If instability is suspected from the physical examination, the initial imaging study is a dynamic ultrasound evaluation of the hip. In addition to static images, the ultrasound evaluation provides a dynamic study to see the degree of instability and in what position the hip is most stable (Fig. 12.17). While a radiograph is less useful prior to the appearance of the ossification center of the femoral head, a radiograph can provide some information to the examiner. A dislocation of the hip can be diagnosed if there is a discontinuity in Shenton's line or if the proximal femoral metaphysis is located outside the inner lower quadrant formed by an intersection of Perkins' and Hilgengreiner's lines (Fig. 12.7). The acetabular index on the affected side is greater than on the normal side, and the metaphyseal-teardrop measurement is increased with a dysplastic hip (Fig. 12.18).

If the diagnosis of hip instability is made, referral should be made to an orthopaedist for definitive care. Generally, if the diagnosis is made in the first few months of life, closed reduction and use of a Pavlik harness or hip spica cast to maintain reduction for 3 to 4 months should produce a good result and normal hip function. The Pavlik harness or hip spica cast hold the hip reduced in a position of more than 90° flexion and moder-

Figure 12.16. As hip abduction is attempted by the examiner, the long finger over the greater trochanter pushes anteriorly to try to lift the femoral head over the posterior lip of the acetabulum and reduce the hip. A positive Ortolani test is present when a palpable "clunk" is noted by the examiner as the hip reduces. A high-pitched "click" at full abduction should not be considered a positive Ortolani test and is probably due to the fascia lata slipping over the greater trochanter in this position.

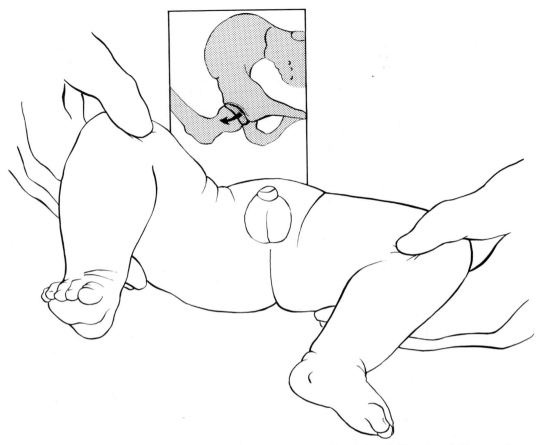

Figure 12.15. The Ortolani test is used to determine if a dislocated hip can be readily reduced. Since the femoral head is dislocated at rest, hip abduction is limited on the affected side.

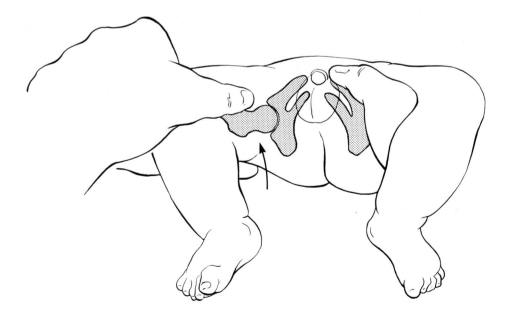

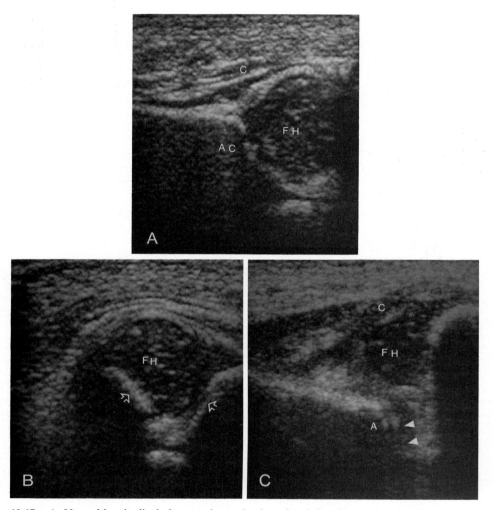

Figure 12.17.   **A,** Normal longitudinal ultrasound examination of an infant hip at 4 weeks of age is shown. The acetabulum (*AC*), femoral head (*FH*), and joint capsule (*C*) are marked. Note the congruence of the femoral head and acetabulum. **B,** Normal transverse ultrasound of the hip of a 4-week-old infant shows anterior and posterior walls of the acetabulum (*open arrows*) and the femoral head located within the acetabulum (*FH*). **C,** Superiorly and laterally dislocated femoral head (*FH*) in an infant shows stretched capsule (*C*), laterally dislocated femoral head (*FH*), and the acetabulum (*A*) with the articular surface indicated by *arrowheads*.

ate abduction. If a hip spica cast is needed, special car seat modifications are available for transport (Fig. 12.19).

The use of triple diapers to treat a dislocated hip is insufficient treatment. While extra diapers allow for hip abduction, there is inadequate flexion to lead to hip reduction. Flexion of the hip is needed to relax the iliopsoas tendon, which passes over the

anterior hip capsule and blocks reduction of the femoral head into the acetabulum if the hip remains relatively extended.

From a legal perspective, the most important feature of DDH for the primary care physician seeing infants for periodic well-baby examinations is to examine the hip thoroughly at each visit and to document the examination, especially the degree of

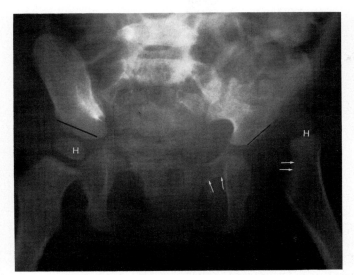

Figure 12.18. Anteroposterior radiograph of the pelvis shows a dislocated left hip in an 8-month-old infant. The dislocation is superior and lateral, and a small femoral head (*H*) is present. The acetabular index is elevated (*solid line*), and Shenton's line (*small white arrows*) is disrupted.

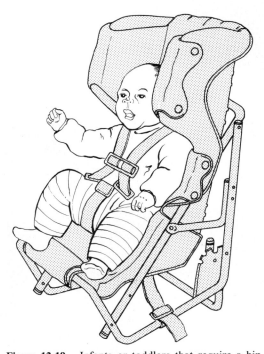

Figure 12.19. Infants or toddlers that require a hip spica cast as treatment for developmental dysplasia of the hip, in which the hip is flexed to 90°, should be placed in a car safety seat, as shown, when transported while in the cast. A similar seat can be used for infants or young children treated for a femoral fracture with a flexed-hip spica cast.

abduction present and the stability or instability of the hips being examined. While a child may develop a hip dislocation after the neonatal period, legal defense can less easily be mounted unless documentation of adequate periodic examination is included in the examining physician's records.

If the diagnosis of DDH is not made in the newborn period, the next most common time of diagnosis is when the child begins to walk. At this time, the child will present with a painless limp. At this age, the primary physical examination finding is limited abduction of the affected hip. The Ortolani test is negative, since it is unusual to be able to reduce a dislocated hip that has been out of the acetabulum for more than 4 to 6 months. The leg will be shorter than the opposite side. Radiographs will allow the diagnosis to be made, since the proximal femoral ossification center is generally present by this time. However, in a dislocated hip, the femoral head ossification center is small and slower to develop compared to the reduced hip. The acetabular index will be greater on the affected side (Figs. 12.20 and 12.21).

If the diagnosis of a hip dislocation is not made until walking age, closed reduction and casting for 4 months may be successful,

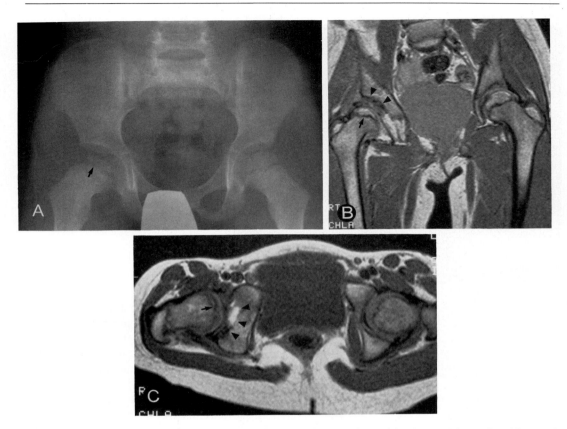

Figure 12.20.   A, After relocation of a dislocated hip on the right, the femoral head (*arrow*) is small and flattened. Partial avascular necrosis of the femoral head has likely occurred at the time of reduction. **B,** MR scan in the coronal plane of this patient shows a hypoplastic femoral head (*arrow*) and a shallow, irregular, poorly formed acetabular surface. **C,** MR scan in axial plane shows a shallow, noncupped acetabulum that is not fully formed (*arrowheads*) and a small femoral head (*arrow*). Compare this with the normal left side.

Figure 12.21.   A coronal MR scan of a dislocated hip that could not be reduced is shown. The femoral head (*FH*) is dislocated and the labrum (*arrow*) is infolded, preventing relocation of the hip. Surgical treatment is needed. (*A*, acetabulum.)

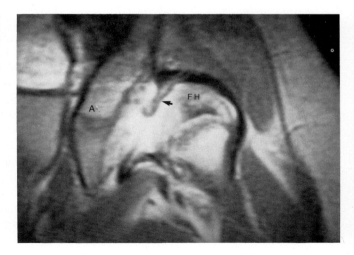

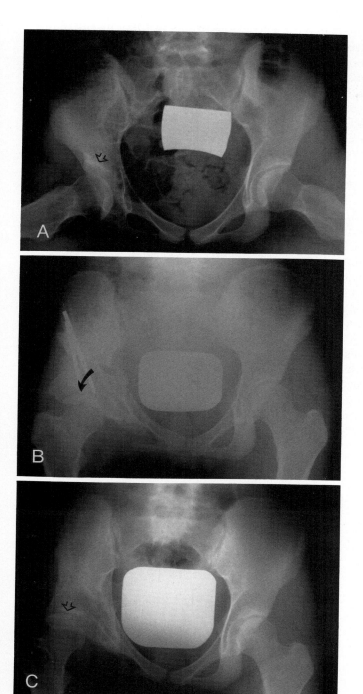

Figure 12.22. **A,** Right hip dysplasia in an adolescent. Note the shallow acetabulum (*open arrow*). **B,** Triple pelvic osteotomy has resulted in improved hip position with a horizontal acetabular roof (*curved arrow*). **C,** After the pelvic osteotomy has healed, the hip is contained within the reconstructed acetabulum and pain has been relieved.

but about two-thirds of these children will require some surgery, either to adequately reduce the hip or to facilitate acetabular development. If the hip is not accurately reduced at a young age, pelvic reconstructive surgery may be needed later (Fig. 12.22).

If a child has bilateral hip dislocation, the diagnosis may be more difficult, since symmetrical findings are present on examination. Here again, limitation of abduction is the major physical finding to note. A waddling gait is seen due to bilateral gluteus medius weakness. If the diagnosis of bilateral hip dislocation is not made by age 3 or 4 years, the child may be noted to have a significant increase in lumbar lordosis secondary to the bilateral flexion contractures present with bilateral hip dislocation. While surgical treatment at age 4 is often successful, the results are seldom as good as if the dislocations had been diagnosed and treated earlier. Beyond the age of 6 years, bilateral hip dislocations are usually left dislocated, since surgical treatment often leads to more stiffness and pain than if no treatment is given (Fig. 12.23). Total hip replacement is usually needed in patients with untreated hip dislocation in their fourth or fifth decade.

Septic Arthritis of the Hip and Proximal Femoral Osteomyelitis

While bone and joint infections are common in the infant and young child, infections in the hip area have some features that deserve special mention. Early diagnosis and treatment of hip infection are needed to prevent disabling consequences.

An infant with a hip infection usually presents with a history of unwillingness to move the leg or of pain with leg movement. In the neonate or infant, the child may be irritable and may often have a low-grade fever. In the ambulatory child, the most common presenting complaint is a limp or refusal of the child to walk or stand. In older children, fever is usually higher.

Anatomically, the hip capsule inserts distally into the base of the femoral neck. This intracapsular location of the femoral metaphysis results in co-existence of femoral neck osteomyelitis and hip septic arthritis.

Physical findings include fever, soft tissue swelling in the hip area and proximal thigh, and limitation of hip motion. Internal rotation of the hip is limited and painful, and the child may hold the hip in a position of flexion, abduction, and external rotation.

Figure 12.23. Frontal radiograph of a 10-year-old child with gait disturbance shows bilaterally dislocated femoral heads. Reduction is not indicated at this age.

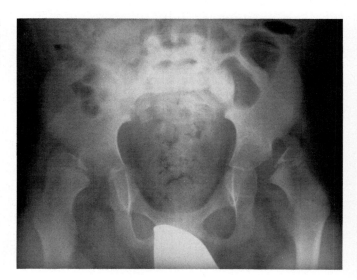

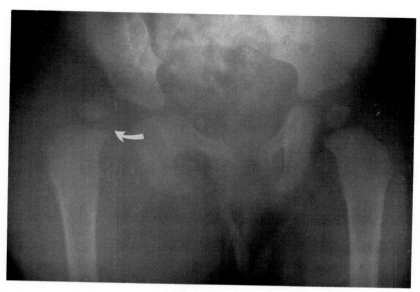

Figure 12.24. Anteroposterior radiograph of the pelvis of a 6-month-old infant, who was crying with movement of the right leg, shows dislocation of the right hip (*arrow*) secondary to a large joint effusion and septic arthritis.

Serum laboratory studies generally show an elevated white blood cell count and an elevated erythrocyte sedimentation rate. Radiographs of the pelvis and hip are generally normal if the clinical course has been less than 1 week. If there is a large accumulation of purulent material within the hip joint, lateral subluxation of the femoral head from the acetabulum is seen on the radiographs (Fig. 12.24). A technetium-99 bone scan will show increased blood flow in the early stages with septic arthritis, and will demonstrate increased bone cell uptake in the proximal femur if osteomyelitis is present.

The diagnosis of septic arthritis of the hip is generally made on clinical grounds, supplemented by an aspiration of the hip. Hip aspiration may be performed through the medial, anterior, or lateral approach, using fluoroscopy or ultrasound to guide the needle insertion (Fig. 12.25). Ultrasound examination of the affected hip can detect the presence of an effusion prior to attempted aspiration. If the aspiration is productive of purulent fluid, the diagnosis of septic arthritis is confirmed. This fluid is sent for a white blood cell count, a Gram stain, and multiple cultures.

If the hip aspirate fluid has a white cell count of 50,000 or more and/or the Gram stain is positive for organisms, the diagnosis of septic arthritis is confirmed. All hips with the diagnosis of septic arthritis require surgical drainage, since failure to adequately drain the hip joint will lead quickly to irreversible damage to the femoral head cartilage. At the time of hip joint drainage the femoral neck is drilled to drain a possible femoral neck osteomyelitis. Appropriate parenteral antibiotics are used for at least 2 weeks to treat a septic arthritis, while at least 3 weeks of antibiotics are needed if a coexisting osteomyelitis is present. As with osteomyelitis and septic arthritis in other parts of the body, the most common causative organism is *Staphylococcus aureus.*

If treated expeditiously and adequately, there should be no long-term sequelae of septic arthritis of the hip. The most serious after-effects are seen in children with neonatal infection of the hip that was undiagnosed. Usually, these are in children in the

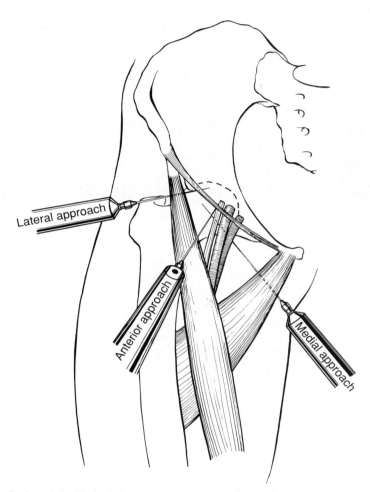

Figure 12.25. Aspiration of the hip is an important diagnostic procedure whenever septic arthritis of the hip is suspected. Aseptic technique is used and aspiration is usually guided by fluoroscopy. The anterior approach is just inferior to the inguinal ligament and 1 to 2 cm lateral to the palpable femoral artery. The medial approach enters just posterior to the adductor longus tendon in the proximal thigh. The lateral approach runs parallel to the femoral neck to enter the hip capsule. Use of fluoroscopy to guide correct needle placement provides valuable assistance.

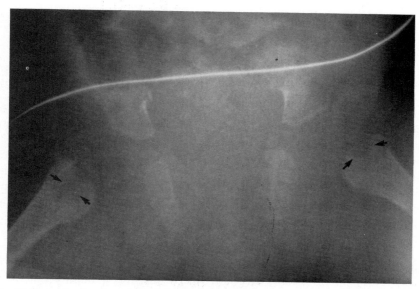

Figure 12.26. Radiograph of a 5-week-old infant in the neonatal intensive care unit shows bilateral femoral metaphyseal osteomyelitis (*arrows*) discovered incidentally on an abdomen film.

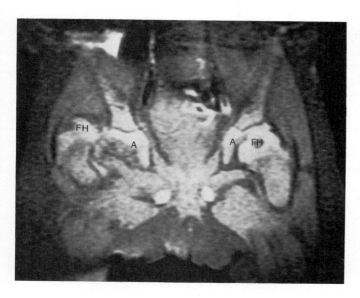

Figure 12.27. MR image of a 4-month-old infant managed in intensive care for several weeks shows right femoral head (*FH*) dislocation secondary to previous septic arthritis. (*A*, acetabulum.)

neonatal intensive care unit who were very ill with sepsis and who had a coexistent hip infection that either was not diagnosed or was diagnosed after substantial cartilage damage had occurred (Fig. 12.26). In neonates in the intensive care unit, it is important to monitor the extremities daily for swelling or other signs of hip joint infection, to allow for early treatment (Fig. 12.27).

Congenital Coxa Vara

While the normal neck-shaft angle of the proximal femur is approximately 135°, some children are born with a varus deformity of this region, with a neck-shaft angle of 90° to 100°.

The physical examination will show diminished hip abduction, and the child usually walks with a Trendelenburg gait. Pain is usually absent. Radiographs demonstrate a neck-shaft angle of less than 115°, together with an inverted V-shaped radiolucency or medial fragmentation at the femoral neck (Fig. 12.28).

Coxa vara may be the only abnormality seen or this condition may be associated with a congenital short femur. Leg lengths should be carefully evaluated prior to treatment.

Congenital coxa vara will not resolve spontaneously. Surgical osteotomy of the proximal femur to restore a more normal neck-shaft angle is generally curative.

Varus deformity of the femoral neck may occur in later childhood in a variety of conditions that predispose this region to recurrent nondisplaced fractures of the proximal femoral region that result in a varus alignment. These conditions include fibrous dysplasia, osteogenesis imperfecta, Gaucher's disease, and other more generalized conditions that affect bone strength. Osteotomy

may be needed to realign the proximal femur and hip in these children.

Congenital Short Femur or Proximal Femoral Focal Deficiency (PFFD)

Congenital deficiency of the femur may be present at birth in varying degrees of severity. The most mild form consists of modest femoral shortening with a normal hip, while the most severe form has only a small portion of the distal femur with no proximal femur or hip joint. Conditions associated with congenital short femur include coxa vara, fibular underdevelopment or absence, and foot anomalies.

On physical examination, the leg length discrepancy is generally noted at birth by the presence of extra thigh folds and a short thigh on the affected side. A skin dimple is often present in the mid-thigh region. In mildly affected children, hip abduction is normal or slightly limited, while in severe cases, gross hip instability is present. The knee is also affected, with excessive anteroposterior laxity present due to deficiency of the tibial spine and cruciate ligaments.

Radiographs at birth will allow partial identification of the femoral defect present,

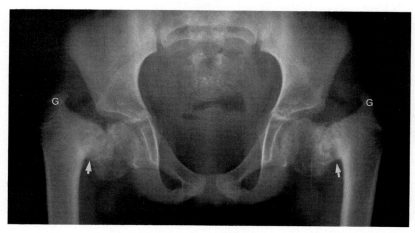

Figure 12.28. Radiograph of a 5-year-old child with limitation of abduction shows bilateral coxa vara deformity of the femoral necks (*arrows*). Femoral heads are unusually spherical, and the greater trochanters (*G*) are located very high. The angle between the femoral neck and shaft is reduced to less than 90°. A valgus femoral osteotomy should be performed for this child.

but the proximal femoral segments often have a delay in ossification. If a well-formed acetabulum is present, there is likely a cartilaginous femoral head within it, even though it is not seen on radiography. Ultrasound examination can be useful in this setting but a MR study should more clearly define what is present and what is absent in the proximal femur and hip.

In general, an estimation of the total leg length discrepancy expected at the completion of growth will help the parents decide on which treatment course to follow. If the limb is 30% short at birth, it will continue with this relative growth inhibition, being 30% shorter than the normal limb at maturity. In such a case, a discrepancy of 7 or 8 cm at birth will likely be greater than 20 cm at maturity.

The treatment options are primarily amputation with prosthetic use or limb lengthening of the short femur and tibia. In the mild forms, femoral lengthening is appropriate, perhaps combined with a distal femoral epiphysiodesis on the normal side to gain full limb equality. In more severe cases of femoral deficiency, in which the femoral portion is very short, the child is best treated with knee fusion and foot removal, essentially becoming a long above-knee amputee with good prosthetic function. While it is difficult for parents to accept an amputation in their young child, it is important for the physician to be realistic in discussing the options for the treatment of this congenital problem. Of all the situations in which limb lengthening is used, treatment of a congenital short femur, in which the soft tissues of the limb are also congenitally shortened, is the most difficult and prone to complications.

Transient or Toxic Synovitis

Although the cause remains unclear, transient synovitis of the hip between the ages of 3 and 5 years remains the most common single cause of hip pain and limp in

children. While this synovitis will resolve without sequelae, it is important to differentiate this from more serious conditions affecting the hip, in particular septic arthritis.

Several possible causes of transient synovitis have been postulated. Minor trauma, allergic reaction, and viral (especially coxsackie B) illness have all been proposed but remain unproven.

The typical child with transient synovitis is between the ages of 3 and 5 years. Hip pain and limp above this age range should generally be considered to be some other hip disorder. The parents will note the child limping or the child will be reluctant to walk or move the affected leg. A low-grade fever may be present, but the child is often afebrile.

After the limp or refusal to walk has lasted for a day or two, medical attention is generally sought. Physical examination will demonstrate limited internal rotation of the affected hip. The child will prefer to hold the hip flexed, abducted, and externally rotated. Minimal or no soft tissue swelling is present in the proximal thigh and buttocks.

The primary condition in the differential diagnosis of transient synovitis is bacterial septic arthritis or femoral osteomyelitis. Other conditions to be considered are acute rheumatic fever and juvenile rheumatoid arthritis, although rheumatoid arthritis in children usually presents with knee or ankle swelling and pain.

In transient synovitis of the hip, radiographs of the pelvis and hips are normal. The white blood cell count may be normal or mildly elevated. The erythrocyte sedimentation rate often is minimally elevated. Ultrasound evaluation will demonstrate a variable amount of fluid within the hip capsule. If hip aspiration is performed, the fluid obtained is yellowish, has a good mucin clot, and has a white blood cell count below $20,000/mm^3$. A technetium-99 bone scan will show increased blood flow in the early stage but normal static images, reflecting no increased bone uptake of the isotope.

The number of the above tests needed to be comfortable with the diagnosis of transient synovitis will vary with each child. The primary goal here is to differentiate transient synovitis from an early septic arthritis or proximal femoral osteomyelitis. In general, an anteroposterior pelvis radiograph, CBC, and sedimentation rate should be obtained. If the white blood cell count and the sedimentation rate are quite elevated and the child has a high fever with marked limitation of hip motion, the hip should be aspirated. The hip aspirate should be evaluated by a cell count, a Gram stain, and multiple cultures.

Once the diagnosis of bacterial infection in the hip has been excluded to the examiner's satisfaction, the young child can be diagnosed as having transient synovitis. Bed rest is needed to allow this synovitis to resolve. Anti-inflammatory agents are not needed. Skin traction may be used, not to distract the hip joint itself, but to anchor the child in bed. Daily evaluation of hip movement is preferred to assess the response to the bed rest.

In general, as the name of the condition implies, the synovitis is transient, resolving within 3 to 5 days from the institution of rest. No long-term restriction of activity should be needed. Less than 10% of the children will have a second episode. If synovitis becomes recurrent, other diagnoses need to be considered.

Legg-Perthes Disease

Legg-Perthes disease, also known as Legg-Calvé-Perthes disease, was described independently in 1909 by Legg in the United States, Perthes in Germany, and Calvé in France. Originally described as a nontuberculous infection of the hip, this condition is now known to be caused not by infection but by avascular necrosis of the ossification center of the femoral head.

Legg-Perthes disease occurs in about one of every 750 children. It most commonly af-

fects boys and primarily occurs between the ages of 4 and 10 years. Taken as a group, boys with Legg-Perthes disease are in the lower percentiles of height for age and may have some delay in their bone age.

Pathologic specimens from children with Legg-Perthes disease demonstrate avascular necrosis of the bone in the femoral head interspersed with healing bone. It is thought that Legg-Perthes disease is the result of repeated trauma to the hip in active boys, in some way causing partial ischemia to the bone of the femoral head. In animal experiments, repeated injury to the femoral circumflex arteries is needed to produce histologic and radiographic findings similar to Legg-Perthes disease in a child, something a single episode of ischemia in dogs does not produce.

Pain with movement of the hip and a limp are the usual presenting complaints. Pain may radiate down the anterior or medial thigh toward the knee. No swelling is present, and tenderness to palpation is not seen. As with transient synovitis, internal rotation is limited. (**Remember**: examine the child in the prone position to measure internal rotation.) Hip abduction is also decreased compared to the other hip, and a mild flexion contracture is often present. It is not unusual to have atrophy of the thigh on the affected side, a finding best confirmed by tape measurement of the circumference of both thighs at the same measured point 10 to 15 cm cephalad to the patella. Gluteus medius weakness is present and the child will have both a positive Trendelenburg sign and a Trendelenburg gait. Because pain is frequently present, an antalgic gait may also be noted.

The CBC and sedimentation rate are normal, as are the routine serum chemistry studies. Thyroid function tests may be obtained to screen for possible hypothyroidism, since similar radiographic findings may be present bilaterally with thyroid disease, in which epiphyses may appear fragmented. Both an anteroposterior neutral and a

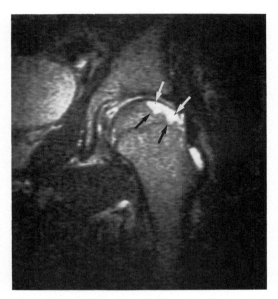

Figure 12.29. T2-weighted MR study of a hip in a child with pain for 4 weeks shows an irregular region of high signal (*arrows*) corresponding to early avascular necrosis and corresponding to a region of decreased isotope uptake on the bone scan. Radiographs and T1-weighted images were normal.

frog-leg lateral radiograph of the pelvis should be obtained as the initial imaging evaluation. The first radiographic finding noted is a smaller ossified femoral head on the affected side, due to the temporary cessation of bone growth and ossification that results from bone ischemia. The articular cartilage space or joint space will appear thicker than the normal hip for the same reason. In this early stage, a bone scan will demonstrate decreased bone uptake in either the entire proximal femoral epiphysis or in the lateral portion. Early avascular necrosis will appear as increased signal on T2-weighted MR images long before changes are visible on routine radiographic studies (Fig. 12.29). MR is an excellent way to make the diagnosis of avascular necrosis and to follow the patient for cartilaginous changes of the femoral head and acetabulum, for femoral head coverage, and for healing (Fig. 12.30).

Radiographic changes appear sequen-

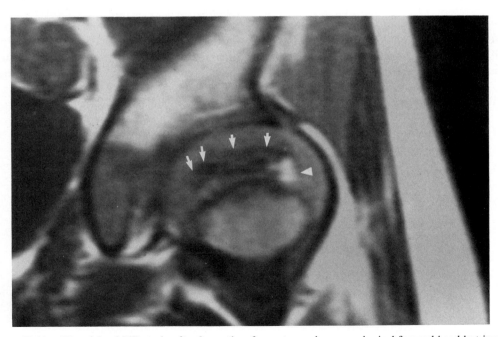

Figure 12.30. T1-weighted MR study after 2 months of symptoms shows a spherical femoral head but irregular regions of low signal (*arrows*), which indicate regions of avascular necrosis and collapse. High-signal area (*arrowhead*) represents hemorrhage.

tially as the length of time since the initial onset of Legg-Perthes disease passes. In some instances, these radiographic changes are present at the time of initial diagnosis, indicating that the ischemia has been present for some time. After the radiographic finding of a smaller ossification area of the femoral head, the next discrete radiographic change is the appearance of a radiodense or sclerotic femoral head, due to the lack of vascularity and lack of normal bone resorption. Subsequently small, crescentic subchondral lucencies appear, which represent fractures of the bone just below the articular surface. During early revascularization the resultant bone resorption produces more radiolucency and fragmentation (Fig. 12.31). Usually, after the femoral head has healed, the affected femoral head is larger than the unaffected hip and the neck is short and thick. The term "coxa magna" is used to describe this radiographic finding. The entire time needed to complete this sequence of radiographic changes is approximately 18 to 24 months.

The differential diagnosis in a child with these radiographic findings is rather limited. If bilateral sclerosis or fragmentation of the femoral head is present, conditions to con-

sider include multiple epiphyseal dysplasia, Meyer's disease (dysplasia of both capital femoral epiphyses only), and hypothyroidism. The diagnosis of multiple epiphyseal dysplasia can be established by radiographs of other epiphyses, especially the knee, shoulder, and wrist. Bilateral disease is seen in less than 20% of children affected with Legg-Perthes disease.

In the young child in whom there is substantial femoral head cartilage at the onset of the disease, Legg-Perthes disease is self-limited and will heal. The primary goals of treatment are threefold: first, to resolve the synovitis of the hip and improve the range of motion; second, to decide if enough of the femoral head is involved to warrant further treatment; and third, in those that need further treatment, to provide a type of therapy that allows the femoral head to be well contained within the acetabulum as healing occurs, so the hip joint will be congruent after healing is complete.

Resolution of the synovitis is accomplished by 7 to 10 days of bed rest, with resultant improvement in abduction and internal rotation. The decision regarding further treatment begins with an assessment of the percentage of femoral head involvement

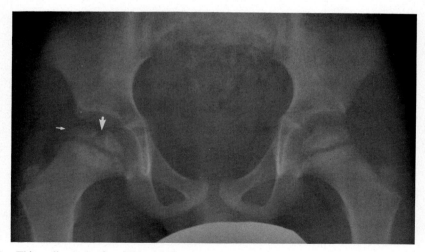

Figure 12.31. This radiograph of a child with Legg-Perthes disease involving the entire femoral head shows a small, flattened, fragmented right femoral head with areas of sclerosis and fractures (*arrows*). The metaphysis is widened.

with avascular necrosis. If less than 50% of the femoral head is avascular, treatment consists only of maintaining good range of motion of the hip until the radiographs demonstrate healing. If more than 50% of the femoral head is involved, treatment consists of either an abduction brace or osteotomy of the proximal femur or ilium to allow the femoral head to fit well into the acetabulum in a "contained" position as healing proceeds. An abduction brace is usually used under the age of 7 years, while surgery is more common in older children.

The prognosis for this condition is usually good. Children with less than half the femoral head involved should have a nearly normal hip. Children under the age of 6 have an excellent likelihood of a very good result. The children with the worst long-term results are those who are 10 years old or older at the time of diagnosis and those with severe flattening of the superior aspect of the femoral head prior to the initiation of treatment, so the femoral head fits the acetabulum in a noncongruous manner.

Slipped Capital Femoral Epiphysis

The most common hip disorder of preadolescent and adolescent children is a slipped capital femoral epiphysis; this should be suspected whenever a child in this age range has limitation of motion, a limp, or pain in the hip or anterior thigh. Obesity is present in 80% of children with this disorder.

Anatomically, a slipped capital femoral epiphysis is analogous to a Salter-Harris type I fracture in this region. Slippage occurs through the zone of cellular hypertrophy of the physis. Obesity is a contributing factor, as is delay in the development of secondary sex characteristics. In the early adolescent period, the fibrous structure that surrounds the physis becomes thin, providing less resistance to slippage through the physis than at a younger age. It is postulated that, if a child is obese, the added forces on the proximal femoral physis cannot be supported and a slip occurs. Absence of sex hormones, which seal the physis, enhances this effect. It is also known that slipped capital femoral epiphysis is more common in children with femoral retroversion, which is present in children who walk with their feet turned outward. The femoral epiphysis slips posteriorly and inferiorly on the proximal femoral neck.

Generally this condition presents in a chronic manner, with a history of limp or of hip or thigh pain following activity beginning several weeks or months prior to seeking medical attention. Less common are children who have sudden severe hip pain with activity (acute type) or sudden severe hip pain after having had a few weeks of mild hip discomfort (acute on chronic type). In children with either the acute or acute on chronic type, the diagnosis is easily made by radiographs, and surgical treatment is utilized in managing this acute fracture.

More difficult to diagnose early is the chronic type of slip. It is important to recognize this disorder early for the best result, because once an acute slip or fracture has occurred, the chance for a resultant normal hip drops significantly.

Physical examination of a child with a possible chronic slipped capital femoral epiphysis begins with observation of the child lying supine on the examination table. At rest the affected leg is usually more externally rotated than the normal side. Internal rotation is decreased when the hip is extended and flexed. When the hip is flexed with the child supine, the leg will go into a position of external rotation, a physical finding strongly suggestive of a slipped capital femoral epiphysis. Abduction of the affected hip is decreased. A positive Trendelenburg test and gait are present, and the child will usually walk with the painful leg rotated outward.

Definitive diagnosis can be made by frontal radiographs of the pelvis with the hips in the neutral and frog-leg positions. If this diagnosis is under consideration, it is essential to obtain both views. On the neutral anteroposterior view, one finding is diminished height of the epiphysis on the slipped side compared to the normal hip. Also, the physis on the involved side appears wider and irregular (Fig. 12.32A) on the frog-leg position radiographs. A line drawn along the anterior superior femoral neck cortex should normally transect the edge of the epiphysis; if this line passes anteriorly to the femoral epiphysis, a slip is present. A line drawn along the posteroinferior femoral neck will normally miss the edge of the epiphysis, but will intersect the epiphysis edge in a slip of the epiphysis (Figs. 12.32**B**, 12.33).

Once the diagnosis of slipped capital fem-

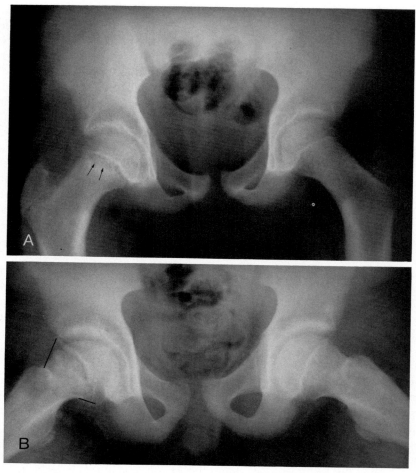

Figure 12.32.   A, Anteroposterior neutral view of the pelvis of a 13-year-old girl with limp shows a slightly shortened right femoral head and widened physis (*arrows*), consistent with a mild slipped capital femoral epiphysis. **B,** The frog-leg view shows posteromedial slip of the femoral epiphysis with lack of intersection of the lateral femoral neck line and intersection of the medial femoral neck line.

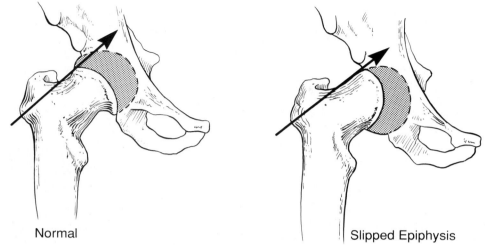

Normal   Slipped Epiphysis

Figure 12.33. On the anteroposterior radiograph of the normal hip, a line drawn along the superior femoral neck will transect the superior-lateral edge of the femoral epiphysis. If a slipped capital femoral epiphysis is present, this line will pass lateral to the femoral epiphysis. Specifically looking at this line on this radiograph will allow the diagnosis of a mild slip that at first was not obvious.

oral epiphysis is made, the child should be admitted to the hospital for surgical treatment. Surgical pinning of a mild slip will allow closure of the proximal femoral physis and prevent further deformity; these teenagers should end up with a nearly normal hip. However, if a mild slip progresses to a complete slip, the outlook is much worse. Complications seen in more marked slips, and especially in the acute or the acute on chronic types, are avascular necrosis of the femoral epiphysis or chondrolysis, both conditions that lead to permanent limitation of motion, often with pain.

As a final note, if a teenager presents with a complaint of anterior knee pain, the hip may be the source of the pain. If the examination of the knee does not yield much in the way of physical findings, the hip warrants examination, especially a check of internal rotation of the hip. Remember that the femoral nerve that innervates a portion of the hip joint may radiate pain originating in the hip to the anterior thigh as far distally as the patellar region.

Fracture of the Femoral Neck

Generally resulting from significant trauma to the knee or outstretched leg, a fracture of the femoral neck in children poses a number of problems. If any displacement occurs at the fracture site, the femoral circumflex arteries, which run in the hip capsule, may be torn or severely stretched.

The first complication is avascular necrosis to either the femoral head or the femoral neck cephalad to the fracture site. Since avascular necrosis may become apparent only several months after the injury, children with this fracture require at least 2 years' follow-up after the injury to assess for avascular changes (Fig. 12.34).

The second problem with this fracture is the tendency of the proximal fracture fragment to move into a varus position during cast treatment. Even if this fracture is nondisplaced, surgical treatment with internal fixation of the fracture is preferred to prevent the development of coxa vara, which will occur even in a hip spica cast.

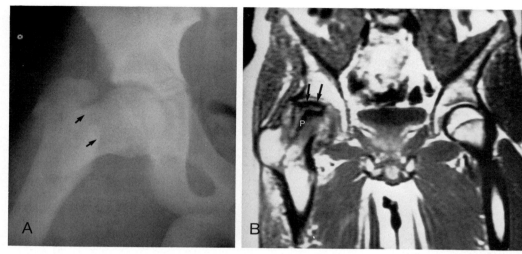

Figure 12.34. **A,** Anteroposterior hip radiograph of a twelve-year-old boy after a bicycle accident shows an acute femoral neck fracture (*arrows*). **B,** The acute fracture was pinned. Two years later, an MR study shows extensive avascular necrosis of the femoral head, a common complication after this fracture. Low-signal, dark areas (*arrows*) indicate absence of bone marrow. The pin tract is also noted (*P*).

Femoral Shaft Fracture

Fractures of the femoral shaft generally result from either a vehicular accident or a long fall, although child abuse should always be suspected in infants with this injury. Although some do occur in collision-type sports, femoral shaft fractures are relatively uncommon in sports compared to vehicular accidents.

The presence of a femoral shaft fracture is virtually always diagnosed at the scene of the accident or injury. Neurovascular function distal to the fracture should be documented and a traction splint should be applied for transport of the child to a hospital or emergency room. In the emergency room, popliteal and pedal pulses are again examined and sciatic nerve function is determined. Since displaced femoral fractures usually result from a severe injury, a full-body examination is needed to diagnose any associated injuries.

Radiographs are needed to determine the location and type of femoral shaft fracture as well as the amount of shortening or angulation present. The hip and the knee must be included in the radiographic assessment, as joint injury adjacent to a femoral shaft fracture is not unusual.

The extent of concurrent soft-tissue injury can often be estimated from the radiograph. If the fracture is a spiral or oblique fracture with little shortening of the femur at the fracture site, it is likely that this fracture is from a low-velocity injury. Characteristic of a high-velocity injury is a femoral shaft fracture that is shortened an inch or more, is comminuted, and is markedly displaced.

Hospitalization with placement of the child in lower-extremity traction is the usual initial treatment for a child with a femoral shaft fracture. Hemorrhage into the thigh from the fracture is common but usually does not require blood transfusion replacement. However, this thigh hematoma is considered to be the source of a fever to 38°C that is commonly present for the first few days after this injury.

In nondisplaced or minimally displaced fractures in infants and toddlers, a hip spica cast can be applied within a few days of the injury and the child can be discharged from the hospital, provided the child is stable and the infant's injury has been judged not to have resulted from child abuse. The cast is left on from 4 weeks for infants to 7 or 8 weeks in older children, and healing time is directly related to the age of the child.

If displacement of the fracture has occurred, the thigh muscles contract, leading to shortening of the femur with overriding of the fracture fragments. Traction is needed to partially regain the normal femoral length, with a residual 5 to 10 mm of overlap at the fracture site preferred to allow for approximately 1 cm of bone overgrowth expected as a result of the fracture. This traction may be provided either by skin or pin techniques and is used until enough early fracture healing has occurred to place the child in a hip spica cast until healing is complete.

Most children under the age of 10 years with a femoral shaft fracture are treated by traction and casting. Care must be taken during the treatment period to avoid excessive femoral shortening or angulation, but nonunion is rare. In children with multiple fractures, open fractures, and associated head injuries, operative treatment with internal or external fixation of the fracture may be preferable.

Over the age of 10 years, operative treatment of femoral shaft fractures is more common, with intramedullary internal fixation being used most often. Surgical treatment generally avoids the need for a cast, allows for a shorter hospital stay, promotes earlier weight bearing, allows the child or adolescent to attend school, and has a lower incidence of angular or shortening malunions. Healing of the fracture may be slower with internal fixation treatment. These internal fixation devices are usually removed surgically after fracture healing is complete.

The primary problems following a femoral shaft fracture are rotational or angular malunion, excessive shortening at the fracture site, and persistent thigh muscle weakness. Since varus and valgus angulation does not remodel well in the mid or distal femur after fracture healing, osteotomy may be needed to correct excessive angular malunion, especially in older children. Since the majority of femoral overgrowth following fracture is usually complete within 18 months from the time of injury, if there is more than a 2-cm leg length discrepancy at that time, surgical procedures to equalize the legs may be indicated.

Even after the children and teenagers have returned to active sports activity a few months after femoral fracture healing, quadriceps and hamstring muscle weakness may persist for several months. Insufficient attention is generally directed toward thigh muscle strengthening after cast removal in children, but if this residual weakness persists, it will predispose the child to muscle or joint injury during sports activities. Although formal muscle testing, such as with the Cybex machine, is possible, a simple method to assess the return to normal muscle size (and by inference strength) is by tape measure assessment of the thigh circumference of the injured leg compared to the normal side at the same level above the knee.

Suggested Readings

Bialik, V., Fishman, J., Katzir, J., et al.: Clinical assessment of hip instability in the newborn by an orthopedic surgeon and a pediatrician. J. Pediatr. Orthop. 703-705, 1986.

Bialik, V., Reuveni, A., Pery, M., et al.: Ultrasonography in developmental displacement of the hip: A critical analysis of our results. J. Pediatr. Orthop. 9:154-156, 1989.

Bos, C.F., Bloem, J.L., Obermann, W.R., et al.: Magnetic resonance imaging in congenital dislocation of the hip. J. Bone Joint Surg. 70B:174-178, 1988.

Carney, B.T., Weinstein, S.L., and Noble, J.: Long-term follow-up of slipped capital femoral epiphysis. J. Bone Joint Surg. 73A:667-674, 1991.

Catterall, A.: The natural history of Perthes disease. J. Bone Joint Surg. 53B:37-53, 1971.

Chung, S.M.: The arterial supply of the developing proximal end of the human femur. J. Bone Joint Surg. 58A:961-970, 1976.

Epps, C.H., Jr.: Current concept review: Proximal femoral focal deficiency. J. Bone Joint Surg. 65A: 867-870, 1983.

Galbraith, R.T., Gelberman, R.H., Hajek, P.C., et al.: Obesity and decreased femoral anteversion in adolescence. J. Orthop. Res. 5:523-528, 1987.

Hadlow, V.: Neonatal screening for congenital dislocation of the hip: A prospective 21-year survey. J. Bone Joint Surg. 70B:740-743, 1988.

Hensinger, R.N.: Congenital dislocation of the hip. CIBA Clin. Symp. 31:3-31, 1979.

Haueisen, D.C., Weiner, D.S., Weiner, S.D., et al.: The characterization of "transient synovitis of the hip" in children. J. Pediatr. Orthop. 6:11-17, 1986.

Herring, J.A.: Legg-Calve-Perthes disease: A review of current knowledge. In Barr, J.S., Jr. (ed): American Academy of Orthopaedic Surgeons Instructional Course Lectures, XXXVIII. Park Ridge, IL, American Academy of Orthopaedic Surgeons. pp. 309-315, 1989.

Ilfeld, W., Westin, G.W., and Makin, M.: Missed or developmental dislocation of the hip. Clin. Orthop. 203:276-281, 1986.

Kalamchi, A. and MacFarlane, R., III: The Pavlik harness: results in patients over three months of age. J. Pediatr. Orthop. 2:3-8, 1982.

McHale, K.A. and Corbett, D.: Noncompliance with Pavlik harness treatment of the infantile hip problems. J. Pediatr. Orthop. 9:649-652, 1989.

Rockwood, C.A., Jr., Wilkins, K.E., and King, R.E. (eds.): Fractures in Children, Volume 3. Philadelphia, J.B. Lippincott, 1984.

Shapiro, F.: Fractures of the femoral shaft in children: The overgrowth phenomenon. Acta Orthop. Scand. 52:649-655, 1981.

Sponseller, P.D., Desai, S.S., and Millis, M.B.: Comparison of femoral and innominate osteotomies for the treatment of Legg-Calve-Perthes disease. J. Bone Joint Surg. 70A:1131-1139, 1988.

Tredwell, S.J. and Davis, L.A.: Prospective study of congenital dislocation of the hip. J. Pediatr. Orthop. 9:157-159, 1989.

Viljanto, J., Kiviluoto, H., and Paananen, M.: Remodelling after femoral shaft fracture in children. Act Chir. Scand. 141:360-365, 1975.

Weinstein, J.N., Kuo, K.N., and Millar, E.A.: Congenital coxa vara: A retrospective review. J. Pediatr. Orthop. 4:70-77, 1984.

Zahrawi, F.B., Stephens, T.L., Spencer, G.E., et al.: Comparative study of pinning in situ and open epiphysiodesis in 105 patients with slipped capital femoral epiphyses. Clin. Orthop. 177:160-168, 1983.

13
Knee

Functioning primarily as a hinge joint with movement in flexion and extension, the knee is nonetheless complex, with several soft tissue structures both inside and outside the joint working to provide stability in a wide variety of knee positions. Largely due to the number of these stabilizing soft tissue structures, the knee is a commonly injured area in almost all sports.

Anatomy

The medial and lateral femoral condyles articulate with the tibial plateau, providing the basic bony components of the knee joint. The tibial plateau has a shallow medial and lateral concavity on its surface to fit the convex contour of the respective femoral condyles. Generally the medial femoral condyle extends farther distally than does the lateral condyle, such that a slight valgus position at the knee is most often noted. As the proximal fibula lies just lateral and slightly distal to the femoral-tibial articulation, the fibula here contributes a site for ligament and tendon insertion rather than being involved in the knee joint articulation.

There are four primary ligaments in the normal knee. The medial collateral ligament extends from the distal femoral epiphysis to the proximal tibial epiphysis and metaphysis, serving to protect against valgus stress at the knee. The lateral collateral ligament runs from the lateral distal femoral epiphysis to the proximal fibula and tibia, protecting against excessive varus movement of the knee. The anterior and posterior cru-

ciate ligaments are intra-articular, being covered by synovium and providing internal check reins against too much anterior or posterior movement of the tibia on the femur. The anterior cruciate ligament courses from the medial aspect of the lateral femoral condyle in the intercondylar notch to the anteromedial portion of the central tibial plateau, while the posterior cruciate ligament runs from the medial femoral condyle to a posterolateral portion of the central tibial plateau (Fig.13.1).

Two other primary soft tissue structures within the knee joint are the medial and lateral menisci, composed of hyaline cartilage. The menisci are wedge-shaped on cross-sectional view and allow a closer fit of the distal femoral condyles to the tibial plateau while sharing some of the mechanical forces across the knee joint, protecting the articular cartilage from damage. When viewed from the top, the medial meniscus is C-shaped, being open on the portion adjacent to the cruciate ligaments, while the lateral meniscus is more doughnut-shaped. Small ligaments attach to the menisci to allow some normal meniscal movement as the knee moves in normal activity and sports. A special feature of the menisci that has an impact on healing after injury is the lack of vascular supply to the central two-thirds of the menisci, with nourishment provided to this segment of cartilage by synovial fluid.

The patella is a sesamoid bone that is located within the distal end of the quadriceps muscle and tendon, with articular cartilage on the inferior surface only. The inferior

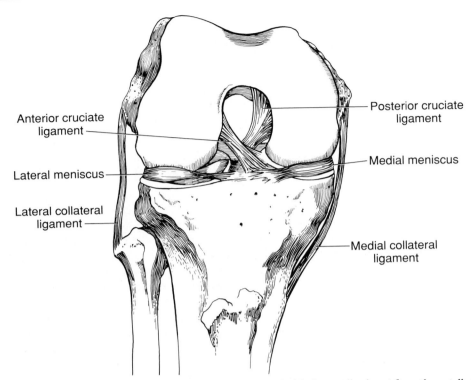

Figure 13.1.   This diagram, with the knee in a flexed position and with the patella absent from the patellar groove of the distal femur, illustrates the primary soft-tissue structures in the knee joint. The collateral ligaments protect against varus and valgus stresses primarily, while the cruciate ligaments provide primary protection from rotational and translational forces. The menisci, wedge-shaped on cross-section, provide a closer fit of the femoral condyles on the tibial plateau and share a portion of the weight-bearing forces across the knee. An injury to any of these soft-tissue structures may involve others.

surface is somewhat V-shaped to fit into the patellofemoral groove on the anterior aspect of the distal femur, between the two condyles. As the knee is flexed and extended, the patella normally moves cephalad and caudad in this groove. Anatomic variations in either the patellar shape or the depth of this groove may lead to knee pain. The primary purpose of the patella is to keep the patellar tendon farther away from the axis of rotation of the knee joint, in this way increasing the moment arm for the quadriceps so contraction of the quadriceps will provide more power for extending the knee than would be the case if the tendon were closer to the knee center.

Several muscles are important to move and help stabilize the knee. The quadriceps muscle is composed of the vastus medialis, vastus intermedius, vastus lateralis, and rectus femoris and is the primary extensor of the knee, attaching to the anterior proximal tibia at the tibial tubercle. The main knee flexors are the hamstring muscles (biceps femoris, semimembranosus, semitendinosus, and gracilis), which arise from the ischial area of the pelvis and insert onto the proximal tibia and fibula. The gracilis and semitendinosus muscles join the sartorius muscle to form the pes anserinus (or "duck-foot"), which inserts onto the anteromedial tibial metaphysis. The semimembranosus muscle inserts onto the posteromedial tibial epiphysis, while the biceps femoris muscle inserts laterally to the proximal tibia and fibula. The tensor fascia femo-

ris muscle of the proximal lateral thigh becomes the fascia lata in the distal half of the
thigh to insert onto the proximal tibia and
fibula, acting as a stabilizer of the lateral
side of the knee joint. Because so many
muscles are important in the smooth normal
function of the knee joint, weakness in these
muscles will significantly impair joint
function.

The major neurovascular structures in
the knee region lie posteriorly, in the popliteal area. The femoral artery courses down
the medial thigh, passing posterior to the
distal femur at the adductor tubercle, becoming the popliteal artery. Just distal to
the knee joint, the popliteal artery trifurcates to form the anterior tibial, peroneal,
and posterior tibial arteries. The anterior

tibial artery pierces the interosseous membrane here and runs in the anterior compartment of the leg to form the dorsalis pedis
artery in the ankle and foot. The peroneal
artery terminates in the lateral compartment, while the posterior tibial artery
courses in the deep posterior compartment,
passing into the foot just posterior to the
medial malleolus (Fig. 13.2).

The common peroneal and posterior tibial nerves are the major neural structures
passing the knee. Arising from the sciatic
nerve, the common peroneal nerve passes
posterior to the biceps femoris tendon at the
knee, then runs around the lateral aspect of
the proximal fibula before splitting to form
the superficial and deep peroneal nerves.
The deep peroneal nerve remains in the an-

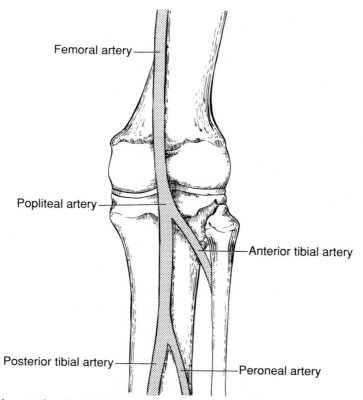

Femoral artery

Popliteal artery

Anterior tibial artery

Posterior tibial artery

Peroneal artery

Figure 13.2. In this posterior view of the knee region, the popliteal artery trifurcates into the three primary
arteries to the lower leg and foot. Since the anterior tibial artery pierces the interosseous membrane to lie in the
anterior portion of the leg, there is little mobility of the arteries at this location, making these vessels prone to
injury with fractures here.

terior compartment with the anterior tibial artery, while the superficial peroneal nerve follows the peroneal muscles laterally. While the peroneal nerve innervates the foot and toe dorsiflexors and foot evertors, the posterior tibial nerve provides motor function for toe and foot plantarflexion as well as inversion of the foot. Dorsal foot sensation is largely from the peroneal nerve, while plantar sensation results from an intact posterior tibial nerve. Injury to nerves at the knee level can be localized best by evaluation of foot and ankle motor and sensory function.

The synovial lining of the knee joint anteriorly extends proximal to the patella in the suprapatellar region. Since this region communicates freely with the rest of the intra-articular area, fluid within the knee joint will present as swelling above the knee.

The primary bursa of importance in the knee is the prepatellar bursa, located between the anterior knee skin and the patella. Normally this is a potential space that can become fluid-filled if inflamed.

Physical Examination

Because of the superficial location of most of the components that form the knee joint, careful physical examination will usually allow for an appropriate diagnosis, provided the anatomy of this region is remembered.

OBSERVATION

Compare both knees first to see if they are symmetrical in appearance. Is swelling present so that the normal hollow areas noted adjacent to the patella are no longer obvious? Look for bruising, which may provide a clue to the direction of the force causing the knee injury. With the knee flexed 60° to 90°, view the joint from the side; is the tibia located more posteriorly on the injured side, indicating a posterior cruciate ligament injury?

PALPATION

Palpation for areas of tenderness is extremely important in the examination of the knee. Tenderness over a specific anatomical structure generally means an injury has occurred in that location.

In the growing child, palpation over the physis of the distal femur and proximal tibia may cause pain, a possible indication of a physeal fracture. The medial and lateral joint lines can generally be easily located; tenderness over the joint line itself may mean a meniscal injury is present. Palpation of the tibial and femoral attachments of the collateral ligaments may detect a partial tear of one of these ligaments. The tibial tubercle is palpated for tenderness, a finding present primarily in Osgood-Schlatter's disease. Finally, the patella is examined on all sides of its anterior surface for possible tenderness.

Palpation of the knee joint for possible effusion completes this portion of the examination. Ballottement of fluid in the suprapatellar area or adjacent to the patella means a significant effusion is present. With smaller effusions, a fluid wave may be produced.

RANGE OF MOTION

The range of motion should be the same on both knees. Full extension should be present, with approximately 140° of flexion, noted on the record as 0° to 140° of motion. With the knee fully extended, the tibia does not normally rotate on the femur, but with the knee flexed, external and internal rotation movements normally occur.

LIGAMENT ASSESSMENT

Each of the four major ligaments of the knee need to be evaluated separately. The medial collateral ligament is examined by applying a valgus stress to the knee, first in a fully extended position and then in a position of 10° to 20° of flexion. Lateral collateral ligament integrity is assessed by varus stress with the knee in the same positions as for the medial collateral ligament.

Cruciate ligament function is evaluated

by the Lachman test or the drawer test. The Lachman test is performed by stabilizing the distal femur with one hand while the other grasps the tibia proximally, then applying stress in an anterior-posterior direction with the knee in nearly full extension. The drawer sign is assessed by flexing the knee 90° with the foot on the examination table. Both hands then grasp the proximal leg and attempt to draw the tibia forward on the femur. Both anterior and posterior cruciate ligament injuries will have increased anteroposterior movement to stress examination. By looking at the flexed knee from the side, a posterior cruciate injury can be diagnosed if the tibia rests in a more posterior position than on the uninjured side.

There is a good deal of individual variability in the normal laxity of knee ligaments. If excessive laxity appears to be present, check other joints of the upper extremity for hypermobility. Instability should not be diagnosed unless there is significantly more laxity present with stress evaluation of one or more ligaments on the injured side than on the normal side.

MENISCUS EVALUATION

Tenderness to palpation directly over the medial or lateral joint line is usually the first hint of a meniscus injury. The examiner should then keep a finger on the joint line as the knee is flexed and extended, first with the tibia externally rotated on the femur, then with the tibia internally rotated. If a palpable click is noted at the joint line with this maneuver, this is confirmatory evidence of a probable torn meniscus.

PATELLA EVALUATION

The patella is first evaluated with the knee fully extended and the quadriceps relaxed, the position in which the patella is the most mobile to passive manipulation. Pain with any passive movement of the patella is noted. The patella is then pushed laterally to assess for possible lateral subluxation; if the patient feels like the patella is about to

dislocate, he will often grab the examiner's hand to stop this lateral movement, resulting in a positive "apprehension sign" of patellar instability.

With the child then sitting on the edge of the examining table with both knees flexed, active extension at the knee is attempted. Pain present with this maneuver usually indicates a patellofemoral problem, particularly in a teenager. If pain is not produced by active extension, the child next slowly extends each leg while the examiner notes the manner in which the patella tracks in the patellofemoral groove as the knee becomes fully extended. As a further component of evaluating the patellofemoral joint, the amount of knee valgus and femoral anteversion is also noted. Finally, the Q angle, formed by the intersection of one line from the mid-anterior thigh to the patella and another line from the mid-patella to the tibial tubercle, is assessed. A normal Q angle is under 20°, while larger Q angles denote a tendency toward lateral patellar subluxation.

POPLITEAL AREA EVALUATION

The popliteal area is best evaluated with the child prone and the knee fully extended or even slightly hyperextended. A popliteal cyst is always present in the same location, between the semimembranosus muscle and the medial head of the gastrocnemius muscle. A cystic structure here is usually nontender and should be measured for baseline evaluation information. A mass in the popliteal area at a more lateral location should be evaluated further as a possible soft tissue tumor.

Imaging Studies

RADIOGRAPHY

The standard initial imaging studies for knee evaluation are anteroposterior and lateral radiographs. In a growing child, the physis should be carefully observed for possible injury to the distal femur or proximal tibia. If a fracture is suspected from physical examination and is not seen on these two projections, oblique positioning for radiographs of the knee should be obtained. With these four views, the majority of bone lesions can be diagnosed. The lateral radiograph is more useful than the anteroposterior view for assessment of the patellar position and for evaluation of the tibial tubercle area.

Anteroposterior radiographs of the knee with either valgus or varus stress applied may be helpful to differentiate a distal femoral physeal fracture from a ligament injury. If physical findings suggest knee instability after an injury, anteroposterior and lateral radiographs are carefully evaluated for possible fracture. If none is seen, the physician (not the radiologic technologist) should carefully apply lateral or medial stress as in a physical examination maneuver while the radiograph is obtained to show the location of the instability.

The "tunnel view" and the "sunrise view" are used in children suspected of having a specific knee problem. The tunnel view radiograph is obtained by flexing the knee approximately 20° during an anteroposterior radiograph. This more clearly visualizes the articular surfaces of the femoral condyle involved with osteochondritis dissecans. The sunrise view is used to evaluate for possible patellofemoral joint pathology. In this radiograph, the x-ray beam is aimed tangentially to the anterior aspect of the flexed knee joint to visualize the position of the patella within the patellofemoral groove of the distal femur. The most information about the patellar position can be obtained if radiographs are obtained at positions of 30°, 60°, and 90° of flexion, but if a single view is obtained, the knee is flexed 45°.

After the age of 5 or 6 years, the normal alignment of the femur relative to the tibia at the knee is a position of approximately 7° valgus on a standing anteroposterior radiograph. When evaluating a child for angular deformity due to problems at the knee level, the child should be standing and the antero-posterior radiograph should include the hip, knee, and ankle for the most accurate measurement. (Measurement methods for angular deformity assessment are described in Chapter 17.)

MAGNETIC RESONANCE IMAGING

Magnetic resonance (MR) scanning of the knee permits evaluation of all the soft tissue structures of the knee not seen with radiography, including the menisci, knee ligaments, physeal cartilage, and articular cartilage as well as the subchondral bone and bone marrow of the femur and tibia.

With the high degree of resolution and tissue specificity of this modality, minimal cartilage abnormalities may be visualized by MR that are not seen by direct visualization through arthroscopy. The interpretation of the MR observations must be correlated with the physical examination and the child's symptoms before a treatment plan is devised.

Evaluation of a Knee Effusion

If a knee effusion is present on physical examination, it is useful to determine from the child or parents whether this is acute or whether recurrent effusions have occurred.

If the effusion develops quickly after an injury, acute bleeding into the knee should be considered the cause. This bleeding may occur from a bony fracture or a tear in the vascular synovial lining of the knee. Aspiration of the knee may be performed by insertion of a needle below the lateral or medial patella to relieve the pain of a stretched knee capsule, to make examination of the knee easier, and to assess for a possible intra-articular fracture. If fat globules are present within the bloody aspirate, an intra-articular fracture should be diagnosed unless proven otherwise by arthroscopy or other means. In the skeletally mature teenager, an acute hemarthrosis after injury (especially of the hyperextension variety) is most often a sign of an anterior cruciate ligament tear.

If the effusion has developed more slowly or is recurrent, fluid aspiration will aid in establishing the diagnosis. The aspirated fluid is visually assessed for color and clarity, as well as for its viscosity. The quality of mucin clot is noted. Laboratory studies should include a cell count, Gram stain, and cultures for bacteria and fungi. If joint fluid glucose and protein studies are obtained, serum glucose and protein studies are also ordered for comparison. Evaluation for crystals may be performed, but crystalline causes of joint effusion in children are much less common than in adults.

Disorders of the Knee

OSGOOD-SCHLATTER DISEASE

A common self-limited condition in active children between the ages of 11 and 14 years, Osgood-Schlatter disease presents with pain on the anterior aspect of the lower knee after sports or running activities.

Either one or both knees may be involved, but when it is bilateral, one side is usually more symptomatic. The pain typically arises during or shortly after activity.

The symptoms and signs of this condition arise as a result of repeated microfractures in the apophyseal cartilage between the proximal tibia and the secondary ossification center onto which the patellar tendon attaches. These cartilaginous microfractures occur as a result of repeated extension of the knee associated with many sports, as the cartilage is less able to resist this stress than is bone or tendon. Inflammation at the site of injury follows, resulting in pain and tenderness. The response of the cartilage to this injury is calcification of the area of cartilage involved. If activity is not restricted and microfractures continue over a period of several months, this abnormal cartilage calcification will lead to enlargement of the tibial tubercle (Fig. 13.3). When the secondary ossification center of the tibial tubercle

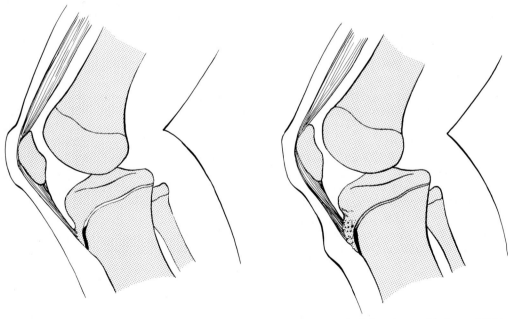

Figure 13.3.   This drawing illustrates the lateral view of a normal knee on the left and one with Osgood-Schlatter disease on the right. The patellar tendon attaches to the tibial tubercle apophysis in the immature child. Repetitive pull on this site during sports activity in this age group will result in microfractures in this cartilage attachment. As healing of these microfractures occurs, enlargement of the tibial tubercle region occurs and a tender bump is palpable at this site.

fuses to the proximal tibia near skeletal maturity, the tibial tubercle may be enlarged, but symptoms virtually always disappear since there is no longer cartilage present at this site to be injured with repetitive knee extension.

The diagnosis of Osgood-Schlatter disease is made by physical examination. Tenderness to palpation directly over the tibial tubercle is the *sine qua non* of this condition. The tibial tubercle may be more prominent on the affected side. Pain is usually exacerbated by attempts at knee extension against resistance or by full passive knee flexion. No effusion should be seen, and other findings of knee abnormality should be absent.

Anteroposterior and lateral radiographs are obtained at initial presentation to rule out other bone lesions in the proximal tibia that might be causing this pain and tenderness. Serial radiographs are not needed once the diagnosis is made. The anteroposterior radiograph is normal. The lateral radiograph may be normal or may demonstrate a pattern of fragmentation of the ossified portions of the tibial tubercle (Fig. 13.4). After skeletal maturity, the tibial tubercle may be larger than on the unaffected side. In unusual cases when pain with activity persists even after skeletal maturity, a small separate ossicle may be seen.

Treatment for Osgood-Schlatter disease consists of activity restriction as needed and an explanation of the self-limited nature of this condition to the child and parents. The amount of activity restriction needed is dependent on the severity of the symptoms. If pain is only intermittently present, athletic activities can be continued, with a stretching program for quadriceps and hamstrings used prior to sports participation and perhaps use of an ice compress over the tibial tubercle for 10 to 15 minutes after playing. If the knee pain interferes with sleep, school work, or other daily activities, sports should be temporarily discontinued and a knee immobilizer should be used to restrict knee

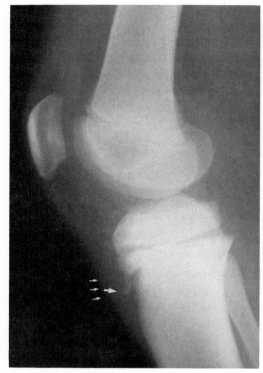

Figure 13.4. A lateral knee radiograph of a child with Osgood-Schlatter's disease shows "fragmentation" of the anterior tibial tubercle (*arrow*) and soft-tissue swelling (*small arrows*) at the site of pain and tenderness.

movement. Full-weight bearing may be continued, and crutches are usually not needed. Isometric quadriceps exercises are continued to limit muscle atrophy with immobilization. Several weeks of restricted activity may be needed in the more severe cases. When pain relief has occurred, the child may return to sports activities only after the quadriceps and hamstring strength on the affected side is as good as or better than the normal thigh. Stretching should continue to be done prior to athletic activities.

While those with mild or moderate Osgood-Schlatter disease may continue to play sports despite occasional and mild pain, the author strongly believes that if pain medication is used or daily activities are affected, restriction of sports activity is needed. Injection of the tibial tubercle with corticosteroids to decrease inflammation here is contraindicated.

Enlargement of the tibial tubercle is the principal after-effect of this condition. This enlargement is a cosmetic problem only, unless the patient kneels often, in which case pain may be noted over this prominence. Surgery is recommended only in the rare cases when pain persists after skeletal maturity and a loose ossicle at this site is seen on a lateral radiograph.

PATELLOFEMORAL MALALIGNMENT DISORDERS

Malalignment at the patellofemoral joint is a common cause of anterior knee pain in teenagers, especially teenage girls. This category includes the conditions of patellar chondromalacia, lateral patellar subluxation, and recurrent patellar dislocation.

Although the term "chondromalacia" is commonly used to describe patellofemoral pain without patellar instability, actual chondromalacia (or "softening of the articular cartilage") occurs much less commonly in teenagers than in adults, with arthroscopy commonly showing normal patellar cartilage in the teenager. Because permanent damage to the patellar articular cartilage is unusual in teenagers, this condition generally resolves with time and does not appear to be a major cause of adult degenerative arthritis of the patellofemoral joint. Lateral subluxation of the patella denotes a lateral drift or positioning of the patella associated with anterior knee pain. Recurrent dislocation of the patella always occurs in the lateral direction and may be caused by either abnormal anatomic features or a prior traumatic patellar dislocation. Symptoms of anterior knee pain may be very similar for all of these conditions.

Pain is present either to the side of the patella or inferior to the patellar pole. Pain is often noted going up or coming down stairs, as the quadriceps muscles contract to stabilize the knee and support the body. Pain may be noted in the first few steps after sitting for awhile with the knees flexed, such as in a car or theater. The knee may have the feeling of "giving way" from pain or instability, and the patient may actually fall. Specific sports aggravate this pain, such as swimming the breaststroke, cycling, or repetitive squatting exercises.

Several factors appear to predispose the teenager to anterior knee pain. The patellofemoral groove in the distal femur may be unusually shallow, providing less guidance for the patella during knee flexion and extension. Excessive knee valgus or increased femoral anteversion both cause the tibial tubercle to be positioned laterally to its normal position, leading to lateral patellar subluxation as the quadriceps muscle contracts. Quadriceps weakness leads to less stable tracking of the patella in its groove, while quadriceps fibrosis may lead to patella dislocation over time. When any of these anatomic variations are present, pain in the patellofemoral region is more likely to occur with activity.

Positive physical findings in this condition are limited to the anterior aspect of the knee. An effusion may be present but generally is not. Tenderness to palpation is most often noted on the lateral or medial aspect of the patella. With the knee fully extended, an attempt to passively move the patella laterally may be resisted by the patient because of pain or the sensation of patellar instability, constituting a positive "apprehension test." Passive compression of the patella against the anterior femur usually causes pain. If the patient actively contracts the quadriceps while the examiner holds the patella from moving, pain is usually produced, but a similar maneuver may cause pain in a normal knee.

The knee should be observed as the child actively extends the knee from a 90° flexed position. As the knee approaches full extension, the patella may drift laterally as it disengages from the tracking guidance of the patellofemoral groove. With this lateral subluxation, the tibial tubercle is often laterally placed, either from increased knee valgus or from femoral anteversion. This degree of lateral placement of the tibial tubercle is related to the tendency for lateral patellar subluxation and can be measured by the Q angle.

Because pain is present with muscle testing, the strength of the quadriceps is difficult to assess properly. If pain precludes this strength testing, measurement of the thigh circumference at the same point above the patella on both legs will provide some clue as to the muscle weakness that may have resulted from this knee pain. If the teenager has had complaints of knee pain for several weeks and has no thigh atrophy, the pain almost certainly has not been severe and has not caused activity limitation, despite the history.

Radiographic studies are useful in determining the type of problem present and the treatment plan needed. If anterior knee pain is the main problem, anteroposterior, lateral, and sunrise view radiographs should be obtained, with at least the sunrise view being bilateral to compare with the asymptomatic side.

The anteroposterior radiograph usually appears normal, though the patella may be noted to be slightly laterally situated. The amount of knee valgus can be estimated from this film. On the lateral radiograph, the patella is often positioned more cephalad than normal, the so-called "patella alta." The degree of cephalad positioning of the patella is measured by the ratio between the length of the infrapatellar ligament (from the patella to the tibial tubercle) and the length of the bony patella. If this ratio exceeds 1.2, patella alta is present.

The sunrise view may demonstrate the patella either tilted or positioned laterally in the patellofemoral groove. In more marked subluxation or recurrent dislocation, the patellofemoral groove may be very shallow, providing little tracking guidance for the patella. The sunrise view at 45° or more flexion may be normal even if lateral subluxation is noted at the end of knee extension, in which case a repeat sunrise view at 30° flexion will often demonstrate the lateral subluxation.

Treatment for a patellofemoral disorder depends on several factors. While correction of anatomic variations, such as excessive knock-knees or femoral anteversion, require femoral osteotomy, the initial treatment for virtually all teenage patellar problems consists of quadriceps and hamstring muscle strengthening, stretching prior to sports participation, and avoidance of repetitive and excessive knee flexion. A short course of anti-inflammatory medication may be given but long-term treatment should not be used. An elastic knee support with a patellar cut-out will not hold the patella "reduced" but may provide the teenager with the subjective sensation of improved knee stability. Most will respond to this conservative regimen of treatment, but some anterior knee pain may persist for months before resolving.

If significant symptoms persist after a few to several months of thigh muscle strengthening and stretching, surgical treatment may be considered. Arthroscopy evaluation can be used to assess for other intra-articular knee pathology and assess the condition of the inferior articular surface of the patella. If the remainder of the knee appears normal, a lateral retinacular release can be performed to allow the patella to track more medially with knee motion. While this release allows for improved patellar movement, muscle strengthening is mandatory to attain better tracking and allow for pain relief. Surgical distal advancement of the vastus medialis may be used with lateral retinacular release to better balance patellar movement, particularly when patellar dislocation recurs. Though rarely used in the growing child, osteotomy of the tibial tubercle, the femur, or the tibia is used to realign the patellar mechanism if soft-tissue procedures are insufficient.

MEDIAL PLICA SYNDROME

Anterior knee pain may also be caused by the medial plica syndrome, with symptoms similar to those with patellofemoral malalignment syndromes.

This syndrome appears to be caused by inflammation of the medial plica of the knee, a fibrocartilaginous band of tissue normally running over the anterior surface of the medial femoral condyle. If this plica is larger than normal or is torn, anterior knee pain results, though it remains unclear why some have pain and others do not with the same arthroscopic findings.

Pain secondary to a plica may be considered if conservative treatment for patellofemoral pain has been unsuccessful. Arthroscopy is needed to make this diagnosis and this plica (remember this is basically a normal structure) has likely been implicated too often as the cause of anterior knee pain of unclear etiology. At arthroscopy, this plica can be partially excised without apparent later sequelae.

OSTEOCHONDRITIS DISSECANS

Osteochondritis dissecans occurs in the subchondral bone and overlying articular cartilage of the distal femoral condyles. Even though only one knee may be symptomatic, radiographs of both knees may show similar abnormalities, leading some to propose that this condition is caused by a localized abnormality in the vascular or end-artery anatomy in the involved area. Others have proposed that this lesion results from repeated trauma of the tibial spine abutting against the femoral condyle.

With osteochondritis dissecans, the child usually complains of poorly localized knee pain during and after activity. Symptoms usually appear in the pre-teenager or adolescent involved in sports. A history of a specific injury leading to this pain is generally absent.

Physical findings may be ill-defined. An effusion is sometimes present but more often is absent. Pain with full passive flexion is often seen. With the knee in the almost fully flexed position, palpation directly over the articular end of the femoral condyles frequently produces pain at the site of the bony lesion. If the involved piece of bone has separated from the femoral condyle and has formed a loose body, an effusion is common, and locking of the knee in a flexed position with incomplete knee extension may be demonstrated on examination.

The diagnosis of osteochondritis dissecans is confirmed by radiographs of the knee (Fig. 13.5). The most common location is on the medial aspect of the lateral femoral condyle, on the side of the intercondylar notch. However, this lesion may occur at any position on the femoral condyles and may be either large or quite small. If the osteochondritic segment has detached from the femoral condyle and formed a cartilaginous loose body, a radiolucent defect is noted in the femoral condyle. The loose body may or may not be seen on radiographs, depending on the amount of bone within the loose body.

The initial treatment for osteochondritis dissecans is activity restriction and use of a knee immobilizer until symptoms improve or resolve. Isometric exercises are continued to maintain thigh muscle strength. A cast is unnecessary and will cause more muscle atrophy than a knee immobilizer. The end point of treatment in this condition is not so much complete healing (as seen on radiographs) but resolution of knee pain. Even if the radiographs continue to show this lesion, participation in sports is allowed provided pain remains absent.

If knee pain persists despite a few to several months of limited activity, arthroscopic evaluation is indicated. At the time of arthroscopy, the articular cartilage over the involved area usually is slightly depressed and somewhat duller in appearance than the normal adjacent articular cartilage. By use of a probe, this area is palpated to determine if the involved area is movable. If no motion is seen at this site, no further treatment is

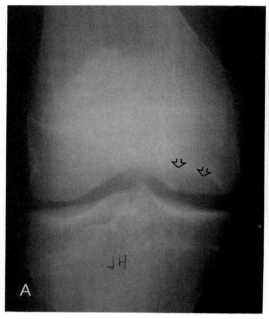

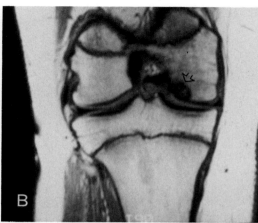

Figure 13.5. **A,** On an anteroposterior knee radiograph, osteochondritis dissecans is seen as a lucent defect (*arrows*) in the subchondral bone of the medial condyle of the femur. **B,** A T1-weighted MR scan shows a low-signal defect (*arrow*) of the subchondral bone of the medial condyle of the femur in this same child.

needed and activity restriction is continued. If motion of this fragment exists with probing, this lesion is either removed or pinned in place. If the segment is removed, fibrocartilage slowly fills in the defect as healing occurs. If a loose body is present from prior detachment of this involved segment, the loose body is removed to avoid further damage to the remaining articular cartilage.

POPLITEAL CYST

A cyst in the popliteal area can be found at any age. This mass is usually an incidental finding by the parents, such as during a bath or when dressing the child. The child generally has no knee pain or limp.

A popliteal cyst always arises from the same location at the posterior aspect of the knee joint. Unlike for adult patients with a popliteal cyst, in whom coexisting intraarticular pathology is present is the majority of cases, a popliteal cyst in a child appears to arise *de novo* and is rarely associated with intra-articular disorders. The base of the cyst initially appears to communicate with the knee joint, but free movement of

the cyst contents back into the knee joint does not occur. This cyst is filled with a clear, jelly-like material as is seen in a ganglion in the wrist area. As the cyst enlarges, it courses between the semimembranosus tendon and the medial head of the gastrocnemius muscle to reach a subfascial position in which it is palpable.

The characteristic physical finding here is a nontender mass in the medial aspect of the popliteal area. With the knee fully extended, this cyst is made most prominent for measurement. Knee motion is not impaired and there are no abnormal findings in the examination of the anterior knee. If the mass is very tender, enlarges rapidly, or is on the lateral aspect of the popliteal region, further workup for a possible soft tissue tumor should be pursued.

Radiographs of the knee are normal except for the presence of a soft-tissue mass on the lateral view. Ultrasound examination clearly indicates a fluid-filled cyst with a wide or narrow neck connecting it to the capsule.

Once the diagnosis of a popliteal cyst has

been made, the child should have the cyst measured for documentation of the size at the first evaluation. Subsequent examination is appropriate in 1 year or if symptoms develop. In the young child, a large percentage of popliteal cysts disappear with no specific treatment, perhaps by rupturing during normal childhood activity. If the cyst is still present by age 8 or 9 or if it has enlarged to an extent that causes symptoms with knee movement, surgical excision is indicated. Even if removed, popliteal cysts may recur.

If a popliteal cyst does develop in a teenager and is associated with any meniscal or ligament injury that causes a chronic knee effusion, treatment of the anterior intra-articular knee abnormality should be the first priority. In a teenage athlete, once the cause of the chronic effusion is corrected, the popliteal cyst will generally resolve without excision, as is often seen in the adult population.

CONGENITAL KNEE DISLOCATION OR SUBLUXATION

Hyperextension of the knees secondary to the intrauterine position of the fetus, usually associated with a breech presentation, may result in anterior dislocation or subluxation of the tibia on the femur. The deformity is obvious at the time of delivery.

Physical examination reveals striking hyperextension of the knees with marked limitation of knee flexion. If subluxation is present, there is more knee flexion possible than if dislocation has occurred. Careful evaluation of the hips is needed because of a high likelihood of congenital hip dislocation in conjunction with the dislocated knees.

Lateral radiographs of the knees will establish the degree of subluxation or dislocation present. Even though the distal femoral and proximal tibial ossification centers may not be present, the relationship of the femoral shaft to the tibial shaft will permit the determination of the degree of displacement present at the knee. Ultrasound examination of the hips should be routinely obtained

in infants with congenital knee dislocation to evaluate for coexisting hip dislocation.

If knee subluxation is present, treatment is usually successful with serial casting, gradually increasing the amount of knee flexion with each successive cast until over 90° is obtained. The amount of knee hyperextension decreases as the flexion increases. Night-time splinting in flexion may be needed for several months, though knee stability and motion are generally satisfactorily regained.

If the knee is dislocated, there is often an associated fixed contracture of the quadriceps muscle and an attenuation of the cruciate ligaments. Surgical lengthening of the quadriceps is needed to reduce many of these dislocations. In children with actual dislocation, some instability of the knee often persists even after treatment.

DISCOID LATERAL MENISCUS

The most common congenital abnormality of the menisci is a discoid lateral meniscus. During fetal development, the lateral meniscus generally develops with a central open area that is present to accommodate the lateral femoral condyle. Instead of being shaped like a doughnut, the discoid lateral meniscus is shaped like a pancake: circular and with normal peripheral contours, but solid in the center.

This condition is not diagnosed at birth, since a discoid lateral meniscus can be present with a normal knee examination. During childhood, symptoms may arise, usually after an injury to the discoid meniscus, which is vulnerable to cartilage tears with normal childhood activity. Usually the child notes a clicking of the knee with or without associated knee pain.

Examination reveals primarily a palpable clunk at the lateral joint line as the knee is flexed and extended. This clunk may also be produced by certain rotational movements with the knee flexed. This clunk is produced by displacement of the entire lateral meniscus or a torn segment of the meniscus as it is squeezed between the lateral femoral condyle and the tibial plateau. Tenderness may be noted at the lateral joint line, particularly if a fresh tear of the meniscus is present.

Radiographs are usually interpreted as normal, but the lateral cartilage space may be wider than normal if carefully measured. Arthrography of the knee (Fig. 13.6A) will confirm the diagnosis, as will magnetic resonance imaging (Fig. 13.6B). Both of these studies will also determine whether or not a tear or degenerative change in the discoid meniscus is present.

If a ''clunk'' is felt and heard with knee movement, but no pain or knee effusion is present, periodic examination can be performed with no active treatment or restriction of activity. However, if pain or a knee effusion is present, the torn portion of the meniscus should be surgically removed to prevent ongoing injury to the articular carti-

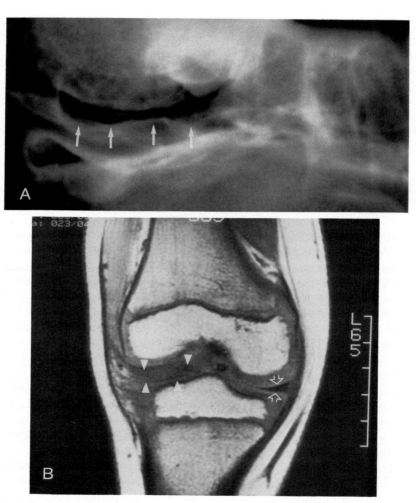

Figure 13.6. **A,** A discoid lateral meniscus (*arrows*) is seen on a knee arthrogram as a thick, disc-shaped negative defect surrounded by contrast material. A normal lateral meniscus appears as a peripheral wedge-shaped structure. **B,** An MR scan shows a discoid lateral meniscus (*arrowheads*) with intermediate signal indicating chronic degenerative change. Compare this to the wedge-shaped medial meniscus (*open arrows*). The normal lateral meniscus should appear wedge shaped in this view.

lage of the femoral condyle. If surgery is needed the peripheral rim of the lateral meniscus is retained if at all possible, since total meniscectomy in childhood often leads to premature degenerative arthritis of the knee.

Traumatic Disorders of the Knee

Traumatic injury of the knee may affect the bone, the articular cartilage, the ligaments, or the menisci. Often, when a knee injury occurs, several of these structures are involved. As a general rule, menisci and ligaments tend to be injured together, while in the case of a fracture, a solitary injury is more common.

DISTAL FEMORAL PHYSEAL FRACTURE

A fracture through the distal femoral physis results from a lateral or medial blow to the knee area. Since the knee ligaments are generally stronger than the physeal cartilage, a physeal fracture occurs in a growing child more often than a collateral ligament tear.

The physical examination demonstrates swelling about the knee with marked pain on attempted movement. No attempt should be made to check the knee range of motion. The point of maximal tenderness is over the physis at the metaphyseal region of the distal femur. Gentle attempts at assessing collateral ligament integrity may demonstrate instability. Particularly if deformity is present at the fracture site, careful evaluation of the neurovascular status of the leg and foot is completed. If this examination is the primary one, a splint should be applied and the child transported to the hospital.

Anteroposterior and lateral radiographs will generally confirm this diagnosis, with mild to marked displacement of the distal femoral physis. However, even if the radiographs are normal, if the examination reveals tenderness over the physis, the diagnosis of a nondisplaced Salter-Harris type I physeal fracture should be made.

Treatment of a nondisplaced physeal fracture consists of 4 weeks of cast immobilization. If this fracture is displaced, operative reduction may be needed to obtain and maintain anatomic reduction, with casting postoperatively.

All growing children with physeal fractures of the distal femur need to be observed for several years after the injury or until skeletal maturity. Although in other long bones, Salter-Harris type I and II fractures rarely lead to growth disturbances, in the distal femur even these fractures commonly cause complete or partial growth arrest at this site. Since this physis accounts for approximately 40% of the growth of the lower extremity, premature closure of this physis will lead to a significant leg length discrepancy.

TIBIAL SPINE FRACTURE

Also known as the intercondylar eminence of the tibia, the tibial spine is the distal site of attachment for the anterior cruciate ligament. If an injury occurs with rotation and knee hyperextension, the anterior cruciate ligament may tear or the tibial spine may fracture. While cruciate ligament tears occur commonly in the skeletally mature teenager by this mechanism, tibial spine fractures are the usual result in the growing child.

Generally, tibial spine fractures occur in children between the ages of 8 and 14 years. Over half of these injuries take place when the child is riding a bicycle. The primary findings on physical examination are pain with movement and an acute knee effusion. If a child in this age group presents with knee swelling and pain after a bicycle accident, a tibial spine fracture should be the diagnosis until proved otherwise.

Anteroposterior and lateral radiographs of the knee will demonstrate the fracture as a radiolucent line extending transversely through the tibial spine. As articular cartilage cannot be seen on radiographs, the size of the fracture fragment is always larger than the radiograph appears to show. If displacement of the fracture is seen on the radiographs, it is possible that the meniscus is interposed into the fracture site. Although MR imaging is not routinely ordered, MR will show the size of the fracture fragment and possible ligament injury.

Treatment of a nondisplaced tibial spine fracture consists of 4 to 6 weeks of immobilization in a long leg cast. If the fracture is displaced, closed reduction is attempted by extending the knee. If closed reduction is unsuccessful, open surgical reduction is needed. Either treatment is followed by immobilization in a long leg cast.

Although these fractures generally heal uneventfully, later follow-up of children with these fractures has shown minimal anterior cruciate instability, indicating that there is often some minor tearing of the anterior cruciate ligament at the same time the tibial spine fracture occurs.

TIBIAL TUBERCLE FRACTURE

A fracture of the tibial tubercle usually occurs in a teenager who is nearing skeletal maturity. Usually the proximal tibial physis begins to close posteriorly, and closure proceeds anteriorly. In this setting, hyperextension of the knee may lead to a fracture through the cartilaginous physis at the tibial tubercle and anterior tibia. The fracture may be intra-articular (similar to a Salter-Harris type III fracture) or may exit through the tibial tubercle itself. While some teenagers with this fracture have had prior symptoms of Osgood-Schlatter disease, the majority have not.

Marked tenderness over the tibial tubercle is found on examination. Pain is present on attempts to actively extend the knee; if the fracture is displaced, active extension of the knee is not possible.

The lateral radiograph will demonstrate the type of fracture present, in particular whether or not the fracture extends into the knee joint. The fracture fragment attached to the patellar tendon will be seen to be displaced anteriorly at the fracture site.

Operative treatment is usually needed to treat this fracture adequately. If the fracture is intra-articular, open reduction and internal fixation are needed for anatomic reduction. However, even if the fracture does not extend into the joint, internal fixation is generally needed to counteract the pull of the patellar tendon and to prevent further displacement of the fracture fragment later. Casting for 4 to 6 weeks after reduction allows adequate healing.

OSTEOCHONDRAL OR CHONDRAL FRACTURE

Chondral and osteochondral fractures of the articular cartilage of the knee may be difficult to detect and diagnose. The chondral or osteochondral fracture fragment is often quite small and, since it contains little or no bone, is difficult or impossible to see on plain radiographs. This injury should be suspected especially after an acute traumatic patellar dislocation. For some reason, this injury is more often seen in soccer players than in other athletes.

Acute knee swelling will occur following this fracture as a result of intra-articular bleeding from the fracture site. Tenderness may be present over the patella or femoral condyle, but the knee effusion is usually too great to allow for clear localization of maximal tenderness. Knee movement is painful.

Unless there is a large enough piece of bone that has detached with the cartilage fragment to allow radiographic visualization, the radiographs are normal except for the knee effusion present. A sunrise view should be attempted to visualize the inferior surface of the patella.

A tentative diagnosis of chondral or osteochondral fracture can be reached if the bloody fluid aspirated from the knee joint contains fat globules. Bloody effusions from injury to intra-articular soft tissue structures do not contain fat, but if the bleeding results from a fracture into the bone marrow, fat will be present.

If fat is present on inspection of a bloody aspirate, further evaluation of the articular surface is indicated, either by magnetic resonance imaging or by arthroscopy. If the diagnosis of chondral or osteochondral fracture is confirmed, surgical treatment is needed. If the fracture fragment is small and emanates from a nonweight-bearing portion of the articular cartilage, it is generally excised. If this piece is large, surgical replacement with internal fixation is indicated.

Failure to diagnose a chondral or osteochondral fracture of the knee in a timely fashion will lead to restriction of knee motion and, perhaps, ongoing articular cartilage injury from the loose body retained within the joint.

PROXIMAL TIBIAL PHYSEAL FRACTURE

Physeal fractures of the proximal tibia are uncommon but are important to recognize because of the neurovascular problems that are often associated with this injury. Even if the fracture appears minimally displaced on the radiographs, popliteal artery injury may occur.

Forced hyperextension of the knee is the cause of this fracture. While in the adult this hyperextension will lead to a knee dislocation, in the growing child a physeal fracture will result, with the tibia distal to the physis being displaced anteriorly. As this anterior displacement occurs, the popliteal artery is stretched (Fig. 13.7). The more the anterior displacement at the fracture site, the higher the risk of distal leg ischemia.

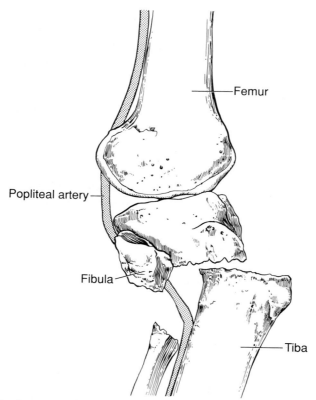

Figure 13.7. The popliteal artery is frequently injured at the time of a displaced fracture through the proximal tibial physis, by stretching as shown in the diagram. An arteriogram of the popliteal area and close observation for a developing compartment syndrome of the leg is indicated when treating a displaced fracture here.

Marked swelling and pain are present around the fracture site. Careful documentation of the presence or absence of the pedal pulses, foot warmth, foot sensation, and toe movement at the initial examination is essential to allow for later comparison in the hours after this injury.

Radiographs will demonstrate the amount of displacement at the fracture site. However, it must be remembered that significantly greater displacement usually occurs in physeal fractures than is seen on the initial radiograph, after the distal fracture fragment has recoiled from its most extreme position of displacement.

Because arterial injury is so commonly associated with a displaced proximal tibial physeal fracture, the author advocates femoral and popliteal arteriography evaluation of the vessels adjacent to the site of the displaced fracture for all patients with this injury. If the arteriogram is abnormal, vascular surgery is performed. Even if the arteriogram is normal, the child requires careful evaluation for the possible development of a compartment syndrome in the leg. (See Chapter 14 on compartment syndromes.)

Urgent operative reduction is generally needed for displaced fractures at this location, with arterial surgery performed at the same time if needed. If either clinical evaluation or direct pressure measurement of the muscle compartments in the leg is indicative of an early compartment syndrome, fasciotomy of the four compartments of the leg is also performed.

As with the distal femur, physeal fractures in the proximal tibia have a propensity to lead to premature physeal closure in the injured area. Follow-up for angular deformity or leg length difference is needed for 2 to 3 years after this fracture.

ACUTE DISLOCATION OF THE PATELLA

Acute patellar dislocation occurs as a result of a sports injury or a fall, usually in the adolescent age group. Dislocation is essentially always in the lateral direction, with the patella coming to rest along the lateral aspect of the lateral femoral condyle.

Initial examination reveals the laterally displaced patella. Pain is present on attempted knee movement, and the leg is preferentially held immobile by the patient. Reduction of this dislocation can generally take place on the playing field by the team doctor, the trainer, or the teenager himself manually pushing the patella medially with the knee fully extended. After patellar reduction has been accomplished, the pain is partially relieved and palpation along the medial aspect of the patella can sometimes determine the amount of medial retinaculum injury associated with this dislocation.

Anteroposterior, lateral, and sunrise-view radiographs of the knee should be obtained after patellar reduction to look for a possible associated osteochondral fracture of the patella or the lateral femoral condyle. If the radiographs show no osteochondral fracture, the bloody effusion from the knee should be aspirated and inspected for fat globules, whose presence would indicate that a chondral or osteochondral fracture had occurred at the time of the patellar dislocation.

If no fracture is present, cylinder cast immobilization with the knee in nearly full extension may allow adequate healing of the injured soft tissues on the medial side of the patella. However, if redislocation occurs later, surgery is needed to tighten the stretched-out medial patellar retinaculum. Another option at the time of the acute dislocation is to surgically repair the torn medial retinaculum, primarily to prevent later dislocation.

PATELLA FRACTURE

Although they are common in adults, transverse or comminuted patellar fractures are uncommon in children. When a patellar fracture does occur in a child, the fracture is generally through the cartilaginous portion of a bipartite patella or through the cartilage at the inferior patellar pole.

With fractures through the bone and cartilage junction in a bipartite patella, pain and tenderness are present on the superolateral aspect of the patella. The bipartite patella can be easily seen on an anteroposterior radiograph of the knee. Since this fracture is generally nondisplaced, the correlation of tenderness in the region of the bipartite patella segment establishes this diagnosis. Treatment is by knee immobilizer until pain and tenderness resolve. Surgery is needed only if displacement of the bipartite segment occurs at the time of injury and interferes with knee motion.

It may be difficult to diagnose the patellar "sleeve fracture," which occurs through the cartilage on the inferior pole of the patella. This fracture is most common in 8- to 12-year-old children. Physical examination will detect tenderness to palpation at the inferior patellar pole, with localized swelling here. Anteroposterior and lateral radiographs of the knee will generally demonstrate a small area of irregular ossification at the inferior patella. While this fracture may contain only a small amount of bone visible by radiography, the distal fracture fragment also includes a large piece of inferior patellar articular cartilage and adjacent retinaculum. Failure to diagnose this "sleeve fracture" will lead to abnormal enlargement of the patella, since the gap formed at the time of the fracture will fill in with bone as healing occurs. Because of this, prompt operative treatment is recommended for these displaced inferior patella fractures.

In the teenager involved with sports such as basketball, tenderness at the inferior edge of the patella may develop as a result of athletic activity. This condition, known as "jumper's knee" or Sinding-Larsen-Johansen syndrome, results from small repeated avulsion fractures at this site, leading to a chronic injury of the patellar tendon. Point tenderness is present at the distal patellar pole. Radiographs may reveal irregular or ectopic ossification within the patellar tendon here.

Normal irregular ossification of the patella is common. As many as six separate ossification centers may be present in the patella, making the differentiation between irregular ossification and a fracture difficult. The rule of thumb is simple: if tenderness is present over these regions, treat the child with short-term immobilization assuming a nondisplaced fracture has occurred.

LIGAMENT INJURY

Although the stability of the knee is dependent on intact ligaments, strong muscles, and normal bony elements, when a sudden or unexpected injury to the knee occurs, the muscles may not have time to react, putting all the stress on the ligaments. If the force of the injury exceeds the strength of the ligaments, partial or complete tearing of one or more of the knee ligaments results.

In a suspected knee ligament injury, a good history of the type of injury incurred and the position of the leg at the time of injury will help point the examiner to the most likely injured areas. If a player is tackled from the lateral side, the medial collateral and anterior cruciate ligaments are most at risk. If the force has struck the tibia from the front, the posterior cruciate ligament will often be damaged. If the knee is fully extended and the athlete rotates the body with the foot planted, the anterior cruciate ligament is most apt to be injured. MR studies are extremely helpful in the assessment of ligament injuries in the knee (Fig. 13.8).

Ligament injuries are commonly grouped into three grades of injury. Mild or first degree sprains result from minor tearing of the ligament. Pain and tenderness are present at the site of injury, as well as localized swell-

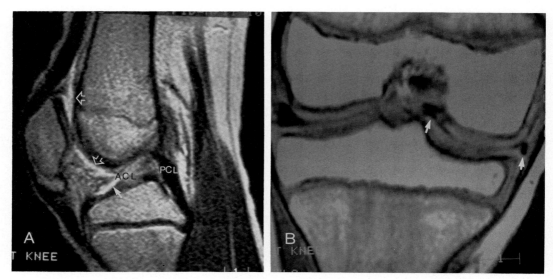

Figure 13.8.   A, A sagittal MR scan of an injured knee shows blood (*solid arrow*) in a fragmented anterior cruciate ligament (*ACL*). The posterior cruciate ligament (*PCL*) is slack. Blood is also present in the joint (*open arrows*). **B,** A coronal MR scan of the same knee shows a torn medial meniscus (*two white arrows*) with displacement of the torn portion into the center of the knee joint.

ing, but no instability of the joint is noted on physical examination. Temporary immobilization of the joint and restriction of activity will allow rapid healing. If athletic activity is reinstituted too quickly, further trauma will turn a first-degree sprain into a more severe ligament injury. With time and adequate activity restriction, full healing is anticipated.

Moderate or second-degree sprains of knee ligaments result if a larger number of ligament fibers are torn, though this injury is still not a complete ligament rupture. Pain and tenderness are greater than with a mild sprain, as is the localized swelling. Bleeding into the joint or adjacent soft tissue often occurs, and restriction of knee motion is present due to the pain. Mild laxity may be noted when testing ligament stability. Immobilization and activity restriction are needed for longer periods than with mild sprains. Prior to beginning sports participation again, complete rehabilitation of lower-extremity muscles is needed to help protect this ligament from re-injury, a common problem with moderate sprains, especially

if even mild ligament instability persists. In some instances, a protective knee brace is needed during sports activities.

Severe or third-degree sprains of the knee ligaments are diagnosed when a total rupture of the ligament has occurred. Pain is marked and obvious instability of the knee is present on physical examination. Radiographs obtained while the knee ligament is being stressed will demonstrate excessive movement. Associated injury to the menisci may be present. Although in some instances an appropriate knee brace may control the instability, surgical treatment is commonly needed to repair a completely torn ligament. Postoperative protection and rehabilitation may require several months until muscle strength is adequate and ligament tensile strength has returned to nearly normal to allow return to sport. If a completely torn ligament is left untreated and the knee instability persists, early degenerative arthritis of the knee is likely to result.

In addition to the severity of the ligament injury, the number of knee ligaments injured has an effect on the prognosis for returning to sports activities. If either collateral ligament alone is torn, recovery is generally quite good with adequate treatment. If one of the cruciate ligaments is also torn in addition to the collateral ligament, instability is greater and full recovery without surgery is less likely, since with cruciate ligament injury, tears of the knee capsule or menisci may be present as well.

If a history of a prior knee ligament injury is elicited at the time of a preparticipation physical examination for high school sports, careful knee evaluation is needed. If instability, pain, or swelling with activity persists as a result of a prior injury, sports requiring sudden changes of direction while running or collision-type sports should generally be avoided, and the teenager should be encouraged to pursue other sport activities less likely to lead to another ligament injury. Each time a ligament sustains an injury, the more likely it is that damage will be permanent, resulting in early degenerative arthritis of the knee. The use of prophylactic knee braces has not been demonstrated to lessen the incidence of football knee injury and may lead to more foot and ankle injuries.

MENISCUS INJURY

Injury to the menisci may occur at the same time as ligament injury or may occur as an isolated problem. In children and teenagers, this injury usually occurs when the body is rotated or twisted at the flexed knee with the foot planted on the ground. This rotation causes the somewhat mobile meniscus to be squeezed between the rotating femur and the intact tibia, leading most often to a longitudinal tear through the meniscus. Horizontal tears occurring through degenerating and aging menisci are the most common type in adults but seldom occur in young patients.

The longitudinal tear in the meniscus may be either through the midportion of the cartilage or along the periphery. The larger the tear, the more likely the torn portion will displace with knee movement. As the knee is flexed, the torn inner portion displaces into the middle of the knee joint. This displaced fragment reduces from the inner joint with knee extension and rotation. As this movement takes place, a palpable clunk will be felt at the joint line adjacent to the injured meniscus and will be noted by the patient. If the torn fragment moves into the middle of the joint and does not reduce, the knee will become "locked," and the patient will be unable to extend the knee until it is "unlocked" with rotation at the knee. These physical findings are nearly pathognomonic for a meniscal injury requiring surgical treatment.

In addition to the findings noted above, a child with a torn medial or lateral meniscus will have tenderness to palpation over the joint line on the injured side. An effusion is usually present. Even if the knee is not fully "locked," the child may lack the final few degrees of full flexion or extension. If the injury is chronic, quadriceps atrophy is usually present.

Radiographs of the knee with only a torn meniscus are normal, with the exception of a possible knee effusion. An arthrogram, performed by injecting radiopaque dye into the knee joint, will demonstrate a meniscal tear, but MR studies are now performed more often to visualize the menisci (Fig. 13.9). The MR image is a very sensitive study for demonstrating even mild injury to the menisci and will clearly show large tears in the meniscal cartilage. The MR image is much superior to the arthrogram in evaluating the integrity of the knee ligaments at the same time.

If a moderate or large tear in the meniscus is demonstrated, surgical treatment is indicated. If the tear is at the periphery of the meniscus, the meniscus should be surgically repaired. Since the peripheral third of the meniscus has a blood supply, healing can be expected after repair and short-term knee immobilization. If the meniscal tear is in the central region or along the inner edge of the meniscus, both of which are avascular

Figure 13.9. In this MR study there is a horizontal tear (*arrow*) through the anterior horn of the medial meniscus (*open arrows*).

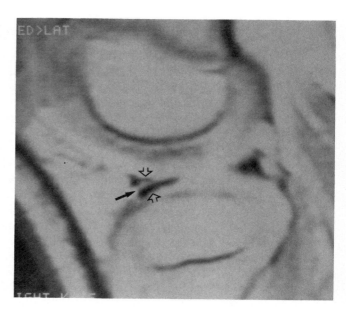

areas dependent on synovial fluid for nutrition, the tear will not heal even if repaired surgically. In these locations, trimming away the torn inner segment of the meniscus, usually through the arthroscope, is the treatment of choice. A decade or two ago, any tear of the meniscus was treated with excision of the entire meniscus, but this treatment is now known to be associated with early onset of degenerative arthritis of the knee in adult life. The torn portion needs to be treated, but total meniscectomy should be avoided if possible.

Following surgical treatment of a meniscal tear, limitation of activity is needed for periods of a few weeks to several weeks. If only a small piece of meniscus on the inner rim has been torn and subsequently been trimmed by arthroscopic surgery, rehabilitation can be started within a day or two of the surgery. However, if the meniscus tear has been repaired, soft-tissue healing is needed before vigorous muscle strengthening is begun. Regardless of the type of meniscal injury treated, thorough strengthening of the lower-extremity muscles must be completed, knee range of motion must be full, and knee effusion should be absent prior to return to sports activities.

BURSITIS

Several bursae are present in the knee area, each of which can become inflamed during activity. Infections may occur in these bursae, and care must be taken to differentiate infection from inflammation. Two of the most commonly involved bursae are the prepatellar bursa and the pes anserinus bursa.

Prepatellar Bursitis

The prepatellar bursa lies superficial to the patella, covered only by skin and subcutaneous tissue. Though less common than chronic bursitis at this site, acute bursitis occurs here following direct trauma to the front of the patella.

Initial treatment consists of the application of ice and a compression dressing, while resting the extremity from activity. Aspiration may be needed if a sizable effusion results, but surgery is rarely needed for acute bursitis. If recurrent direct trauma is expected, knee pads should be worn.

Chronic prepatellar bursitis is the result of repeated mild trauma to the bursal area at this location. Inflammation occurs, which in turn leads to fluid collection within the bursa. Pain will vary and at times will be absent. Aspiration and the application of a pressure dressing may cure this condition. If re-accumulation of fluid occurs, injection of corticosteroids into the bursa after repeat aspiration may help seal the bursal sac walls together and prevent further recurrence. (Corticosteroids should *not* be injected into the adjacent patellar tendon or knee joint.) If the bursa has been stretched excessively by fluid collection, surgical excision of the bursal sac may be needed. Knee padding can sometimes prevent the recurrence of bursal swelling here.

Pes Anserinus Bursitis

The pes anserinus tendinous attachment is formed by the sartorius, gracilis, and semi-tendinosus tendons as they insert onto the proximal tibia medial to the patellar tendon and tibial tubercle. The medial collateral ligament lies directly beneath these tendons with a bursa interposed.

Inflammation of this bursa can occur with direct trauma or with repetitive movements of the knee. Tenderness is present about 1 or 2 cm below the joint line over this bursa. Rotational movements of the flexed knee will increase the pain. Stress testing of the medial collateral ligament will generally not produce pain and will help to differentiate this inflammation from a ligament injury.

In a young child or adolescent, an osteochondroma commonly occurs in the proximal medial tibia location. If it is large enough, the bony exostosis can cause this bursa to become inflamed as the pes anserinus tendons move repeatedly over this prominence. In a child with pain at this site, check carefully for an early osteochondroma or enchondroma, both of which should be seen on radiographs of the knee.

Treatment of pes anserinus bursitis in-cludes rest, application of ice, and administration of oral anti-inflammatory agents as needed. Corticosteroid injection in this region in a child is not recommended. Excision of a bone exostosis at this site may be needed if conservative treatment does not relieve the pain and tenderness.

FASCIA LATA SYNDROME

Although a true bursa does not generally exist in this location, inflammation may develop at the region of the lateral femoral condyle from repetitive movement of the fascia lata over this condyle. This condition is found primarily in joggers and long-distance runners.

Pain and tenderness to palpation over the lateral aspect of the lateral femoral condyle generally will confirm this diagnosis. The stability of the lateral collateral ligament should be checked to ensure that this pain is not from an injury to the proximal end of this ligament. Radiographs of the knee are normal.

Conservative treatment is generally successful. Rest is initially used with oral non-steroidal anti-inflammatory medication. After the pain is gone, careful attention to pre-exercise stretching will diminish the likelihood of recurrent pain when resuming running activity. Surgical treatment is rarely indicated.

Suggested Readings

Baxter, M.P.: Assessment of normal pediatric knee ligament laxity using the genucom. J. Pediatr. Orthop. 8:546-550, 1988.

Baxter, M.P. and Wiley, J.J.: Fractures of the tibial spine in children: an evaluation of knee stability. J. Bone Joint Surg. 70A:228-230, 1988.

Bensahel, H., Dal Monte, A., Hjelstedt, A., et al.: Congenital dislocation of the knee. J. Pediatr. Orthop. 9:174-177, 1989.

Bertin, K.C. and Goble, E.M.: Ligament injuries associated with physeal fractures about the knee. Clin. Orthop. 177:188-195, 1983.

Bradley, J. and Dandy, D.J.: Osteochondritis dissecans and other lesions of the femoral condyle. J. Bone Joint Surg. 71B:518-522, 1989.

Cahill, B.R. and Berg, B.C.: 99m-Technetium phosphate compound joint scintigraphy in the management of juvenile osteochondritis dissecans of the femoral condyles. Am. J. Sports Med. 11:329-335, 1983.

Clark, C.R. and Ogden, J.A.: Development of the menisci of the human joint: Morphological changes and their potential role in childhood meniscal injury. J. Bone Joint Surg. 65A:538-547, 1983.

Dinham, J.M.: Popliteal cysts in children: The case against surgery. J. Bone Joint Surg. 57B:69-71, 1975.

Grace, T.G., Skipper, B.J., Newberry, J.C., et al.: Prophylactic knee braces and injury to the lower extremity. J. Bone Joint Surg. 70A:422-427, 1988.

Hayashi, L.K., Yamaga, H., Ida, K., et.al.: Arthroscopic meniscectomy for discoid lateral meniscus in children. J. Bone Joint Surg. 70A:1495-1500, 1988.

King, A.G.: Meniscal lesions in children and adolescents: A review of the pathology and clinical presentation. Injury 15:105-108, 1983.

Kujala, U.M., Kvist, M., and Heinonen, O.: Osgood-Schlatter's disease in adolescent athletes: Retrospective study of incidence and duration. Am. J. Sports Med. 13:236-241, 1985.

Manzione, M., Pizzutillo, P.D., Peoples, A.B., et al.: Meniscectomy in children: A long term follow-up study. Am. J.Sports Med. 11:111115, 1983.

McCarroll, J.R., Rettig, A.C., and Shelbourne, K.D.: Anterior cruciate ligament injuries in the young athlete with open physes. Am. J. Sports Med. 16:44-47, 1988.

Medlar, R.C. and Lyne, E.D.: Sinding-Larson-Johansson disease: Its etiology and natural history. J. Bone Joint Surg. 60A:1113-1116, 1978.

Riseborough, E.J., Barrett, I.R., and Shapiro, F.: Growth disturbances following distal femoral physeal fracture-separations. J. Bone Joint Surg. 65A:885-893, 1983.

Sandow, M.J. and Goodfellow, J.W.: The natural history of anterior knee pain in adolescents. J. Bone Joint Surg. 67B:36-38, 1985.

Sullivan, J.A. and Grana, W.A.: The Pediatric Athlete. Park Ridge, Ill., American Academy of Orthopaedic Surgeons, 1990.

Suman, R.K., Stother, I.G., and Illingworth, G.: Diagnostic arthroscopy of the knee in children. J. Bone Joint Surg. 66B:535–537, 1984.

14
Lower Leg and Ankle

Sports injuries in children and teenagers occur commonly in the region of the lower leg and ankle. Any running activity places considerable repetitive stress on both the tibia and the ankle and, particularly in the skeletally immature athlete, may lead to injury specific to a growing child.

Anatomy

The tibia and fibula are the skeletal components of the lower leg. The tibia is the prime supporting bone, articulating with the talus at the ankle and the femur at the knee. The fibula, while not essential for weight bearing, serves as the origin or insertion of several muscles and ligaments and contributes to knee and ankle stability. The tibia and fibula are connected by an interosseous membrane, which provides stability and serves as one of the dividers of the muscle compartments of the leg.

The proximal tibial physis accounts for about 60% of the growth of the tibia and about 30% of the growth of the entire leg. When viewed from the lateral side, the proximal tibial physis is continuous anteriorly with the physis below the tibial tubercle. (The proximal tibial articular surface features are described in Chapter 13.)

The distal tibial articular surface is relatively flat and is called the tibial plafond, as it articulates with the superior dome of the talus. The distal tibial physis accounts for approximately 20% of the growth of the lower extremity. On the medial side of the tibial plafond is the medial malleolus, which articulates with the medial aspect of the talus and forms a buttress for the ankle joint on this side.

Proximally, the fibula articulates with the lateral aspect of the tibia to form a joint that allows a small amount of normal rotation. The distal end of the fibula forms the lateral malleolus of the ankle, articulating with the lateral aspect of the talus and providing lateral bony stability.

Several ligaments of the ankle are of major clinical importance. The deltoid ligament is on the anteromedial side of the ankle, just anterior to the medial malleolus, and is composed of deep and superficial portions. The deep deltoid ligament runs from the tibia to the talus, while the superficial portion inserts onto the medial calcaneus. The deltoid ligament is the primary soft-tissue constraint to avoid excessive eversion of the foot at the ankle. The anterior and posterior talofibular ligaments and the calcaneofibular ligament are located on the lateral side and function to resist sudden inversion of the foot at the ankle. The anterior talofibular ligament is just in front of the lateral malleolus, the calcaneofibular ligament is at the tip of the lateral malleolus, and the posterior talofibular ligament is located posteriorly. The anterior and posterior tibiofibular ligaments, also known as the syndesmotic ligaments, stabilize the distal tibia and fibula and prevent divergence of these two bones during ankle movement with walking and running.

The muscles of the lower leg provide control over the movements of the ankle, foot, and toes. Strong fascial structures divide these muscle groups into various compartments containing similarly functioning muscles. There are four major muscle compartments: anterior, lateral, posterior, and deep posterior. The interosseous membrane between the tibia and fibula divide the anterior and lateral compartments from the two posterior ones. Three of the four compartments also contain major arterial, venous, and nerve branches. The nerve and vascular supply of these muscles is generally from the neurovascular structures within that compartment. Because these compartments have strong fascial borders, any incident that will lead to swelling within the compartment may cause serious ischemic injury to the contents of that compartment.

The muscles of the anterior compartment are the tibialis anterior, extensor hallucis longus, and extensor digitorum communis. The latter two muscles dorsiflex or extend the toes, while the tibialis anterior muscle functions mainly as a dorsiflexor of the foot at the ankle. The anterior tibial artery and a branch of the peroneal nerve are located in the anterior compartment.

The muscles of the lateral compartment are the peroneus longus and peroneus brevis, both of which act to evert the foot and provide some foot dorsiflexion. The peroneus brevis inserts onto the base of the fifth metatarsal. The peroneus longus inserts into the plantar medial aspect of the first metatarsal and will pronate the forefoot. The peroneal artery and the deep peroneal nerve are also in the lateral compartment.

The muscles of the deep posterior compartment are the tibialis posterior, providing foot inversion, and the flexor digitorum communis and flexor hallucis longus, providing strong toe flexion and "push-off" when running or walking. The posterior tibial artery and nerve run in this compartment as well.

The posterior compartment consists of the gastrocnemius and soleus muscles, which provide plantar flexion of the foot at the ankle. The strength of the gastrocnemius and the soleus combined is as great as all the other muscles of the leg combined. The posterior compartment muscles are supplied by branches from the posterior tibial artery and nerve.

Physical Examination

Following an injury in this region, the injured leg should be visually compared with the uninjured one. Alignment of the leg is assessed as is localized swelling. The location of an abrasion or bruise will help to determine the likelihood of an important adjacent soft tissue injury.

Especially in the ankle, palpation is an extremely important part of the examination. This is particularly true in trying to differentiate between a physeal fracture and a ligament injury. If tenderness is maximal 1 to 2 cm cephalad to the tip of the lateral or medial malleolus, a physeal fracture can be diagnosed, even if the radiograph shows no displacement here. If the tenderness is mainly *distal* to the malleoli and over the anatomic location of the deltoid ligament (medially) or the talofibular ligaments (laterally), a ligament strain or sprain is the appropriate diagnosis.

With an acute injury, an accurate evaluation of instability is generally precluded because of the pain and swelling present. However, in selected instances, aspiration of the ankle hematoma and infiltration of local anesthetic into the joint can be used to allow a more accurate examination for marked instability, particularly by using the "drawer" test, in which the heel is pulled forward on the tibia.

Even if the ankle is the primary region that appears to be injured, it is important to examine the entire lower leg, particularly the upper fibula, for associated injury.

Assessment for a possible compartment syndrome, in which the internal pressures within one or more compartments may be elevated, is extremely important in any child with a severe contusion to the leg, a tibial or fibular fracture, or a proximal vascular injury. Although the classic descriptions of this syndrome stress the "five P's" (pain, pallor, paresthesias, paralysis, and pulselessness), the appearance of some of these "P's" is indicative that substantial irreversible muscle and/or nerve injury has already occurred. Instead of the "five P's," look first for pain greater than expected or pain that worsens rather than improves over the first 1 or 2 days after injury. Hypesthesia of the dorsum of the toes and marked pain on hyperextension or hyperflexion of the toes are other early signs of elevated compartment pressure. In the majority of compartment syndromes of the leg, pulses are still present in the foot and the foot is warm.

In nontraumatic conditions affecting the lower leg and ankle, evaluation of the child's walking and standing will provide much useful information. Is the progression angle of the foot normal and symmetrical? Is one leg bowed or knock-kneed compared to the other? Check to see if the child can toe-walk (strength of the gastrocnemius) or walk on the heels (strength of the tibialis anterior). If the knee is flexed more on one side than the other during the swing phase of gait, there is likely a partial or complete foot drop, indicating impaired peroneal nerve function. If no gross muscle weakness can be elicited, tape measurement of the calf at the same location on both legs may allow detection of some muscle atrophy or weakness.

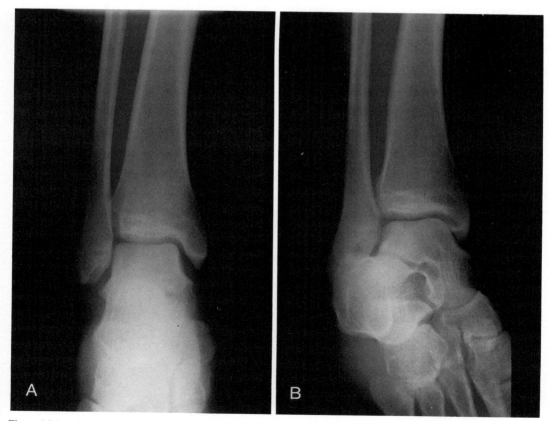

Figure 14.1. **A,** Normal anteroposterior radiograph of an ankle of a skeletally mature teenager. **B,** Normal mortise view radiograph of an ankle of a skeletally mature teenager.

Ankle range of motion should be compared between the affected and normal ankles. Normally, foot dorsiflexion should be approximately 15° above neutral and foot plantar flexion at least 45°. Normal walking

requires 10° of dorsiflexion; if there is less dorsiflexion than this, the child will walk with the foot turned out, in which position it is not necessary to dorsiflex the foot at the ankle throughout the stance phase of gait.

NORMAL RADIOGRAPHIC ANATOMY

Three radiographic views are generally used to assess the ankle for possible traumatic disorders, while two views are usually employed in nontraumatic situations. The anteroposterior and lateral views are standard; the mortise view is obtained by internally rotating the leg 20° compared to the anteroposterior radiograph, since the fibula is positioned posterolateral to the midsagittal line of the tibia. The mortise view is useful to view the entire tibial epiphysis without fibular overlap and to detect any widening of the ankle joint following malleolar fractures (Fig. 14.1).

On the normal anteroposterior view, the distal fibular physis should be positioned at the same level as the tibial plafond or the dome of the talus (Fig. 14.2). The medial malleolus does not fully ossify until late childhood, and more than one ossification center may be present to simulate a fracture (Fig. 14.3). When evaluating physeal fractures of the distal tibia, a comparison radiograph of the normal leg may be very useful. On an anteroposterior radiograph of the en-

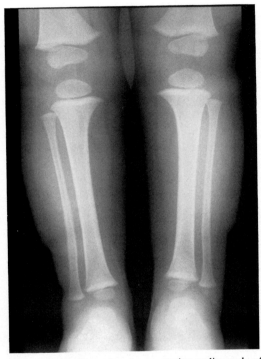

Figure 14.2. Normal anteroposterior radiograph of tibiae, including the knees and ankles. Note that the distal fibular physis is at the level of the tibial plafond.

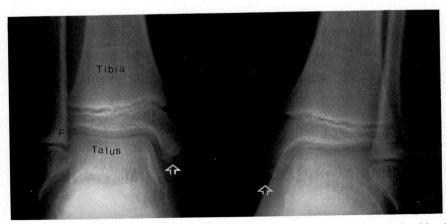

Figure 14.3. Radiograph of the normal ankles of a 10-year-old child shows the articular relationship of the tibia, the talus, and the fibula (*F*). Small, normal accessory ossicles (*open arrows*) are present at the medial malleolus.

tire tibia, the distal tibial plafond is in 0° to 5° valgus compared to the horizontal axis of the proximal tibial articular surfaces.

Traumatic and Sports Injuries

SHIN SPLINTS

This condition, common in teenagers involved with running sports or running for training purposes, is not serious but can interfere significantly with athletic performance. The etiology remains unclear. However, in some cases, athletes have been noted to develop periosteal new bone on the tibia, leading to conjecture that subperiosteal hemorrhage may occur from stress applied with repeated muscle contracture at the origin of that muscle. Other runners have had elevated pressures measured in the muscle compartments of the leg, suggesting that increased tissue pressure and subclinical muscle ischemia may result from this exertional activity.

The runner generally notes the onset of anterior and anterolateral midleg pain during running activity. The muscles in this area may be slightly tender if examined at this time, but pain and tenderness subside quickly with the cessation of running. Pain is rarely present with walking. Range of motion of the ankle and knee are usually normal. Except for occasional cases in which slight periosteal new bone formation is noted in the shaft of the tibia, radiographs are normal. In long-standing cases, the bone scan may show increased activity along much of the anterior proximal tibial shaft, where the muscles originate.

If running is stopped, shin splints will disappear. However, most teenage athletes want to continue to play their sport, and stopping activity is not acceptable. In this case, attention to stretching both the calf and anterolateral muscle groups prior to running is mandatory. Changing the running footwear or the running surface will often relieve this condition. Using a foam pad in the heel of the shoe may be helpful. Applying ice to the leg for a few minutes after running can help decrease any tendency toward muscle edema. With these modifications, shin splints can usually be controlled or relieved sufficiently to allow the teenager to return to sports.

STRESS FRACTURE OF THE TIBIA

A stress fracture of the tibia in a teenage athlete will initially be thought to be shin splints. A stress fracture generally occurs within the first few days of rigorous running as training for a sport and usually occurs in individuals who have not been playing another running sport in the prior months.

A stress fracture of the tibia typically occurs at the junction of the proximal and mid thirds of the tibial shaft. Pain is present a little more proximally than is typical for shin splints, and tenderness is often more on the medial side of the tibia instead of over the anterolateral muscle groups. Pain may be minimal or absent with walking but begins almost immediately after resumption of running activity. Muscle stretching does not lessen the pain with running.

Radiographs will not demonstrate a stress fracture until at least 1 or 2 weeks after the fracture has occurred, since it takes that long for enough periosteal new bone to form at the fracture site to be seen by routine radiography. This new bone formation will lead to the appearance of thickening of the posterior and medial cortex in the proximal to mid tibia, a radiographic picture that is nearly pathognomonic for a stress fracture (Fig. 14.4). A computed tomographic (CT) scan will demonstrate cortical thickening from periosteal new bone with little new bone formation on the endosteal or intramedullary surface.

Once the diagnosis of a tibial stress fracture is made, sports activity must be stopped until healing is complete. Cast immobilization is not necessary or recommended. Crutches may be used initially until pain with weight bearing is absent. Muscle strengthening exercises should be

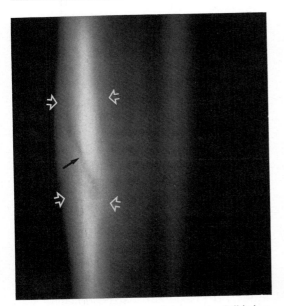

Figure 14.4. This tomogram of the proximal tibia in a teenager with tibial pain for 3 weeks shows marked periosteal thickening (*open arrows*) and a linear stress fracture (*arrow*). The teenager had recently started a job as a valet parker, which necessitated running to retrieve the parked cars.

continued during the period of crutch walking to prevent unnecessary muscle atrophy, so the teenager can return to sports activity in good condition after the stress fracture is healed. Most stress fractures of the tibia should be healed in 6 to 8 weeks.

TODDLER'S FRACTURE

The term "toddler's fracture" has been applied to a spiral fracture of the mid to distal tibia that occurs after mild trauma to a walking child between the ages of 1 and 3 years. The trauma may be as simple as a fall when walking; or the traumatic incident may not have been witnessed, and the parents simply note that the toddler is limping or refusing to walk. In this age group, this fracture should always be included in the differential diagnosis of a limping child.

The child is often unable to tell the examiner where the pain is. Tenderness is present at the mid to distal tibia, as evidenced by increased crying with palpation in this area.

Mild swelling may be present. The child resists attempts of the parents or examiner to place the foot in a weight-bearing position. Because a similar fracture may occur as the result of child abuse, careful examination of the remainder of the body for other evidence of possible abuse is included in the initial evaluation.

Radiographs will generally demonstrate an oblique or spiral fracture involving the mid and distal shaft of the tibia (Fig. 14.5), with almost no displacement. In some instances, the fracture cannot be seen acutely but is noted by the appearance of periosteal new bone formation 1 or 2 weeks later (Fig.

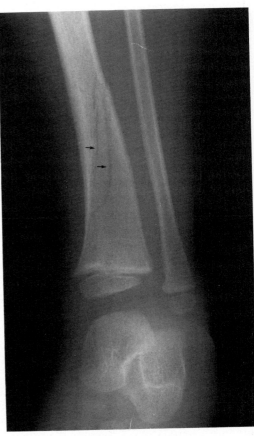

Figure 14.5. This anteroposterior radiograph of the tibia shows an oblique fracture (*arrows*), or toddler's fracture, of the distal tibia in an 18-month-old child who refused to walk after an observed fall.

14.6). In this case, a bone scan will allow earlier diagnosis of a nondisplaced fracture of the tibia. If abuse is suspected, a skeletal survey is obtained to search for other recent or old fractures.

Treatment of a toddler's fracture consists of ruling out the diagnosis of child abuse and applying a long leg walking cast for 3 or 4 weeks. The child will usually begin walking on the cast within a few days of cast application. After fracture healing is complete, the child rapidly returns to full activity. The child may continue walking with the foot turned out for a few weeks, partly due to the habit of walking in the cast and partly due to transient limitation of ankle dorsi-

flexion as a result of the cast. No long-term growth or functional problems are expected as a result of a toddler's fracture.

FRACTURE OF THE PROXIMAL TIBIAL METAPHYSIS

A fracture of the metaphyseal area of the proximal tibia has features that are different from the usual tibial shaft fracture. The primary difference is the tendency for this fracture to develop a progressive valgus deformity after healing has occurred.

The proximal tibial metaphyseal fracture is usually caused by the child being struck on the lateral side of the upper leg, forcing the leg into a valgus position. Physical ex-

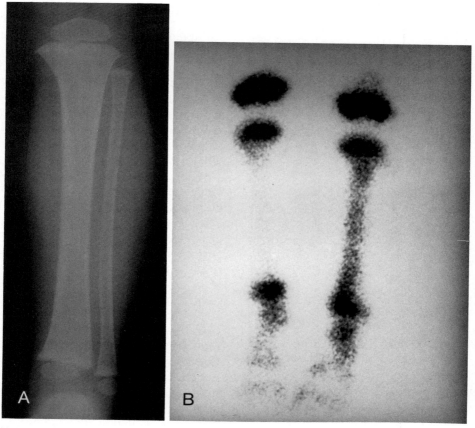

Figure 14.6. **A,** Anteroposterior radiograph of the tibia in a 16-month-old child shows no fracture. The child had refused to walk for 1 week. **B,** The bone scan of the same child shows increased uptake of radioisotope along the length of the tibia, indicating subperiosteal hemorrhage, consistent with the diagnosis of a toddler's fracture.

amination will demonstrate tenderness at the fracture site, but since this fracture is not displaced, deformity will not be apparent. Radiographs will show a nondisplaced fracture of the proximal tibia, sometimes with slight medial opening of the fracture site (Fig. 14.7). The fibula is not fractured.

The initial treatment consists of application of a long leg cast, with an attempt to mold the cast into slight varus. Fracture healing is complete within 4 to 6 weeks after injury. At the time of fracture healing, no angular deformity is noted. However, over the ensuing 12 to 18 months, probably due to overgrowth of the tibia relative to the uninjured fibula, a valgus deformity commonly becomes apparent to the parents and child. Although this valgus deformity may

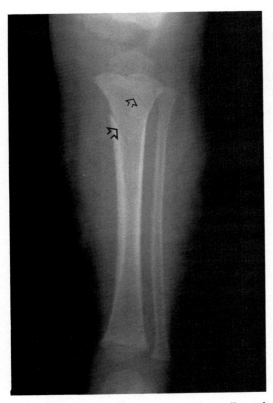

Figure 14.7. An anteroposterior tibial radiograph shows an oblique proximal tibial fracture (*open arrows*) with compression at the fracture site. This type of fracture often later develops a valgus deformity.

be 10° to 20°, no surgical treatment is indicated early, as most of these will remodel back toward a normal alignment within the following 2 to 3 years.

One of the most important features of this fracture is the recognition that a valgus deformity often occurs after healing and the communication of this expectation to the parents of a child with this fracture at the time of the initial treatment.

TIBIAL SHAFT FRACTURE

Fractures of the tibial shaft in children and teenagers more often result from vehicular accidents than from sports activities, but both may cause this injury. The fibular shaft is often fractured as well as the tibia.

If the injury is seen at the accident scene, the playing field, or the emergency room, deformity of the lower leg is often obvious. The skin needs to be carefully inspected for bruises and abrasions, as well as any puncture wound or laceration that would make this an open fracture requiring urgent operative treatment. Distal pulses are evaluated, as is toe movement and sensation. A splint should be applied before transport for radiographs if a splint was not applied at the point of injury.

Radiographs will not only clearly demonstrate the site of the fractures but can also provide clues as to the mechanism of injury (Fig. 14.8). Since a fracture of a long bone generally begins on the tension side (the convex side of a bone that is bent as the result of the force of injury) and propagates at 45° angles to this point, the presence of a triangular-shaped fragment at the fracture site indicates that the injury force came from the same side of the leg as the base of this triangular fragment. Knowing the direction of injury force will lead the examiner to evaluate more carefully the skin and muscle in the area of the leg that was struck by the car or other force causing the fracture.

Closed reduction and application of a long leg cast constitute the general treatment for closed fractures of the tibia and

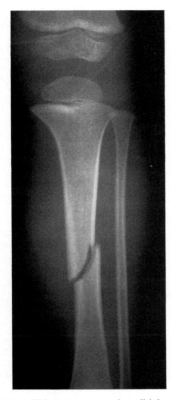

Figure 14.8. This anteroposterior tibial radiograph shows a mid-tibial shaft fracture in a child who was struck on the medial leg by a cart.

fibula. After reduction of displaced fractures of the tibia, elevation of the leg and careful observation for a possible compartment syndrome are needed, especially during the initial 24 hours. As with other fractures, it is important to avoid varus or valgus angulation as the fracture heals. Tibial shaft fractures usually heal in 6 to 8 weeks.

COMPARTMENT SYNDROME OF THE LEG

As noted under Anatomy above, there are four muscle compartments in the lower leg. Each compartment is surrounded by either inelastic fascia or bone, so muscle swelling or hemorrhage into muscle will lead to increased tissue pressures within that compartment. With increasing compartment tissue pressure, the capillary blood flow through the muscles in the compartment decreases; when the tissue pressure outside the capillaries exceeds the capillary blood pressure the capillary blood flow is stopped. Arterial blood continues to flow into the arterial side of the capillary bed to further increase the tissue pressure, and venous outflow becomes blocked as the compartment pressure increases even further. If the compartment muscle tissue pressure exceeds the blood pressure in the arterial branches to these muscles, the arterial flow is also stopped, first on a microscopic level and later with complete loss of arterial blood flow to the foot. This ischemia quickly leads to irreversible muscle and nerve injury if not treated promptly.

The initial physical findings of a developing compartment syndrome are increasingly severe leg pain, hypesthesia over the toes, and marked leg pain with passive hyperextension or hyperflexion of the toes as the involved muscles are stretched. Palpation of the compartments may reveal tense swelling in one or more compartments. In young children or in those with an associated head injury, it will be difficult to accurately assess the child for a possible compartment syndrome. In this situation, a high index of suspicion of a compartment syndrome is necessary and, especially after high-velocity tibial shaft fractures or after fractures with a good deal of soft tissue injury, direct measurement of the compartment pressures is advised.

Direct measurement of compartment tissue pressures is possible by several techniques (Fig. 14.9). Tissue pressures can generally be measured by using an arterial pressure manometer or a central venous pressure manometer. Sterile tubing filled with intravenous fluid is attached to the manometer at one end and an 18-gauge needle is attached at the other. The needle is inserted into the muscle of the compartment in question and the tissue pressure is read on the manometer. More than one needle insertion may be needed to confirm the

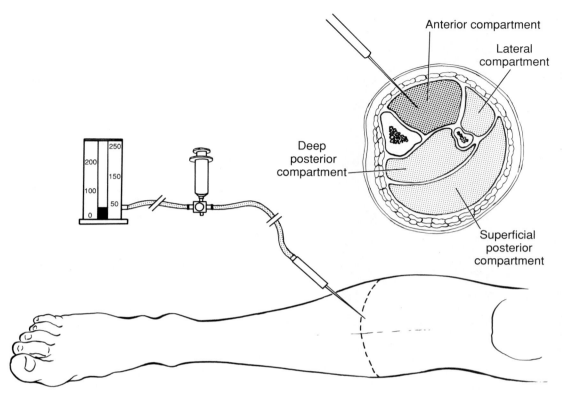

Figure 14.9. Direct measurement of pressures within the muscles of each of the four lower leg compartments is relatively simple to do. The simplest technique begins with aseptic needle insertion into the muscle compartment to be measured. With a fluid-filled line connected to an arterial pressure monitor, the tissue pressure can be readily noted. Fasciotomy is indicated if the compartment pressure is elevated above 30 to 40 mm Hg (see text).

presence of elevated muscle tissue pressure. In general, at least the anterior and the lateral compartments should be tested, but it is preferable to insert the needle into each of the four compartments.

Normal muscle tissue pressures should be below 10 mm Hg. If the muscle pressure is over 30 mm Hg or exceeds two-thirds of the diastolic blood pressure, a fasciotomy (surgical release of the fascial envelope to permit muscle swelling to occur) of the involved compartments should be considered. If the compartment pressure is 30 mm Hg and the child or teenager is in a coma, fasciotomy should be performed. In an alert and cooperative child with compartment pressures of 30 mm Hg, clinical findings should confirm the presence of a compart-

ment syndrome before fasciotomy is recommended, but if the compartment pressure continues to increase, fasciotomy is needed on an emergency basis. Irreversible muscle and nerve damage begins to occur within a few hours of the onset of this elevated compartment pressure and increases with increasing ischemia time. It is important not to be fooled by an intact pedal pulse; arterial blood flow to the foot will not be affected until severe muscle and nerve injury has occurred within the affected compartment, since the tissue pressures have to exceed arterial blood pressure, not only capillary blood pressure, to lead to pulselessness.

If a compartment syndrome is diagnosed, fasciotomy of all four compartments should be performed, generally using a medial and a lateral incision. The incisions are left open for several days until the muscle edema has subsided, at which time skin grafting or delayed wound closure is carried out. Prompt fasciotomy for a compartment syndrome will allow full recovery of muscle function, while a delayed diagnosis may lead to the necessity for a below-knee amputation. The difference between these two outcomes may just be a matter of a few hours, so the presence of a compartment syndrome constitutes a legitimate orthopaedic emergency.

Fractures of the proximal tibial physis, knee dislocations, and displaced proximal tibial shaft fractures are the most common fractures associated with a lower-leg compartment syndrome. If a femoral or popliteal artery injury has led to more than 4 hours of ischemia to the lower leg muscles, a compartment syndrome is a common sequela, and fasciotomy should be performed prophylactically at the time of arterial repair.

DISTAL TIBIAL PHYSEAL FRACTURES

Fractures through the distal tibial physis are relatively common and may occur in a variety of fracture patterns. An accurate assessment of the type of injury present is important, since many of the displaced physeal fractures in this location are best treated surgically. Partial growth arrest at this location following physeal fractures is relatively common, so radiographic follow-up 1 to 2 years after fracture healing is recommended to assess for permanent physeal injury.

Nondisplaced Salter-Harris Type I Fracture

The primary question that arises regarding a child with this injury is whether a ligament sprain or a fracture is present. The ankle is generally mildly swollen and pain is present with attempted weight bearing. The key finding on physical examination is the location of the tenderness to palpation: if the tenderness is worse over the physis than over the ligaments, a physeal fracture is most likely. Radiographs will generally appear normal, though slight widening of the physis may be present (see Fig. 1.5). Treatment with a short leg cast for 3 to 4 weeks will allow complete healing. Growth arrest after a type I fracture in this location is uncommon.

Displaced Salter-Harris Type II Fracture

With this fracture, the epiphysis is usually displaced laterally, with a concomitant fracture of the distal fibular shaft. Deformity is usually obvious and swelling can be marked. Since this is not an intra-articular fracture, closed reduction and casting are attempted initially. However, this fracture has a tendency to slip into a valgus position distally. Many of these fractures require reduction under general anesthesia, and pinning with a smooth Steinmann pin may be needed to maintain the reduction. Immobilization for 3 to 4 weeks with a long leg cast will allow healing.

Salter-Harris Type III or Type IV Fracture of the Medial Malleolus

In the skeletally mature patient, a medial malleolus fracture usually begins at the medial-superior aspect of the ankle mortise and propagates obliquely in a superior and medial direction. If the physis is still open, this type of fracture becomes either a type III or type IV fracture of the distal tibial epiphysis (see Figs. 1.6, 1.7, and 1.8).

It is important not to underestimate the amount of rotation or medial displacement of the medial malleolus on the anteroposterior radiograph here, especially in the young child with incomplete medial malleolus ossification. A comparison view of the normal ankle is helpful in this assessment. A magnetic resonance imaging study will demonstrate this as well but is not generally needed.

Surgical treatment is needed if any displacement of this type of fracture is diagnosed. Because the fracture is intra-articular and the fracture crosses the physis, results are better with surgical management than with closed reduction and casting. Closed reduction and casting of this fracture leads to a much higher incidence of medial physeal growth arrest and angular deformity at the ankle than if surgical treatment is employed.

Salter-Harris Type III Fracture of the Lateral Distal Tibial Epiphysis (Tilleaux Fracture)

This fracture occurs only in the pre-adolescent or adolescent age group, near the time of distal tibial physeal closure. The distal tibial physis begins to close from the medial aspect. If an ankle injury occurs during that period of time, a Salter-Harris type III fracture can result, extending vertically through the mid or lateral aspect of the epiphysis into the physis and then laterally through the portion of the growth plate that has not yet closed.

The diagnosis of this fracture can be difficult. However, if an ankle injury occurs in a child who is mature enough to have started to close off the medial aspect of the distal tibial physis, attention should be drawn to this region for careful assessment. A radiograph with the ankle rotated 20° internally from the anteroposterior position will allow better visualization of the lateral physis here.

Operative reduction and internal fixation are commonly required to adequately treat this intra-articular physeal fracture. Healing occurs in 3 to 4 weeks. Angular deformity does not occur after this fracture, but untreated Tilleaux fractures may lead to premature ankle degenerative arthritis.

Triplane Fracture of the Distal Tibial Physis

This complex fracture is analogous to a Salter-Harris type IV fracture, though it occurs in three planes rather than the usual two planes and therefore may be more diffi-

cult to diagnose accurately. The fracture line extends vertically through the epiphysis, then transversely through a part of the physis, then finally exits vertically through the metaphysis.

Anteroposterior and lateral plain radiographs will demonstrate the fracture. However, a CT scan is often useful to better understand the amount of fracture displacement at the articular cartilage surface and at the physis.

Surgical treatment is needed if more than 1 or 2 mm of displacement at the articular surface is visible on the CT scan or radiographs. Surgery is commonly needed to anatomically reduce the articular surface and the physis. As with other physeal fractures here, healing occurs by 4 weeks after injury. If this fracture is not anatomically reduced, a substantial incidence of premature physeal growth arrest is common.

DISTAL FIBULAR PHYSEAL FRACTURE

Physeal fractures of the distal fibula are essentially always Salter-Harris types I or II. The diagnosis of this fracture can be confused with an adjacent lateral ankle ligament injury. Actually, these two diagnoses can usually be readily separated. If tenderness is maximal 1 or 2 cm cephalad to the tip of the lateral malleolus, a physeal fracture is present. An ankle sprain should be diagnosed only if the tenderness is over the distal tip of the fibula or over the lateral ligament itself.

Radiographs are commonly normal, but a small metaphyseal fragment and slight widening of the physis will confirm the fracture diagnosis. Even with normal radiographs, if the physeal area is tender on examination, a short leg cast should be worn for 3 weeks to allow healing. If growth is arrested as a result of this fracture, the ankle will gradually develop a valgus position as the tibia outgrows the fibula. As with other physeal fractures, a 1- to 2-year follow-up is recommended to enable an early diagnosis of growth arrest when present.

Congenital Disorders

FIBULAR HEMIMELIA

Partial or complete congenital absence of the fibula is a relatively uncommon condition. Even though the fibula is not needed for weight bearing during walking and running, this deformity is often associated with foot and ankle deformities that do limit leg function. Additionally, hypoplasia of the fibula may be associated with a congenital short femur deformity.

Fibular hemimelia varies widely in its severity. With terminal fibular hemimelia, the entire fibula is absent as well as the lateral foot and toes. With the intercalary form of fibular hemimelia, the foot is essentially normal, and variable portions of the fibula are absent. If the distal fibula or lateral malleolus is hypoplastic or absent, the ankle has an insufficient lateral buttress and assumes a valgus position. The tibia is often slightly shorter than on the unaffected side.

Initial radiographs of the leg at birth will demonstrate at least a portion of the congenital deformity. However, there may be a significant amount of fibrocartilaginous anlage for the fibula that is unossified at birth but that will become ossified as the child ages. A magnetic resonance study is useful in this condition to better define what portions of the fibula are present or absent.

Treatment decisions revolve around the effect the hypoplastic or absent fibula has had on the ankle and foot. If the infant is born with the ankle and foot in marked valgus and the lateral part of the foot missing, Syme's amputation is indicated, with preservation of the heel pad at the end of the tibia. Function with prosthetic wear will be nearly normal, including participation in competitive sports, and repeated surgical procedures are not generally needed. If the foot is normal and the ankle is stable, reconstructive procedures to improve the valgus and lengthen the tibia may be indicated. In some cases, the fibrocartilaginous hypoplastic fibula is surgically removed to delay the recurrence of a valgus deformity of the ankle.

Despite the advent of innovative reconstructive techniques proposed and used for this deformity, the parents of a child with this deformity, even of the milder types, should be advised from the time of birth that an amputation of the foot may be needed and will generally result in excellent function. At present, parents seem more willing to accept such an amputation for a male child than for a female child.

TIBIAL HEMIMELIA

Congenital absence of part or all of the tibia is one of the few limb deformities that has a genetic transmission, being inherited in an autosomal-recessive mode. This condition is rare.

At birth, the infant's lower leg is shorter than the normal side and the foot is in varus, with a club foot appearance. The presence or absence of a patella is an important part of the initial examination, since this has ramifications for treatment possibilities. If the initial radiographs of the leg show any ossification of a tibia, a magnetic resonance study should be obtained to establish the amount of cartilaginous tibia present, especially at the proximal end.

Some type of amputation is nearly always the treatment of choice. With complete tibial absence, attempts have been made to transfer the fibula medially to articulate with the femur, a procedure that should not be attempted unless a patella is present. Even if this fibular transfer is "successful" knee motion is never normal and instability or contractures often result later. With complete tibial absence, a knee-disarticulation amputation is usually needed. If a substantial portion of the tibial anlage is present, reconstructive procedures to maintain leg length and perform a more distal amputation may be indicated. Genetic counseling should be provided to parents of an infant with this deformity at birth.

Suggested Readings

Balthazar, D.A. and Pappas, A.M.: Acquired valgus deformity of the tibia in children. J. Pediatr. Orthop. 4:538-541, 1984.

Dunbar, J.S., Owen, H.F., Nogrady, M.B., et al.: Obscure tibial fracture of infants: The toddler's fracture. J. Can. Assoc. Radiol. 15:136-144, 1964.

Engh, C.A., Robinson, R.A., and Milgram, J.: Stress fractures in children. J. Trauma 10:532-541, 1970.

Ertl, J.P., Barrack, R.L., Alexander, A.H., et al.: Triplane fracture of the distal tibial epiphysis: Long-term follow-up. J. Bone Joint Surg. 70A:967-976, 1988.

Gregg, J. and Das, M.: Foot and ankle problems in preadolescent and adolescent athletes. Clin. Sports Med. 1:131-147, 1982.

Hansen, B.A., Greiff, J., and Bergmann, F.: Fractures of the tibia in children. Acta Orthop. Scand. 47:448-453, 1976.

Herring, J.A., Barnhill, B., and Gaffney, C.: Syme amputation: An evaluation of the physical and psychological function in young patients. J. Bone Joint Surg. 68A:573-578, 1986.

Kling, T.F., Jr., Bright, R.W., and Hensinger, R.N.: Distal tibial physeal fractures in children that may require open reduction. J. Bone Joint Surg. 66A:647-657, 1984.

Mubarak, S.J., and Owen, C.A.: Double incision fasciotomy of the leg for decompression in compartment syndromes. J. Bone Joint Surg. 59A:184, 1977.

Rockwood, C.A., Jr., Wilkins, K.E., and King, R.E. (eds.): Fractures in Children, Volume 3. Philadelphia, J.B. Lippincott, 1984.

Schoenecker, P.L., Capelli, A.M., Millar, E.A., et al.: Congenital longitudinal deficiency of the tibia. J. Bone Joint Surg. 71A:278-287, 1989.

Whitesides, T.E., Jr., Haney, T.C., Morimoto, D., and Harada, H.: Tissue pressure measurements as a determinant for the need of fasciotomy. Clin. Orthop. 113:43, 1975.

15
Foot Disorders

A normal foot is essential for normal walking and running. The ability to differentiate between foot conditions that require orthopaedic attention and those that will not lead to functional impairment is useful to the primary care physician. Overtreatment of children with essentially normal foot conditions is as much to be avoided as inadequate treatment of pathologic foot problems.

Anatomy

The foot can be divided into three primary segments: hindfoot, midfoot, and forefoot. Deformity may occur in any of these segments alone or may involve more than one segment (Fig. 15.1).

The talus and the calcaneus are the bones of the hindfoot. The talus articulates proximally with the distal tibia to form the ankle joint. The talocalcaneal joint (often referred to as the subtalar joint), formed by the talus and calcaneus, provides the ability of the foot to invert and evert at the heel, as is needed to smooth the gait when walking on rough or rocky ground. Distally, the talus articulates with the tarsal navicular.

The talus is an unusual bone in that it has no muscular attachments. The proximal or posterior portion of the talus is narrower than the more distal portion. The blood supply to the main body of the talus enters distally at the talus neck region and runs retrograde to supply the body of the talus; consequently, fractures of the talar neck

may disrupt the circulation to the more proximal talus.

The calcaneus is a strong bone that provides the first bony support for the foot when walking, during the heel strike part of the normal gait cycle. The Achilles tendon, formed by the gastrocnemius and soleus muscles, attaches to the posterior aspect of the calcaneus. At this location, in the skeletally immature, a secondary ossification center is present, termed the calcaneal apophysis. No other muscles insert on the calcaneus (Fig. 15.2). In addition to the articulation with the talus noted above, the calcaneus articulates distally with the cuboid bone in the midfoot. On the medial side of the calcaneus, the sustentaculum tali provides some bony support for the talus during weight bearing. On the lateral side of the hindfoot, the hollow area noted in the normal foot is called the sinus tarsi, a region that is often painful to palpation when there is an abnormality of the subtalar joint. At this location, the short toe extensor muscles have their origin.

The midfoot bones consist of the tarsal navicular, cuboid, and the three cuneiforms. The tarsal navicular, positioned between the talus and the medial cuneiform, serves as the insertion of the posterior tibialis tendon on its medial surface. It is at the talonavicular joint that displacement occurs with a clubfoot deformity. The medial cuneiform articulates distally with the base of the first metatarsal and serves as an insertion point for the anterior tibialis tendon. The middle cuneiform articulates distally with

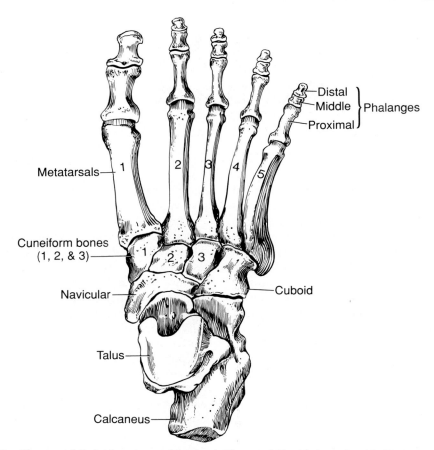

Figure 15.1.   The normal skeletal anatomy of the foot is illustrated (dorsal view). The hindfoot is formed by the talus and calcaneus; the midfoot by the navicular, cuboid, and the three cuneiform bones; and the forefoot by the five metatarsals with their respective phalanges. A line up the long axis of the talus should point toward the first metatarsal and a line up the calcaneus should be directed toward the fifth metatarsal.

the bases of the second and third metatarsal bones. The cuboid articulates distally with the lateral cuneiform and articulates with the fourth and fifth metatarsals.

The forefoot bones include five metatarsals, with distal articulations with their respective phalanges, much like in the hand. Unlike the long bones in the remainder of the extremity, the metatarsals have a growth plate at only one end, proximally in the first metatarsal and distally in the remaining four metatarsals. The peroneus brevis tendon attaches to the base of the fifth metatarsal. The peroneus longus ten-

don inserts into the fifth metatarsal base and continues under the foot to terminate on the plantar aspect of the first metatarsal. The abductor hallucis muscle inserts onto the medial distal aspect of the first metatarsal. The long and short flexors and extensors of the toes attach to the phalanges, as do the intrinsic muscles of the plantar aspect of the foot. Independent motion of individual toes is normally less well developed than in the hand.

Several ligaments or fascial structures are important in the foot. The plantar fascia runs from the plantar aspect of the calca-

neus to the plantar aspect of the first metatarsal and is responsible for maintaining at
least a portion of the normal arch structure
(Fig. 15.2). The deltoid ligament, the major
medial ankle ligament, begins on the distal
tibia, with the deep portion inserting onto
the talus and the superficial portion inserting onto the medial calcaneus. On the lateral
side, the anterior and posterior talofibular
ligaments run between the fibula and the
talus to provide support to the ankle in re-
sisting excessive hindfoot and ankle inversion. The spring ligament is on the medial
plantar aspect of the distal talus and provides support for this region during weight
bearing to help maintain a medial arch. Intermetatarsal ligaments connect the metatarsals distally and prevent splaying of the
foot with weight bearing.

Sensation of the skin on the foot is supplied primarily by the superficial peroneal
and posterior tibial nerves, though smaller
segments are innervated by the sural and
saphenous nerves. In general, the superficial peroneal nerve supplies the dorsum of
the foot and the posterior tibial nerve innervates the sole. When divided into dermatomal innervation, the great toe is supplied
dorsally by the L4 nerve root, the middle
toes by L5, and the lateral toes by S1. The
saphenous nerve usually innervates a portion of the medial heel, while the sural nerve
provides some of the lateral heel sensation.
The motor nerve supply to the intrinsic muscles of the foot is from the posterior tibial
nerve. As a general rule, the deep tendon
reflex at the ankle is a reflection of S1 nerve
root function.

The two major arteries in the foot are the
dorsalis pedis artery, a continuation distally
of the anterior tibial artery, and the posterior tibial artery. Of these two, the posterior
tibial artery is often the predominant blood
supply. These two arteries join together to
form a vascular arch in the foot, so that even
with an injury to one of these vessels, the
blood supply to the foot is generally adequately preserved.

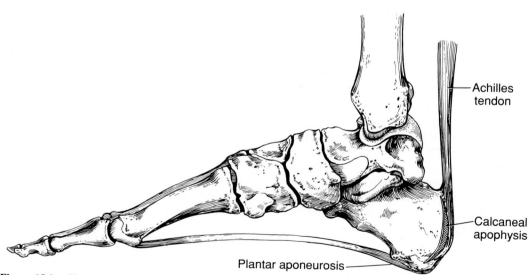

Figure 15.2. The calcaneus provides the site of attachment of the Achilles tendon and the plantar fascia, as
illustrated in this medial view. The Achilles tendon inserts onto the posterior calcaneus and provides strong plantar
flexion of the foot at the ankle. In the skeletally immature child, this attachment is onto the calcaneal apophysis
or secondary ossification center. The plantar fascia runs from the inferior portion of the calcaneus to insert onto
the first metatarsal head, providing support for maintenance of an arch when bearing weight.

Physical Examination

Physical examination of the foot involves identification of foot deformity, evaluation of the foot position in both the supine and standing positions, the dynamic assessment of muscles while walking and by individual testing, and the determination of the neurovascular status of the foot.

OBSERVATION

Are the feet symmetrical in size and shape? Is a toe deformity present? Is the arch higher on one side than the other? With the child standing, observe the child from behind to assess the position of the heel; is it in a neutral position straight down from the calf or is valgus (flat-foot position) or varus present? If valgus of the heel is seen, have the child stand on tip-toes; if the valgus changes to a neutral heel position as an arch forms, no fixed deformity is present. Look on the sole of the foot to see where callosities may be present to demonstrate the areas of the foot that are having pressure applied when walking; normally the heel, the lateral border of the foot, and the metatarsal head regions are the greatest weight-bearing areas of the sole of the foot, and thickening of the plantar skin is present.

Observe the child walking. Normally, the heel strikes the ground first, then the entire foot is on the ground, and finally the heel rises off the ground and the ball of the foot pushes off as the leg swings to the next step. If this normal heel-toe progression is not present on gait observation, check further for muscle weakness, contractures of the ankle, or other foot malfunction. Having the child walk on the heels will assess the function of the anterior tibialis muscle (L4 nerve root or peroneal nerve), while toe walking will assess the strength of the gastrocnemius and soleus muscles (S1 nerve root or posterior tibial nerve). If excessive toe dorsiflexion is seen during the swing phase of gait, suspect some weakness of the anterior tibialis muscle, since this excess toe extensor activity is trying to assist in foot dorsiflexion to clear the foot when swinging forward.

If a high arch, also known as a cavus foot, is seen (particularly if it is seen only on one foot), a careful lower-extremity neurologic examination and a spinal examination are in order, since this high arch is generally a manifestation of imbalance of the muscle function of the foot and toes from an underlying neurologic abnormality, with causes ranging from a peripheral neuropathy to a spinal cord lesion.

PALPATION AND PASSIVE MANIPULATION

If tenderness is present, the exact location is relatively easy to determine, since essentially all foot structures are located just below the skin and are easily palpated. Fractures can be readily located by tenderness to bony palpation or by longitudinal compression along a toe or metatarsal. Passive movement of the foot, ankle, and toes, leading to stretching of an injured or inflamed tendon, will allow localization of these soft-tissue abnormalities.

NEUROLOGIC TESTING

Potential abnormalities of the nerve root levels that contribute to the sciatic nerve (L4 to S2) can be tested quickly by assessing the motor function of the foot and ankle and the sensory status of the foot. Dorsiflexion of the foot at the ankle is primarily accomplished by the anterior tibialis muscle, innervated by L4 and L5. Inversion of the foot by posterior tibialis and great toe dorsiflexion are largely controlled by the L5 nerve root level. Foot eversion is effected by peroneal muscle function, innervated by L5 and S1. Toe walking or foot plantar flexion by the triceps surae muscle relies on S1 and S2 innervation. Abnormalities in sensation over the dermatomal distribution of sensation, as noted in the Anatomy section of this chapter, should be noted. The deep tendon reflex at the knee is primarily related to L4 function and at the ankle to S1 function. The presence or absence of ankle clonus should be tested.

Imaging Studies

The large majority of foot disorders can be adequately assessed and diagnosed by a careful physical examination and by plain radiographs.

As a general rule in a child of walking age and older, standing anteroposterior and lateral radiographs of both feet should be obtained as the initial imaging study for foot evaluation. Since the foot is usually symptomatic when the child is either walking or running, radiographs in the standing position will potentially provide more information than will radiographs obtained with the child lying down.

On the lateral standing radiograph, the angle formed by the intersection of a line drawn along the long axis of the talus and a line along the long axis of the calcaneus should measure between 25° and 45° (Fig. 15.3). A talocalcaneal angle outside this range with the child standing helps to diagnose hindfoot disorders. The angle formed

by lines drawn along the long axis of the first metatarsal and the long axis of the calcaneus on the lateral radiograph is used to quantitate the height of the arch and is useful primarily in evaluating for progression of a pes cavus deformity.

On the anteroposterior standing radiograph, this talocalcaneal angle should measure approximately 25° to 45°, as on the lateral view. Another angle that may be useful is the intermetatarsal angle. In particular, the angle formed by lines drawn up the long axis of the first and second metatarsal shafts, normally measuring under 10°, is useful when assessing a child for bunions (Fig. 15.4). As an indirect measurement of the position of the unossified midfoot bones in the young child, a line along the long axis of the talus should run up the first metatarsal and a line along the long axis of the calcaneus should pass up the fifth metatarsal.

Usually, standing anteroposterior and lateral radiographs of the foot are sufficient to make the appropriate diagnosis. However, special 45° oblique views of the hindfoot and axial views of the calcaneus are useful adjuncts in further evaluating the

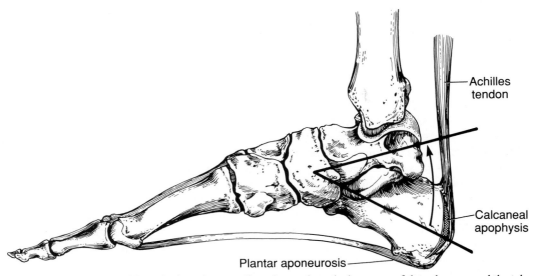

Figure 15.3. When viewed from the lateral aspect, lines drawn along the long axes of the calcaneus and the talus intersect to form an angle, as drawn, that is normally between 25° and 45°.

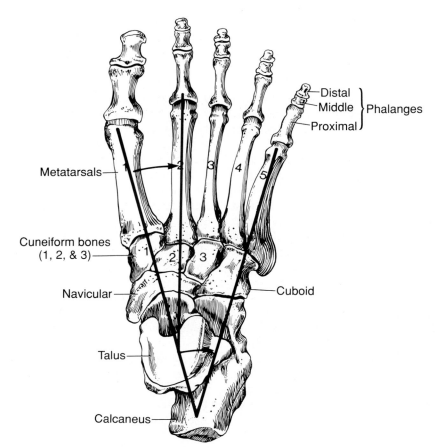

Figure 15.4.   This dorsal view of a foot demonstrates several useful lines to measure on a radiograph. The angle between lines drawn along the first and second metatarsals should normally be less than 10°; in adolescent bunions, this angle is generally larger. A line drawn up the talus should pass into the first metatarsal and a line up the calcaneus should pass into the fifth metatarsal shaft; in the hindfoot, this talocalcaneal angle should be between 25° and 45°.

hindfoot. In conditions of marked valgus foot position, a standing anteroposterior radiograph of the ankle is useful to determine whether the valgus is in the foot or in the ankle. Valgus ankle position is generally limited to children with a neuromuscular disease or with a growth disorder of the fibula.

It is helpful to recall a few facts related to the ossification of some of the bones of the foot. The tarsal navicular, which often has a role in foot deformity, is not ossified until age 3 or 4, so indirect radiographic assessment of its position is needed in the young child. The calcaneal apophysis or secondary ossification center appears by age 8 and fuses with the body of the calcaneus at about age 12 years. The physes of the foot bones are largely closed by a bone age of 12 years, and shoe size should be basically unchanged after this time.

CT scans are used in the foot primarily to assess for possible subtalar joint abnormalities or to further define the extent of bone lesions noted on plain radiographs. Magnetic resonance (MR) studies are excellent in delineating the extent of soft-tissue lesions in the foot and ankle region.

Nontraumatic Foot Disorders

METATARSUS ADDUCTUS

Metatarsus adductus, also referred to as metatarsus varus, is the result of all the metatarsals being directed medially at the junction of the cuneiform bones and the bases of the metatarsal bones. The result of this medial deviation of the forefoot is a kidney bean–shaped foot, with a convex lateral border when viewed from the plantar surface. The midfoot and hindfoot in this condition are normally developed and aligned.

Metatarsus adductus generally results from the intrauterine position of the fetal foot, with the lateral foot border against the uterine wall and the medial foot abutting the shin region. Rarely, congenital bone or soft-tissue deformity may be the cause. Two conditions associated with metatarsus adductus are muscular torticollis and congenital hip dysplasia, so the neck and hips need to be checked carefully when this foot deformity is present.

Metatarsus adductus should be recognizable in the newborn child. Physical examination will reveal an inturned foot. Inspection of the plantar surface will show a convex lateral border and a concave medial border. The heel will be in a neutral position, and ankle motion is normal. Normally, a line along the longitudinal axis of the heel will pass between the second and third toes distally; in metatarsus adductus, this heel bisector line will pass lateral to the third toe, with the severity of the metatarsus adductus classified by noting which of the lateral toes this line passes through (Fig. 15.5).

In addition to estimating the position of this heel bisecting line, the flexibility of the foot deformity is noted. To assess this flexibility, the examiner needs to stabilize the hindfoot by grasping the heel between the thumb and index finger. With the heel stabilized, the forefoot is pushed laterally in an attempt to straighten the foot. The degree of flexibility is the primary determinant of what, if any, treatment is needed.

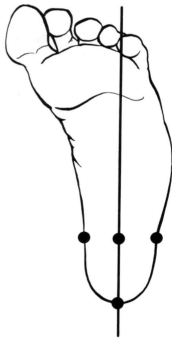

Figure 15.5. The foot illustrated has metatarsus adductus. In the normal foot, a line drawn bisecting the heel, as shown, should pass distally between the second and third toes. In this foot, the line passes more laterally, confirming the diagnosis of metatarsus adductus.

In addition to the most common form of metatarsus adductus resulting from intrauterine molding, other causes of forefoot adduction that may be confused with metatarsus adductus include an atavistic or "searching" great toe noted at the time walking begins, mild clubfoot, or overpull of the posterior tibialis in mild cerebral palsy.

If the forefoot can be overcorrected into valgus so that the lateral foot border becomes concave, the foot is very flexible and will likely require no treatment. With these physical findings, no special shoes are needed and the metatarsus adductus will resolve with growth in virtually all infants.

If the foot with metatarsus adductus can be passively corrected to a neutral position but not into valgus, the foot is termed "moderately flexible." These feet may develop a permanent deformity. However, the initial treatment is to instruct the parents in passive manipulation exercises, by stabilizing the hindfoot and pushing the forefoot laterally, to be performed a few times daily, often at the same time as diaper changes. If, as a result of these stretching exercises, the metatarsus adductus becomes flexible enough to be passively placed into a valgus or overcorrected position, resolution of this condition is expected. If the flexibility does not improve over the first few months with stretching, two or three stretching casts, changed at weekly intervals, will adequately treat this condition. Long-term use of "corrective shoes" is not indicated or needed in this group of children.

If fixed metatarsus adductus deformity persists with attempts at passive correction, active orthopaedic treatment is needed. In the small number of infants that need orthopaedic treatment, the most effective treatment is a series of corrective casts, usually changed weekly for 3 to 6 weeks. Casts are continued until the forefoot can be passively placed in a valgus position and the lateral foot border is straight. After this cast correction has been obtained, reverse-last or straight-last shoes can be used for a few months to help maintain this correction.

Approximately 90% of infants with metatarsus adductus do not need treatment and have gradual resolution of this adducted foot position with growth. These children obviously do not need special shoes or night splints. Reverse-last shoes (shoes that look like they are on the wrong foot) appear to be useful in maintaining the correction obtained by applying casts to feet with stiffer metatarsus adductus, although shoes alone without the casts do not hold the heels tightly enough to allow correction of these feet. In general, reverse-last or straight-last shoes are probably overused by anxious parents and physicians. Remember that nine of 10 feet with metatarsus adductus at birth will improve with no treatment.

If a child had a fixed metatarsus adductus that was not treated with casts as an infant, the child may develop shoe wearing problems in later childhood. The primary problems are callosities over the bony prominence at the base of the fifth metatarsal or over the medial aspect of the first metatarsal head. In some teenagers, this may progress to the formation of a bunion at the medial first metatarsal head as the great toe is pushed laterally (hallux valgus) by the narrowing at the end of most shoes. The cosmetic appearance of the inturned foot, particularly if this affects only one foot, is also of common concern to the child or parents.

Past the age of 1 year, cast correction alone has little effect. Wearing soft-sided shoes or using other shoe modifications may allow relief of pressure over the bone prominences. However, surgical treatment is needed if the metatarsus adductus is severe enough. Although soft-tissue releases at the base of the metatarsals have been used in younger children, corrective osteotomy of all five metatarsals is the most predictably successful surgical procedure to correct residual metatarsus adductus during childhood.

CLUBFOOT DEFORMITY

Largely because it is easier to use than the more technical term talipes equinovarus deformity, the term "clubfoot" is recognized and used by all involved with child care. This term should be reserved for the child with a specific set of physical and radiographic findings and should not be used for a child who has a more mild deformity, such as metatarsus adductus.

A clubfoot has three major components: forefoot and midfoot adductus, heel varus, and heel equinus. The key concept to recall here is that in a child with a clubfoot, the tarsal navicular is located on the medial aspect of the distal talus instead of in its normal position at the distal end of the talus (Fig. 15.6). Since the navicular is located medial to the talus, the remainder of the foot distal to this point is directed medially, re-

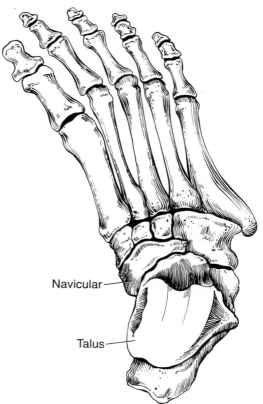

Figure 15.6. In clubfoot deformity, the tarsal navicular has moved medial to the talus, rather than being in the normal position at the end of the talus. This medial navicular movement forces the talus laterally, which in turn pushes the calcaneus into varus and equinus.

sulting in the forefoot and midfoot adductus. (This adduction deformity is different from metatarsus adductus since the medial movement of the distal part of the foot takes place at the talonavicular joint, not at the cuneiform-metatarsal joint.) In this medial position, the navicular forces the talus laterally, which in turn forces the calcaneus downward to assume a varus and plantar-directed position. This hindfoot malalignment results in the equinus and varus position of the heel noted on physical examination. Since these malalignments have been present during at least a part of intrauterine development, contractures occur in the joint capsules, ligaments, and tendons at the foot and ankle, leading to the fixed or rigid clubfoot deformity.

This deformity is common in infants born with neuromuscular conditions, such as spina bifida and arthrogryposis, in which case the cause is assumed to be muscle imbalance resulting from the neurologic or muscular deficit. The etiology of idiopathic clubfoot, occurring in children with no other neurologic or muscular problems, remains unclear.

Several theories have been advanced in an attempt to explain why a clubfoot develops in an otherwise healthy child. The most plausible theories include vascular dysgenesis, asymmetrical skeletal growth in the leg, subclinical neuromuscular disease, and intrauterine position. First, children with clubfoot usually have an abnormal arteriogram of the leg and foot, with absence of one or more of the major terminal branches; perhaps this leads to abnormal development of the soft tissues and bones of the foot, since the clubfoot is always smaller than the normal foot if a unilateral deformity is present. Second, during fetal growth, the fibular side grows longer before the tibial side does. Although the tibial side normally catches up with the lateral side growth, perhaps a minor disturbance at this point in fetal development will lead to a clubfoot position persisting. Third, clinically the calf musculature is always atrophic on the affected side compared to the normal, no matter what treatment is given for the clubfoot; biopsies of calf musculature in children with clubfoot have demonstrated microscopic changes similar to those seen in some neuromuscular diseases. And finally, the effect of the intrauterine position of the foot during fetal growth may play a role in the development of a clubfoot, particularly in unusual clubfeet that are quite readily correctable with casting.

The diagnosis of clubfoot can be readily made at birth. (If the foot is normal at birth and develops an equinovarus deformity later, a thorough search for an underlying spinal cord or peripheral nerve disorder is needed.) The affected foot is shorter than the normal foot and the calf musculature on the affected side has a smaller circumference. The foot is in an equinus position at the ankle and cannot be dorsiflexed to a neutral position. The total amount of ankle movement is less than on the normal side. A skin crease is common at the posterior heel and the medial midfoot regions. When viewed posteriorly, the heel is in varus, and when viewed from the plantar aspect, the lateral foot border is convex and cannot be passively corrected to a neutral position. In fact, the entire foot deformity is quite rigid, with little initial passive correction possible. A careful assessment of the lower back and sacral region for a skin dimple or cutaneous hemangioma is needed in the search for a possible neurologic cause of the clubfoot.

Although they are not usually necessary to make the initial diagnosis of a clubfoot, foot radiographs should be obtained to rule out congenital bone malformations. The lateral radiograph should be obtained while attempting to dorsiflex the foot to simulate weight bearing. In a clubfoot, the talocalcaneal angles on both the anteroposterior and lateral radiographs will be low, often below 10°, on both radiographs (normal is 25° to 45°) (Fig. 15.7). On the lateral view, the distal end of the calcaneus is angled plantarward, correlating with the equinus deformity seen clinically (Fig. 15.8). On the anteroposterior view, the line along the long axis of the talus passes through the fourth or fifth metatarsal shaft instead of the first (Fig. 15.9).

The initial treatment of a clubfoot should begin with corrective cast application in the first day or two after delivery. Prior to the application of a long leg cast, the foot is manipulated to try to improve the foot deformity by moving the navicular from the medial side of the talus to its normal distal

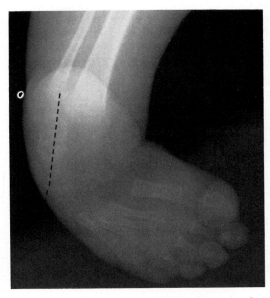

Figure 15.7. This anteroposterior radiograph of a clubfoot deformity shows a talocalcaneal angle of 0° (25° to 45° is normal).

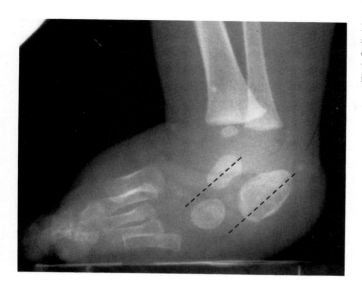

Figure 15.8. Lateral foot radiograph of a clubfoot illustrates the parallel position of the talus and calcaneus with simulated weight bearing. The talocalcaneal angle is near 0°.

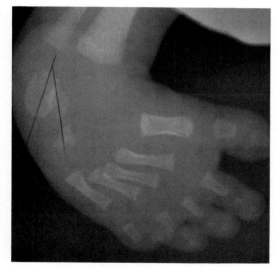

Figure 15.9. This anteroposterior radiograph of a clubfoot demonstrates that a line along the talus points toward the lateral foot, not the first metatarsal.

position. The adduction part of the clubfoot deformity is improved as gradual repositioning of the navicular to a more anatomic position is obtained. After the foot adduction has been improved, the cast is applied each week or two in an attempt to correct the heel varus and equinus.

Several weeks of cast treatment should be attempted, with cast changes each 1 or 2 weeks. After 3 or 4 months of cast treatment, a decision is made either to continue with the cast treatment or to recommend surgical correction at about 6 months of age. Radiographs should be obtained to ensure any apparent clinical correction has resulted in repositioning of the hindfoot bones and has not just molded the pliable soft tissue of an infant's foot. Even if surgical treatment is needed, use of the casts during the first few months of life will have stretched the soft tissue contractures, making surgery easier and safer. Less than 20% of infants with rigid clubfeet at birth can be adequately corrected by nonsurgical means.

Surgical treatment is most commonly performed between the ages of 6 and 12 months of age. Treatment consists of lengthening the Achilles tendon and the posterior tibialis tendon, as well as extensively releasing all the joint capsules of the hindfoot to allow anatomic repositioning of the hindfoot and proximal midfoot bones. Postoperative radiographs will demonstrate a normal realignment of the talocalcaneal angles. Casts are used for 3 or 4 months following surgery to help maintain the corrected position of the foot. In some children, nighttime braces are worn for several months following cast removal, but normal shoes are generally worn during the day.

The functional results of surgery are quite good in about 85% of the children. The affected foot will always be a shoe size or two smaller and the calf muscles will be less developed than on the normal side. The ankle range of motion, though better centered than before surgery, will be less than in the unaffected leg. Despite this, most children will be able to participate fully in desired athletic or work activities. The primary complication of surgical treatment is an excessive flatfoot or valgus position due to overcorrection of the soft-tissue supporting structures of the foot.

A child with a clubfoot in infancy requires periodic follow-up until growth is complete, since recurrent deformity may partially occur as the child grows, making later reconstructive surgery necessary. A rapid recurrence after apparent correction should alert one to assess the lower spinal cord region with an MR study, since conditions such as a spinal cord lipoma, lipomeningocele, or tethered cord may present as a progressive clubfoot deformity.

SUPPLE CALCANEOVALGUS AND FLATFOOT

In the overwhelming majority of times that parents are concerned about the flatfoot appearance of their child's feet, the feet are supple, without fixed deformity, and generally without pain. It is the suppleness or passive mobility of the foot that allows the examiner to differentiate this relatively benign condition from one that will need more extensive orthopaedic care.

This condition is usually noted first by the parents when the child is about a year of age and is just starting to stand and walk. The hindfoot at this age is very supple and can be moved freely into either valgus or varus by passive pressure. When learning to walk, the child usually has a fairly wide-based stance to improve upright balance. In this position, the line of force resulting from body weight passes medial to the ankle and foot, producing a valgus position of the calcaneus when standing. This is not a fixed deformity, and when the foot is not bearing weight the heel is in a neutral position (Fig. 15.10). In this calcaneovalgus position, the foot is everted, with much of the body weight borne on the medial aspect of the foot. The appearance of a flat foot is accen-

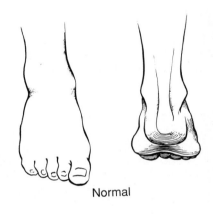

Normal

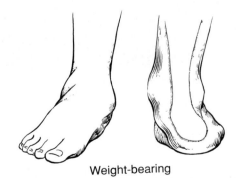

Weight-bearing

Figure 15.10. In a child with a supple calcaneovalgus foot, the foot is normal when not standing or bearing weight. When the child is standing, the heel assumes a valgus position, as illustrated. This is not a fixed foot deformity and rarely requires active treatment or special shoes.

tuated by any external tibial or femoral rotation of the leg and by the relatively large amount of fatty tissue present in the medial foot at this age.

The primary features to note on the physical examination of a child with supple calcaneovalgus are the free mobility of the foot with passive manipulation, normal ankle dorsiflexion, and absence of pain or tenderness. Children with a stiff hindfoot, limited ankle dorsiflexion, and pain have a more serious problem, as discussed in later sections. If the working diagnosis is supple calcaneovalgus, radiographs are not generally obtained, but if obtained they demonstrate loss of a medial arch when standing (Fig. 15.11).

In a child just beginning to walk, initial treatment of this condition consists of explaining the condition to the parents and reassuring them that this is not a serious problem. So-called corrective shoes are not necessary. Annual or biannual examination will generally confirm that improvement occurs within the first year or two of walking, partly through improved stability at the hindfoot and ankle and partly due to placing the feet closer together when standing and walking.

If an older child continues to have some calcaneovalgus of concern to the parents, treatment is rarely instituted unless walking is affected or pain in the foot or calf is present with activity. In these children, as the calcaneus assumes a valgus position, the talus deviates medially and is palpable on the medial aspect of the hindfoot. As the talar head moves medially, the navicular moves laterally, resulting in the loss of any observable arch medially. A standing lateral radiograph of the foot will confirm this loss of the normal arch and may demonstrate a talocalcaneal angle that is greater than 45°.

If the supple heel valgus is marked, the posterior tibialis muscle and tendon, which pass on the medial side of the hindfoot to attach to the tarsal navicular, will demonstrate increased muscular activity to try to support the hindfoot while bearing weight. This may result in fatigue-type pain in the medial calf or ankle area, in which case an orthotic device providing medial arch support can be placed in the shoe to help relieve this muscle overactivity. An argument can also be made that using an orthotic device to place the heel in a neutral position will improve the strength and function of the gastrocnemius by allowing a straighter pull on the Achilles tendon, but the fact remains that most children with mild or moderate

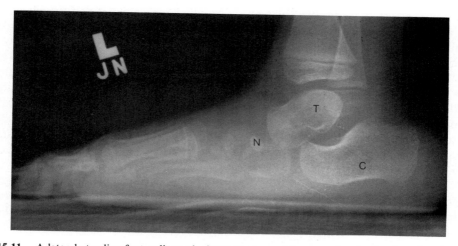

Figure 15.11. A lateral standing foot radiograph shows the loss of the normal arch. *T*, talus; *C*, calcaneus; *N*, navicular.

supple calcaneovalgus are asymptomatic and are able to participate fully in sports using regular footwear.

If an orthotic device is thought to be needed for pain relief in supple calcaneovalgus, the heel must be firmly held by either the orthosis or a firm, snugly fitting shoe heel (not generally possible with athletic shoes). This type of orthotic device should incorporate a heel cup with a medial longitudinal arch support to best provide this heel correction, such as with the UCBL (University of California, Berkeley, Laboratories) orthosis. If only an arch support is used inside a shoe with a loose-fitting heel, radiographs of the foot with the shoe on will show little change in the position of the calcaneus.

If orthotics are ineffective in relieving foot symptoms resulting from a supple calcaneovalgus and flatfoot, surgical treatment may be considered but is not commonly employed in children without neuromuscular or connective tissue disease. Lateral calcaneal lengthening osteotomy can produce arch formation. Fusion of the subtalar joint will stabilize the calcaneus and talus in a neutral position. If foot growth is not complete, an extraarticular subtalar fusion is used to allow further growth, while complete subtalar fusion is employed in teenage patients.

The predisposition to supple calcaneovalgus and flat feet tends to run in families, with either one or both of the parents having a similar condition. There is a higher incidence of supple flat feet in some racial groups. Most adults with these conditions (provided it is a supple and not a rigid foot deformity) do not have pain or other problems, a situation substantiated by the fact that supple flatfoot is no longer a disqualifying condition for military service.

It is important to keep in mind that for most persons this is a benign condition, and the primary care physician should be careful not to overtreat children with this diagnosis. While arch supports and other foot orthotics can be used to relieve pain when present,

there is no evidence that corrective shoes or arch supports will lead to any permanent change in the bony architecture or arch height of the foot.

CONGENITAL VERTICAL TALUS

Although it is uncommon, congenital vertical talus is the most likely cause of a rigid flatfoot in a newborn or young child. This condition, also known as convex pes planus, may occur in otherwise normal children but more often is associated with neuromuscular disorders or syndromes associated with chromosomal abnormalities. The component abnormalities of congenital vertical talus include heel equinus and valgus, midfoot and forefoot abduction, and a "rocker-bottom" appearance to the sole of the foot.

As with a clubfoot, the key anatomic abnormality here occurs at the talonavicular joint. Instead of being displaced medially as in the clubfoot, the tarsal navicular is displaced dorsally in children with congenital vertical talus. The navicular is positioned on the dorsal aspect of the talar neck, forcing the talus plantarward and somewhat medially. In turn, the calcaneus is pushed into an equinus and valgus position (Figs. 15.12 and 15.13).

On observation of the foot, there is no medial arch present and the plantar aspect of the foot is convex, with a "rocker-bottom" appearance. The forefoot may be in a neutral or an abducted position. The most striking feature on passive manipulation of the foot is the rigidity of the deformity present, unlike that seen with supple calcaneovalgus. With congenital vertical talus, the hindfoot has little or no inversion and eversion movement, and the foot is held in a plantarflexed position.

Radiographs will confirm the diagnosis of congenital vertical talus. On a lateral view, the talus is vertically oriented and the calcaneus is also plantarflexed (Fig. 15.14). A line drawn along the long axis of the talus projects well plantar to the long axis of the

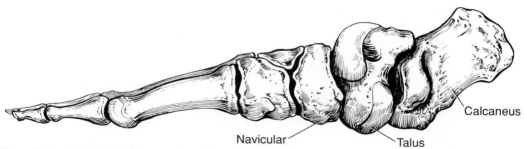

Figure 15.12. This diagram of a lateral view of a foot with a congenital vertical talus illustrates the bony relationships in the midfoot and hindfoot. The navicular is dorsally displaced on the talus, forcing the talus into a vertical position and the calcaneus into an equinus position.

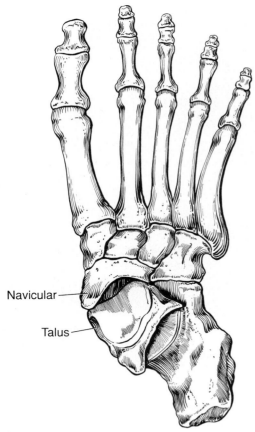

Figure 15.13. The skeletal anatomy of a foot with congenital vertical talus, from the dorsal view, demonstrates the navicular on the dorsal neck of the talus, the talus in a vertical position, and the calcaneus in a valgus and equinus position. The forefoot is in an abducted or valgus position as a result of the navicular moving laterally on the talus at the midfoot level.

first metatarsal, even if a radiograph is obtained with the foot in full plantarflexion. The talocalcaneal angle is greater than 50° on both the lateral and anteroposterior radiographs.

Surgical treatment is needed in children with congenital vertical talus deformity. Stretching casts, holding the foot in the plantarflexed position, are useful to provide soft-tissue stretching prior to surgery at approximately 6 months of age, but the use of casts alone is not effective treatment. The combination of a dorsal talonavicular dislocation and an equinus contracture of the heel cannot be treated appropriately in a nonoperative fashion.

The surgical procedure used here is similar to that employed for a clubfoot deformity. Extensive joint capsular releases, with appropriate tendon lengthenings, allow anatomic repositioning of the hindfoot bones to correct this deformity, though transfer of the anterior tibialis to the talus may be needed to maintain this correction. Postoperative nighttime splinting is often used for several months, but normal shoes are used during the day.

OBLIQUE TALUS

This flatfoot condition is not as flexible as supple calcaneovalgus and not as rigid as congenital vertical talus. The diagnosis of oblique talus is often not made until walking age, at which point the absence of a medial

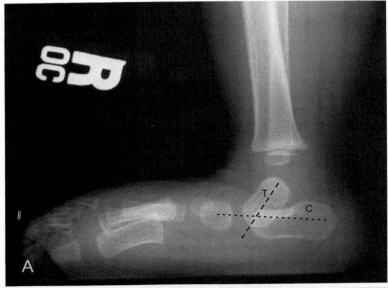

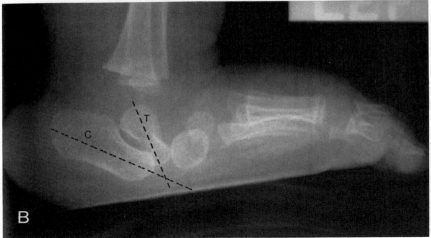

Figure 15.14.   **A,** A lateral foot radiograph shows a congenital vertical talus with the vertically oriented talus (*T*) (*dashed line*), plantarflexion of the calcaneus (*C*) (*dotted lines*), and an increased T-C angle. **B,** A lateral foot radiograph of a congenital vertical talus demonstrates marked equinus of the calcaneus.

arch is noted. While there is a dorsal dislocation of the navicular on the talus in congenital vertical talus, a child with oblique talus has a dorsal subluxation of the navicular at this location, so contact is still present between the articular surfaces of the talus and navicular.

On physical examination, the foot appears flat but does not have a rocker-bottom appearance of the plantar aspect. The forefoot can be passively moved quite easily, though the hindfoot remains in mild equinus. There is more passive subtalar movement possible than with congenital vertical talus.

Lateral radiographs of the foot with the foot in a plantarflexed position allow differentiation of oblique talus from congenital vertical talus. In the neutral position, the line drawn along the long axis of the talus will pass plantar to the first metatarsal in both of these conditions. However, in a child with an oblique talus, as the foot is placed in a plantarflexed position the talonavicular subluxation will reduce so that this talar line will now pass through the long axis of the first metatarsal. In a congenital vertical talus, the radiograph of the foot in a neutral and a plantarflexed position will show no change in this line.

It is most important not to confuse this condition with congenital vertical talus, which requires more extensive surgical treatment. Initial treatment of a child with oblique talus consists of the use of foot orthotics that support the medial longitudinal arch and position the heel in a neutral position. In some cases, limited soft-tissue surgical release in the hindfoot and Achilles tendon lengthening are needed prior to the use of an orthosis.

ACCESSORY NAVICULAR

This condition most commonly presents during childhood or adolescence with a painful flatfoot. Pain is located over the medial aspect of the navicular and is aggravated by activity or sports. The child or the parents have often previously noted a prominence on the medial aspect of the midfoot but generally do not seek medical advice until pain is present.

The tarsal navicular does not begin to ossify until age 3 years and may be formed by more than one ossification center. In some children, the medial aspect of the navicular may be more prominent than usual or may develop into a separate bone or accessory navicular. Since the posterior tibialis tendon normally inserts onto the medial aspect of the navicular, if an accessory navicular is present, the posterior tibialis tendon inserts mainly onto this accessory bone. This tendon insertion is more proximal and plantar than normal and predisposes the child to episodes of pain with activity.

On physical examination, there is a tender bony prominence on the medial aspect of the midfoot and the foot appears to have a lower medial arch than normal. Eversion of the heel or foot will increase the pain at this medial location.

Standing anteroposterior and lateral radiographs will establish the diagnosis of an accessory navicular. A separate ossification center is noted medial to the navicular on the anteroposterior view and in a proximal and plantar position on the lateral view. On the lateral radiograph, the medial arch, as measured by the angle formed by lines drawn up the first metatarsal and the calcaneus, is generally within a normal range, even though the foot appears flat in this condition.

The pain that occurs in association with an accessory navicular is probably best thought of as an overuse syndrome, with resultant inflammation at the site of the aberrant tendon insertion or at the cartilaginous junction between the accessory navicular and the primary navicular.

The initial treatment of pain with this condition is immobilization with a short leg cast for 3 to 6 weeks to allow resolution of the inflammation and relieve the pain. After the pain has resolved, a medial longitudinal arch support can be worn to prevent the recurrence of pain with walking or running activity. If pain recurs, surgical treatment, consisting of removal of the accessory navicular and distal reattachment of the posterior tibialis tendon insertion, is warranted. Treatment of children with an accessory navicular that is asymptomatic is unnecessary.

TARSAL COALITION

The most common cause of a painful, stiff flatfoot after the age of 8 years is tarsal coalition. Although this condition exists from the time of birth, symptoms rarely develop until late childhood or early adolescence. A variety of tarsal coalitions may occur, but all result in limitation of normal hindfoot mobility.

A tarsal coalition results from incomplete formation of the articulation between adjacent hindfoot bones. The two most common types are talocalcaneal and calcaneonavicular coalitions. This condition runs in families and is likely transmitted by an autosomal-dominant type of inheritance. Even though one parent may have a tarsal coalition, symptoms of foot pain may never have been present in that parent and the diagnosis may not have been previously made.

The primary finding on physical examination is the limitation of hindfoot motion with attempts at passive inversion and eversion of the heel. Pain may or may not be present. The heel is generally in valgus, and weight bearing is principally on the medial side of the sole. In about 10 to 20% of patients, spasm of the peroneal tendons may be sufficient to lock the heel in an everted or valgus position that makes passive heel movement impossible, a situation that has led to tarsal coalition being sometimes referred to as peroneal spastic flatfoot.

Although these coalitions are present from the time of fetal development, pain may be absent throughout life. If pain does develop, calcaneonavicular coalitions usually become painful between the ages of 8 and 12 years, while talocalcaneal coalitions are generally symptomatic between the ages of 12 and 15 years. Once pain starts, it is generally aggravated by episodes of increased walking or sports activity.

If limitation of heel inversion and eversion is noted on examination, radiographs of the foot should be obtained. In looking for a tarsal coalition, a complete radiographic series should include standing anteroposterior and lateral views, a 45° oblique radiograph, and an axial view of the heel. Although the coalition cannot usually be seen on the lateral view, beaking of the dorsal edge of the talus at the talonavicular joint is indirect evidence of the presence of a tarsal coalition (Fig. 15.15A). It is presumed that this talar beak formation is a result of cartilage modeling that resulted from increased talonavicular forces due to the absence of normal mobility at adjacent hindfoot joints.

The oblique radiograph will demonstrate a calcaneonavicular coalition well. This coalition may be bony, with complete bone continuity between the calcaneus and the navicular, or fibrous, with narrowing of the normal radiolucent space between these bones. The axial view of the heel is obtained by directing the x-ray beam along the axis of the subtalar joint to visualize the medial and posterior facets of the joint between the talus and the calcaneus. A talocalcaneal coalition is diagnosed if one of these joints is not well visualized on this view.

The axial plane of a computed tomographic (CT) scan is extremely useful in establishing the diagnosis of talocalcaneal coalition and in determining the extent of this coalition prior to surgical treatment. Medial coalitions are most commonly noted at this joint by CT scanning (Fig. 15.15B).

Initially, the pain in a foot with tarsal coalition should be treated with a 6-week trial of immobilization using a short leg cast to relieve the inflammation in the hindfoot region. Since many have tarsal coalition that is never painful, this cast treatment could be the only treatment needed, as the pain may not recur once the inflammation has resolved. If the pain is successfully treated by this cast immobilization method, an orthotic device to support the medial arch may be helpful to prevent the recurrence of pain.

If the cast does not relieve the pain, surgical excision of the bony or fibrous coalition is indicated to help restore normal hindfoot motion. Muscle or fat tissue is inserted in the resection area to prevent reformation of this coalition. The results of resection are better for the calcaneonavicular type of tarsal coalition than for the talocalcaneal type. If pain persists, even after resection of the talocalcaneal coalition, triple arthrodesis is indicated to fuse the talus, calcaneus, navic-

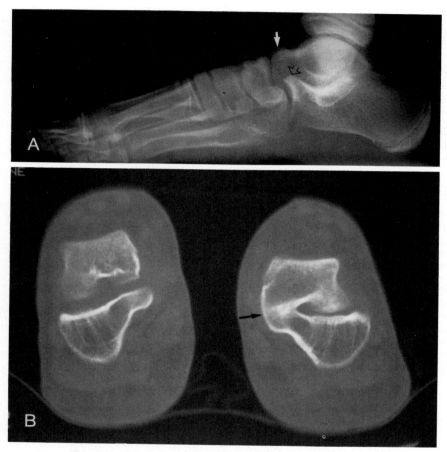

Figure 15.15. **A,** Lateral projection of the foot with tarsal coalition shows beaking of the talus (*arrow*) and calcaneus (*open arrow*), suggesting talonavicular coalition. **B,** A CT scan shows medial bony talocalcaneal coalition (*arrow*). The affected heel is in valgus. Compare with the normal opposite side.

ular, and cuboid together to prevent painful movement in the hindfoot region. While this hindfoot fusion permanently restricts heel inversion and eversion, pain-free activity can be restored.

HALLUX VALGUS, METATARSUS PRIMUS VARUS, AND BUNIONS

A bunion, which is really an inflamed bursa over the medial aspect of the first metatarsal head, results from the use of shoes on a foot with abnormal anatomy of the first metatarsal and the great toe phalanges. Because of the resultant prominence at the first metatarsophalangeal joint, pain results where the shoe comes in contact with this prominence. While bunions are most common in adults, they may develop in some teenagers as well.

The primary reason for the development of bunions in an adolescent is an abnormal medial deviation of the first metatarsal. This may be the result of residual metatarsus adductus of infancy or may be from the presence of metatarsus primus varus. With the first metatarsal deviated medially, the wearing of shoes pushes the great toe laterally. With time, the great toe becomes fixed in this laterally deviated position and is termed a hallux valgus. This leaves the medial aspect of the first metatarsophalangeal joint as the first point of pressure on the shoe, and it is here that a painful bursa or bunion develops. In teenagers, this condition is most commonly seen in those with a pronated forefoot, which further accentuates the prominence at the first metatarsophalangeal joint.

The hallux valgus is easily seen on physical examination. Generally in teenagers, this hallux valgus is worsened by weight bearing, in which position a flatfoot is also commonly seen. Tenderness is present over the bunion on the medial side of the first metatarsal head, where redness of the skin is also often noted. The second toe is often longer than the great toe.

A standing anteroposterior radiograph (Fig. 15.16A) will permit quantitation of the intermetatarsal angle between the first and second metatarsals, as well as the degree of hallux valgus present. Since the intermeta-

Figure 15.16. **A,** Standing anteroposterior radiograph shows increased intermetatarsal angle between the first and second metatarsals, metatarsus primus varus, and hallux valgus (*HV*) (indicated by *dashed lines*). **B,** In this teenager, bunion repair included osteotomy of the first metatarsal (*open arrow*) with alignment of the distal shaft and distal resection of the first metatarsal (*closed arrow*) to relieve the medial prominence.

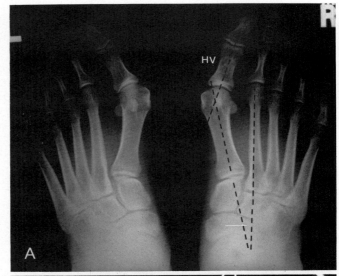

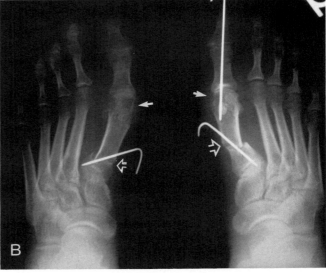

tarsal angle between the first two metatarsals is normally less than 10°, an angle greater than this is termed metatarsus primus varus (Fig. 15.4). The hallux valgus angle is measured by the intersection of a line up the first metatarsal shaft with a line along the long axis of the proximal phalanx of the great toe.

Initially, attempts at footwear modification should be used to relieve the pressure over the first metatarsal head. A medial longitudinal arch support may be useful to prevent excessive pronation of the forefoot, which in turn will diminish the prominence of the first metatarsal head. However, teenage girls will usually be reluctant to wear broad, soft shoes that are not in style and will prefer an attempt at surgical correction.

Surgical treatment consists of a valgus osteotomy at the proximal end of the first metatarsal (Fig. 15.16**B**) to make the first metatarsal more parallel with the second metatarsal shaft, together with resection of a small portion of the medial first metatarsal head and tightening of the medial capsule at this joint to realign the great toe on the end of the first metatarsal. A cast is used for a few weeks until metatarsal union has occurred.

Results of surgical treatment of adolescent bunions are imperfect, with about 50% developing a partial or complete recurrence of this condition. Recurrence is most common if the child has a long second toe or has a flatfoot with heel valgus and forefoot pronation. In teenagers with a flatfoot, the use of a medial longitudinal arch support postoperatively may prevent this recurrence, but most teenage girls do not accept these orthotics readily. In some situations, a calcaneal osteotomy to correct the heel valgus is needed at the same time as the bunion surgery to attempt to ward off a later recurrence.

PES CAVUS ("HIGH-ARCHED FOOT")

Pes cavus is the term used to describe a foot with an abnormally high medial arch.

Anatomically, this appearance of a high arch is caused by a fixed equinus or plantarflexion deformity of the forefoot in relation to the hindfoot.

Approximately 90% of the children with a cavus foot deformity will be found to have an underlying neurologic abnormality as the cause for this foot deformity. The most common causes of cavus foot deformity are peripheral neuropathies, such as Charcot-Marie-Tooth disease, or disorders in the lower spinal cord and cauda equina leading to lumbosacral nerve root dysfunction. *All children with a cavus deformity require a thorough neurologic evaluation to ascertain the cause of the cavus position before this foot deformity is called "idiopathic."*

There are four major types of cavus foot deformity, all resulting from imbalance of the intrinsic and/or extrinsic muscles of the foot. Pure *pes cavus* is diagnosed when the heel is in a neutral position and the forefoot equinus is equal on both the medial and lateral sides. A foot with this deformity will be shorter than normal, and plantar callosities will occur over all the metatarsal heads. With a *cavovarus deformity* the first metatarsal is more plantarflexed than the lateral metatarsals. With standing, the entire foot inverts, including the heel, to allow all metatarsals to bear weight. Even though the foot deformity is primarily in the forefoot, with time the heel may become fixed in this varus or inverted position. A *calcaneocavus deformity* is found mainly in children with prior polio or with spina bifida at the midlumbar level. Because of a lack of function of the gastrocnemius, the calcaneus becomes vertically oriented, raising the forefoot off the ground with weight bearing, resulting in only the heel taking the weight of the body when standing or walking. An *equinocavus deformity*, in which both the forefoot and the hindfoot are in a plantarflexed position, is seen primarily in children with clubfeet from a neurologic cause.

If a cavus foot deformity is noted, a history should be obtained from the family about any other family members that might have a similar foot shape. The family's impression should be sought regarding any worsening that might have occurred, as well as how quickly such changes happened.

The physical examination should concentrate on the neurologic evaluation of the spine and both lower and upper extremities, as well as evaluation of the foot itself. Deep tendon reflexes, muscle strength, and sensory function all should be checked. For example, a child with a peripheral neuropathy due to Charcot-Marie-Tooth disease (one of the more common causes of pes cavus) will have weakness of the peroneal muscles of the foot and may have weakness of the muscles of the hand innervated by the ulnar nerve. The spine needs to be carefully assessed for a possible sacral skin dimple, patches of hair, or other cutaneous markings, all of which may indicate a lower spine and spinal cord lesion that can cause a cavus foot deformity.

When evaluating the foot, the type of cavus (among the four types described above) should be determined. The flexibility or ease of passive correction of the deformity is noted, particularly in the heel region. As a cavus deformity develops, the plantar fascia becomes shortened, in turn leading to a progressive cavus with further foot growth. Even without foot growth, the deformity can worsen as the muscle imbalance becomes more advanced. In the early stages, some passive correction is possible, but the longer the deformity is present, the more rigid it becomes.

In children with a cavovarus deformity, with the medial side of the forefoot in a more plantarflexed position than the lateral side, the heel assumes a varus or inverted position with standing. To determine if this heel varus is a fixed deformity or is only secondary to the forefoot abnormality, the "block test" can be used. The child stands with the lateral half of the foot on a wood block, with the first metatarsal off the edge of the block. If the first metatarsal equinus is the reason

the heel has inverted, the heel should return to a neutral position when the foot is on a block in this position. If the heel remains inverted even with this block test, a fixed deformity is present in the heel as well as in the forefoot.

Associated with a cavus foot deformity and related to the muscle imbalance in the foot is the appearance of *claw toes*. With this deformity, the proximal phalanx moves dorsally while the distal toe becomes more flexed. This leads to a dorsal prominence at the proximal interphalangeal joint, where a callosity often forms due to shoe pressure. In addition, this dorsal movement of the proximal phalanx further depresses the metatarsal head and accentuates the cavus appearance of the foot.

The location of the cavus is best determined from a standing lateral radiograph of the foot; this radiograph is also used to quantitate the amount of cavus present, a measurement that is useful to document progression of the deformity. This "cavus angle," formed by the intersection of lines drawn along the long axis of the first metatarsal shaft and the long axis of the calcaneus, is normally between 30° and 50°.

Special diagnostic studies for pes cavus are largely reserved for the evaluation of the underlying neurologic problem present. Nerve conduction studies and electromyographs, together with an MR study of the lower spine, are the most helpful to discriminate between the large number of neurologic etiologies possible.

Because of the large number of children who have cavus feet caused by a neurologic abnormality, the first step in treatment is to diagnose the exact neurologic condition and to treat it, if either medical or surgical treatment is possible. Unfortunately, many of the neurologic causes of cavus foot deformity are progressive neurologic conditions without a specific treatment or cure.

Shoe inserts may be useful to decrease plantar pain or pain over the heads of the metatarsals with weight bearing. Metatarsal pain can be relieved by a metatarsal pad placed just proximal to the painful metatarsal head in such a way that the pad bears the weight instead of the metatarsal head.

If the cavus deformity continues to worsen or if foot pain is not relieved with shoe inserts, surgical treatment is warranted. Initially, release of the plantar fascia with cast immobilization to correct the cavus deformity can be effective, but with more severe deformity, corrective osteotomies and tendon transfers may be needed.

Pes cavus should be thought of as a marker for a neurologic problem that is usually not diagnosed prior to the appearance of this foot deformity. While high arches can be a normal feature that may run in families, when only one foot has a high arch or if a worsening foot deformity is present, the examiner must be alerted to look into the reason behind this foot abnormality.

CALCANEAL APOPHYSITIS (SEVER'S DISEASE)

Referred to as Sever's disease in the past, this condition, more appropriately termed calcaneal apophysitis, is the most common cause of heel pain in active children between the ages of 9 and 12 years.

The explanation of why pain occurs in the heel area in this age group is akin to the reason for tibial tubercle pain in Osgood-Schlatter disease found in children somewhat older. In the calcaneus, the posterior portion is formed by a secondary ossification center, attached to the main body of the calcaneus by the calcaneal apophysis. The Achilles tendon inserts onto this secondary ossification center rather than onto the main body of the calcaneus (Fig. 15.2). With repetitive stress on this area of tendon insertion, microfractures occur at the apophysis, leading to a localized inflammatory response, the source of the pain and tenderness present here.

This condition generally affects children involved in sports and is seen in boys more than in girls. Pain may be present during participation in the sport or may start shortly after the running activity is completed.

Physical findings are limited to tenderness at the posterior aspect of the heel at any point from the proximal Achilles tendon insertion to the tip of the heel. Pain is worsened by passive ankle dorsiflexion, as this maneuver stretches the gastrocnemius muscle and applies a pull to the calcaneal apophysis.

A lateral radiograph of the foot is normal in this condition. The radiologic diagnosis of Sever's disease was previously made when the secondary ossification center of the calcaneus was fragmented or more radiodense than the rest of the calcaneus. It is now generally recognized that this sclerotic or fragmented appearance is one of a number of normal ossification patterns for this secondary center and should not be used to make the diagnosis of calcaneal apophysitis. Special imaging studies are not used for making this diagnosis.

This condition is a self-limited disorder that resolves when the secondary ossification center fuses with the main calcaneus body at about age 12. Before this age, treatment consists of placing a 0.5-inch foam or felt pad inside the heel of the shoe to elevate the heel enough to eliminate some of the pull of the Achilles tendon on the calcaneal apophysis. The child should stretch the calf muscles prior to engaging in sports activity and may benefit from the application of ice for a short period following exercise. Though this regimen is generally effective, a short leg walking cast can be used for 3 to 6 weeks if pain persists. Surgery is not needed in the treatment of calcaneal apophysitis.

KÖHLER'S DISEASE

Another self-limited condition affecting the young foot is Köhler's disease, characterized by foot pain and radiographic abnormality in the tarsal navicular in children between the ages of 4 and 7 years (Fig. 15.17).

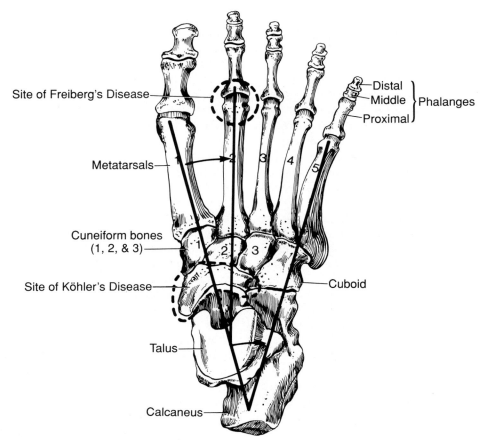

Figure 15.17. Two osteochondritis-like conditions occur at specific locations and at specific ages in children. Köhler's disease occurs in the tarsal navicular between the ages of 4 and 7 years. Freiberg's disease occurs in teenagers at the head of the second metatarsal.

This disorder affects boys more often than girls and is usually first noted because the child is limping. The pain is aggravated by running or other activity. The primary physical finding is midfoot tenderness to palpation, though local edema and increased skin warmth may be noted.

The diagnosis is made by an anteroposterior and lateral radiograph of the foot. The ossification center for the navicular is flattened, is more radiodense than normal, and is often fragmented in appearance. This same finding may be noted bilaterally, even though one foot is free of pain.

If the condition is sufficiently symptomatic, the initial treatment is application of a walking short leg cast for 3 to 6 weeks to decrease the local inflammatory reaction. This may allow complete resolution of symptoms without recurrence. If pain recurs, a second application of a cast followed by application of an orthosis designed to support the midfoot region is often useful in preventing further recurrences.

Children with a radiographic abnormality of the navicular but with no pain need no treatment. The radiographic changes resolve by the time the child is 7 years old.

Surgical treatment is not needed, and no long-term sequelae of Kohler's disease are apparent.

FREIBERG'S DISEASE

Generally occurring in early adolescence, this disorder presents with pain over the metatarsal head region that is greatest when walking or running. There is usually no history of preexisting trauma. The major physical finding is tenderness over the plantar and dorsal aspects of the second metatarsal head (Fig. 15.17).

Anteroposterior and lateral radiographs of the foot establish the diagnosis. Changes of increased sclerosis and partial collapse of the bone of the second metatarsal head can be seen (Fig. 15.18), reminiscent of the radiographic picture seen in other conditions of avascular necrosis of bone. Even though some bone healing may occur over a period of several months, irregularity of the affected metatarsal head will usually persist.

The initial treatment consists of use of an orthotic device inside the shoe to relieve the weight-bearing pressure on the second met-

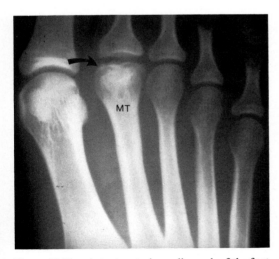

Figure 15.18. Anteroposterior radiograph of the foot with Freiberg's disease in a 15-year-old who had pain when running shows sclerosis and compression of the second metatarsal (*arrow*).

atarsal head. Generally this is effectively done with a metatarsal pad placed just proximal to the second and third metatarsal heads. Running activity should be curtailed. If pain persists or worsens after several months of treatment with this orthotic device and restriction of activity, surgical treatment to relieve the weight-bearing pressure on the second metatarsal head may be warranted.

INGROWN TOENAIL

An ingrown toenail, primarily involving the great toe, is a common problem during late childhood and adolescence. This condition seems to be a particular problem in those involved in sports.

The pain from an ingrown toenail results from localized inflammation and infection at the site of the impingement of the distal toenail on the adjacent skin. Although some toenails seem to have an anatomic predilection to this disorder, the method of cutting the toenail also is a major contributing factor.

On physical examination, the skin adjacent to one side of the nail is red and tender, with a purulent discharge sometimes present. Radiographs are unnecessary.

Treatment consists of care of the localized infection and preventing further impingement of the nail into the skin. Antibiotics are rarely needed. Warm-water soaks two or three times a day help to relieve the inflammation. Usually, a small piece of gauze can be inserted to elevate the nail away from the skin. Placement of this gauze can be facilitated by use of a pointed orangewood stick to lift the edge of the toenail.

Once the acute inflammation and infection have resolved, the teenager should be instructed to always trim the toenail horizontally, leaving the edge of the nail above the level of the adjacent skin. If soaks and nail elevation are ineffective or if this condition recurs, surgical removal of a portion of the nail is effective in curing this condition.

Traumatic Disorders of the Foot

CALCANEUS FRACTURE

Though much less common in children than in adults, a fracture of the calcaneus usually results from a fall in which the heel strikes first upon landing. In the teenager, the presence of a calcaneus fracture should alert the examiner to carefully assess the patient for a thoracolumbar spine compression fracture, a commonly associated injury.

Physical findings include pain with palpation over the heel and often greater localized heel and foot swelling than is seen for other fractures of the foot. Lateral and axial radiographs of the heel will demonstrate the site of fracture and the amount of displacement.

A fracture that is nondisplaced or minimally displaced requires application of a nonwalking short leg cast for 4 to 6 weeks to allow healing. If marked comminution of the calcaneus is present but the subtalar joint is preserved, the cast is applied but it is often several months before swelling has subsided and full weight bearing is completely pain free. If the fracture extends into the subtalar joint and is associated with comminution of the calcaneus, surgery may be needed to realign the articular surface between the talus and the calcaneus in an attempt to delay the onset of degenerative arthritis at this location.

TALUS FRACTURE

A talus fracture is rare but may have serious consequences, the two most common being avascular necrosis and posterior tibial artery injury.

The vascular supply to the talus enters primarily from the distal end, so a fracture through the neck or the body of the talus often leads to avascular necrosis of the main proximal portion of the talus that articulates with the tibia at the ankle joint. This can occur with minimally displaced fractures as well as with those that are severely displaced.

If a child has a fracture-dislocation of the talus, the displaced part of the talus may produce compression of the posterior tibial artery, in turn leading to ischemia of the distal foot. This injury requires urgent attention to reduce the fracture-dislocation and relieve the ischemia.

Radiographs are important for the initial diagnosis of this fracture and for later serial evaluation to assess for possible avascular necrosis. Standard anteroposterior and lateral radiographs will usually demonstrate the fracture site initially, but a bone scan may be needed in pathologic fractures (Fig. 15.19). If no avascular necrosis has occurred, the anteroposterior radiograph of the ankle obtained 6 weeks or more after the fracture will demonstrate a radiolucent line just below the subchondral bone of the talus body. If avascular necrosis has occurred, this radiolucent line will be absent and the avascular bone of the body of the talus will become increasingly radiodense in the ensuing months.

Treatment of a minimally displaced fracture consists of the application of a cast. Weight bearing is not allowed until the fracture is healed and a determination has been made regarding the presence or absence of avascular necrosis. Displaced fractures usually require surgical treatment. If avascular necrosis of the talus occurs, limited weight bearing is needed for several months in an attempt to prevent collapse of the talus as bone healing slowly proceeds.

METATARSAL FRACTURES

Fractures of the metatarsals can be divided into those that affect the fifth metatarsal and those that affect the other four metatarsals.

Fifth Metatarsal Fractures

Fifth metatarsal fractures primarily occur in the proximal third of the metatarsal. The two most common types result from a sudden or forced inversion of the

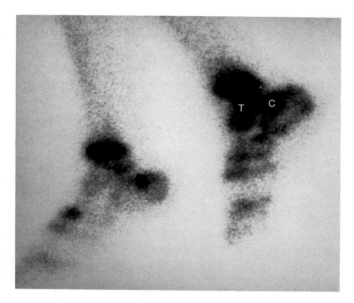

Figure 15.19. Bone scan of a talus fracture in a child with leukemia who experienced sudden pain after a jump shows increased uptake in the talus and superior calcaneus (*T, C*) secondary to compression fractures.

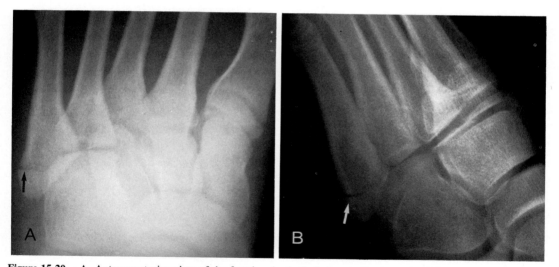

Figure 15.20. **A,** Anteroposterior view of the foot in a basketball player after inversion injury shows transverse fracture of the fifth metatarsal (*arrow*) just distal to the peroneus brevis attachment. **B,** Oblique view of the foot provides a better view of the fifth metatarsal fracture (*arrow*).

foot or ankle, frequently during athletic activity.

The most common type is an avulsion fracture through the base of the fifth metatarsal, just distal to the peroneus brevis tendon insertion. This injury occurs if the ankle or foot is inverted suddenly, resulting in this tendon pulling off a proximal piece of bone at this location. The primary physical finding is tenderness at the base of the fifth metatarsal with pain on attempted passive inversion of the foot.

Anteroposterior (Fig. 15.20A) and lateral radiographs of the foot will generally demonstrate the fracture site, but a 45° oblique view (Fig. 15.20**B**) may be needed if no displacement has occurred. Since a secondary ossification center occurs at or near the site of this fracture, a comparison view of the uninjured foot may be useful.

Treatment of a fracture at the base of the fifth metatarsal consists of application of a short leg walking cast for 3 weeks. Even if the radiograph still shows the persistence of the fracture line, the fracture is healed if the injured area is no longer tender.

The second type of proximal fifth metatarsal fracture is a transverse fracture 1 to 2 cm distal to the peroneus brevis insertion at the base of the metatarsal. Resulting from sudden foot inversion, this fracture occurs mainly in teenagers and often when playing basketball. Tenderness is present directly over the fracture site on physical examination. Radiographs of the foot will establish this diagnosis.

Although a short leg cast is used for this fracture, it is usually necessary for the patient to wear the cast for 6 weeks to complete healing. If the fracture is displaced, surgical treatment is preferred. If a nonunion results at this site after cast treatment alone, operative treatment is required to obtain union.

Other Metatarsal Shaft Fractures

Shaft fractures of the other metatarsals are all treated in a similar manner. These injuries are usually caused by a direct force to the dorsum of the foot, often resulting in more than one metatarsal being fractured.

If one metatarsal fracture is noted, carefully examine the adjacent metatarsals as well. Tenderness will be present over a fracture site but may be difficult to clearly define in a young child. If longitudinal compression of a toe on the metatarsal produces forefoot pain, a fracture is likely present; if this compression is painless, the metatarsal is probably not fractured.

Metatarsal shaft fractures are visualized well by anteroposterior, lateral, or oblique radiographs (Fig. 15.21). Treatment with a short leg walking cast for 3 weeks will permit healing to occur, and normal activity can be resumed. Surgical treatment is needed to treat some displaced fractures, particularly those involving the first and second metatarsals.

PHALANGEAL FRACTURES

Fractures of the phalanges of the toes are common occurrences, usually resulting from stubbing the toe (Fig. 15.22) or from a crushing force on the dorsum of the foot. Swelling and tenderness are present. Ecchymosis is visible within the first day or

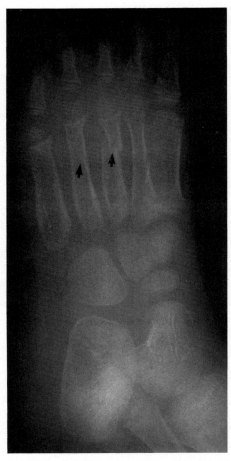

Figure 15.21 Transverse fracture (*arrows*) of the third and fourth metatarsals resulted from a box dropping on the child's foot.

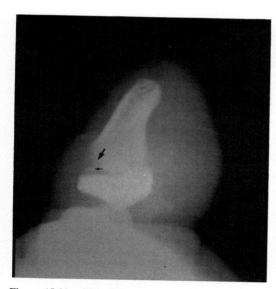

Figure 15.22. This Salter-Harris type II fracture of the physis (*small arrow*) of the distal phalanx of the first toe resulted from a stubbed toe. Nail avulsion occurred at the time of the injury, and osteomyelitis resulted (*larger arrow*) where bone destruction occurred.

two on the injured toe, and the toenail may have a subungual hematoma. Unless a crushing injury has occurred, the fracture is relatively nondisplaced on the anteroposterior and lateral radiographs.

Treatment consists of relative immobilization of the injured toe and the use of firm-soled shoes to limit toe movement when walking. Immobilization of the injured toe is generally adequately accomplished by taping this toe to the adjacent toe(s) for 2 or 3 weeks. A cast can be used but is usually unnecessary. To prevent pain from dorsiflexion of the toe when walking, use a wood-soled fracture shoe or firm-soled shoe, in addition to the tape immobilization.

Suggested Readings

Coleman, S.S. and Chestnut, W.J.: A simple test for hindfoot flexibility in the cavovarus foot. Clin. Orthop. 123:60–62, 1977.

Cowell, H.R. and Wein, B.K.: Genetic aspects of club foot. J. Bone Joint Surg. 62A:1381-1384, 1980.

Cummings, R.J., and Lovell, W.W.: Operative treatment of congenital idiopathic club foot. J. Bone Joint Surg. 70A:1108-1112, 1988.

Gray, D.H. and Katz, J.M.: A histochemical study of muscle in club foot. J. Bone Joint Surg. 63B:417-423, 1981.

Herzenberg, J.E., Goldner, J.L., Martinez, S., et al.: Computerized tomography of talocalcaneal tarsal coalition: A clinical and anatomic study. Foot Ankle 6:273-288, 1986.

Mann, R.A.: Decision-making in bunion surgery. In Greene, W.B. (ed.): American Academy of Orthopaedic Surgeons Instructional Course Lectures, XXXIX. Park Ridge, Ill., American Academy of Orthopaedic Surgeons, pp. 3-13, 1990.

Mosier, K.M. and Asher, M.: Tarsal coalition and peroneal spastic flat foot; A review. J. Bone Joint Surg. 66A:976-984, 1984.

Rushforth, G.F.: The natural history of hooked forefoot. J. Bone Joint Surg. 60B:530-532, 1978.

Scranton, P.E., Jr.: Treatment of symptomatic talocalcaneal coalition. J. Bone Joint Surg. 69A:533-539, 1987.

Seimon, L.P.: Surgical correction of congenital vertical talus under the age of 2 years. J. Pediatr. Orthop. 7:405-411, 1987.

Staheli, L.T., Chew, D.E., and Corbett, M.: The longitudinal arch: A survey of eight hundred and eighty-two feet in normal children and adults. J. Bone Joint Surg. 69A:426-428, 1987.

Vanderwilde, R., Staheli, L.T., Chew, D.E., et al.: Measurements on radiographs of the foot in normal infants and children. J. Bone Joint Surg. 70A:407-415, 1988.

Wenger, D.R., Mauldin, D., Speck, G., et al.: Corrective shoes and inserts as treatment for flexible flatfoot in infants and children. J. Bone Joint Surg. 71A:800-810, 1989.

Williams, G.A. and Cowell, H.R.: Kohler's disease of the tarsal navicular. Clin. Orthop. 158:53-58, 1981.

16
Septic Arthritis and Osteomyelitis

Infections of the long bones of the extremities and adjacent joints are relatively common occurrences during infancy and early childhood. The incidence of orthopaedic infections decreases substantially during the teenage years. An infant or young child who has any alteration of extremity function, such as refusal to walk or refusal to move an arm, should be suspected of having an infection and should be evaluated thoroughly for this possibility. Failure to accurately diagnose and treat osteomyelitis or septic arthritis in a timely fashion may lead to irreparable damage to the joint articular cartilage, the growth plates, or the bone itself.

Etiology

SEPTIC ARTHRITIS

Septic arthritis in childhood usually results from one of three primary causes. The most common cause is hematogenous spread of infection, related to a bacteremia or septicemia produced by an infection or manipulation at a distant site. The joint capsule is very vascular, and bacterial emboli lodge in the vessels of the capsule; clinical infection subsequently occurs as bacteria multiply and white blood cells accumulate within the joint.

Second, septic arthritis may develop from contiguous spread of infection from the adjacent bone affected by osteomyelitis. If osteomyelitis is not adequately treated at an early stage, pus accumulates in the me-taphyseal region and spreads into the joint either by direct passage through the physis and epiphysis into the joint or by rupture through the adjacent cortex and subperiosteal region of the metaphysis into the joint space. Any joint in which the joint capsule attaches onto the metaphysis so that the metaphysis is intracapsular is at risk for early development of septic arthritis in conjunction with an osteomyelitis.

Third, septic arthritis may result from intra-articular injury in which the joint space is contaminated as a result of trauma. This is seen in patients with puncture wounds of a superficial joint, most commonly the knee joint. Even though an object (such as a needle or large wood splinter) that caused the puncture wound is thought to have been removed, incomplete removal of a foreign body or inoculation of the joint with bacteria at the time of the puncture wound may lead to septic arthritis.

OSTEOMYELITIS

Hematogenous spread of bacteria to bone is the most common etiology for osteomyelitis in children. The bacteremia or septicemia may occur during systemic illness with high fevers or may even occur during common activities such as tooth brushing. If the bolus of bacteria to the bone is too great for natural host defense mechanisms, infection ensues.

The role of trauma in childhood osteomyelitis is not yet fully defined. Frequently a child presents with an early bone infection and a history of a recent injury to the affected region. This may be twisting of the leg or arm or a bruise over this region. It has been demonstrated in a rabbit model that a nondisplaced physeal fracture in the tibial region is a significant predisposing factor in the development of experimental osteomyelitis. Trauma likely leads to localized hematoma formation or other susceptibility, allowing osteomyelitis to develop when bacteremia occurs. The lesson for the physician is that even in the presence of a history of trauma, an early bone infection may be present in a child, particularly if some fever is present.

Another important etiology of osteomyelitis is bone infection following an open fracture or a puncture wound. As a general rule, all open fractures should be irrigated and debrided in the operating room within a few hours of the time of injury. Failure to do so predisposes to acute and chronic osteomyelitis.

The same is true of puncture wounds that come in contact with bone. The most common infection following puncture wounds is a *Pseudomonas aeruginosa* osteomyelitis of the calcaneus occurring after a child steps on a nail. Typically the wound is treated with local cleansing and a broad-spectrum antibiotic. However, inoculation of *Pseudomonas* into the calcaneus results from the nail passing through a tennis shoe (from which *Pseudomonas* cultures are frequently positive). Children with puncture wounds of the feet must be carefully observed for this infection (Fig. 16.1). If infection occurs despite appropriate local wound care, irrigation, debridement, and administration of *Pseudomonas*-specific antibiotics are required for adequate treatment.

Children with a suppressed immune system must be closely monitored for possible osteomyelitis. These children are susceptible to generalized sepsis and are less able to wall off infection or to muster an adequate host response to generalized or local infection.

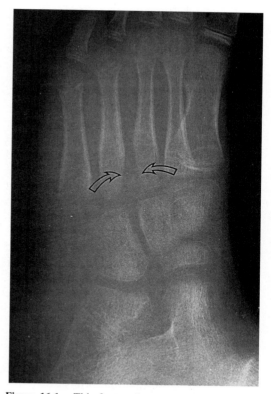

Figure 16.1. This foot radiograph demonstrates osteomyelitis involving the third and fourth metatarsals (*arrows*) 2 weeks after a puncture wound with a nail.

Anatomical Considerations

The anatomical distribution of infection of bone or joints varies as the vascular supply of the epiphysis and metaphysis changes with maturation. This anatomical difference between children less than 12 to 18 months of age and those over 18 months of age is useful in assessing the co-existence of metaphyseal osteomyelitis and septic arthritis.

Before the age of 18 months, there is vascular communication between the metaphysis and the epiphysis. Before significant ossification of the epiphysis occurs, communication is via cartilage canals. As epiphyseal ossification advances, there is continued communication with cartilage canals and with vessels that cross the physis. Because of direct communication between the metaphysis and epiphysis, co-existence of a septic arthritis and osteomyelitis is common. Infections initially begin in the highly vascular metaphyseal region and pass into the epiphysis, then into the joint space.

After the age of 18 months, vascular communication across the growth plate ceases. The vascular supply of the epiphysis is mostly provided by arteries that course in the joint capsule. With maturity the blood vessels of the metaphyseal region, which in the neonate cross into the epiphysis, form a loop and turn back on themselves on reaching the zone of provisional calcification of the growth plate. This loop-like arrangement results in slowing of the blood flow velocity in this area, and increases the likelihood that bacteria will lodge in the metaphysis and develop multiple bone microabscesses, leading to osteomyelitis.

Because there is no vascular communication across the growth plate in the older child, osteomyelitis and septic arthritis coexist less often than in the neonate. However, these conditions can co-exist in specific joints, such as the hip and the shoulder, in which the joint capsule inserts low onto the metaphysis and the metaphysis is intra-articular. If metaphyseal osteomyelitis is not treated in a timely fashion, infection will also destroy and cross the growth plate. The epiphyseal surface may be destroyed sec-

ondary to the effect of bacteria and products of leukocytes released into the joint space as well as from the effect of ischemia from increased intracapsular pressure.

The important point to remember is that in all children with osteomyelitis below the age of 18 months, co-existing septic arthritis of the joint can occur easily. In the neonatal age group, physical examination and imaging studies to delineate these conditions are warranted. In the older child osteomyelitis and septic arthritis generally do not co-exist, as each of these conditions usually occurs by itself.

Pathophysiology of Osteomyelitis

Acute osteomyelitis in children is the result of hematogenous spread of bacteria into bone. However, septicemia or bacteremia alone is generally insufficient to produce bone infection. If bacteremia alone caused osteomyelitis, multifocal bone infection would occur rather than focal involvement of a single bone. It is only in the neonate that involvement of more than one bone is commonly seen. Furthermore, acute osteomyelitis is a childhood disease, rarely seen in the skeletally mature teenager or adult. A predisposing factor in addition to bacteremia must be responsible for osteomyelitis.

The additional factor most commonly im-

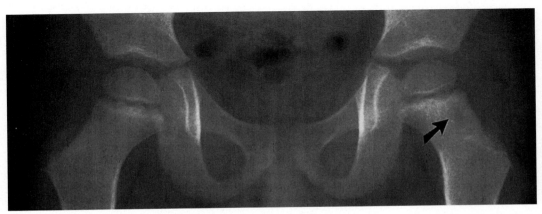

Figure 16.2. Anteroposterior pelvis radiograph shows focal femoral metaphyseal osteomyelitis with local bone destruction (*arrow*) in a 16-month-old child.

plicated is trauma to the area that later develops infection. The trauma may be a subclinical injury to the growth plate resulting from a fall or sports activity. Though this minor injury is not detected clinically, it is believed that a hematoma forms at the site of a physeal microfracture. When bacteremia occurs, the hematoma acts as an inoculum, allowing bacterial growth. The slow, loop-like circulation in the region of the hematoma increases the risk that bacteria will lodge in this region (Fig. 16.2).

When infection begins in the metaphysis, there is rapid bacterial multiplication and a rapid host response with delivery of white blood cells to this region. The formation of micro-abscesses leads to destruction of bony trabecula in this region, and the infection spreads down the shaft of the long bone into the diaphysis and also spreads laterally, rupturing through the cortical margin (Fig. 16.3). Since the cortex of a young child is relatively thin and porous, medullary infection can extend through the porous cortex, producing periosteal elevation and subsequent subperiosteal abscess. If the infection remains untreated, the increasing volume of bacteria and white blood cells within the enclosed space of medullary bone can lead to a sufficient increase in pressure for the vascular supply to this segment of bone to be compromised, with resultant bone ischemia. Additionally, as the abscess spreads within the bone, destruction of the adjacent growth plate can occur, with consequent extension of infection into the epiphyseal region. In some cases in which treatment has been inadequate, a segment of necrotic bone (termed a sequestrum) is walled off by new bone formation (termed an involucrum), and a chronic draining sinus will occur and persist until the necrotic bone has been removed.

It is evident from the manner in which osteomyelitis spreads that the earlier the diagnosis is made, the lower the probability of permanent injury to bone, cartilage, and growth plate.

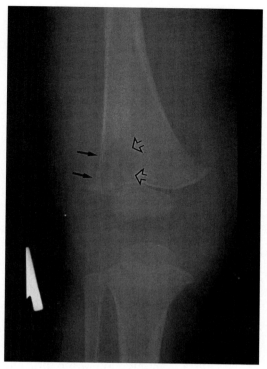

Figure 16.3. Distal femoral metaphyseal osteomyelitis in a 12-month-old child is shown with metaphyseal destruction (*open arrows*) and cephalad spread into the diaphysis, as well as thinning of the lateral cortex (*arrows*). Note also the soft tissue swelling present.

Clinical Presentation

The clinical presentations of septic arthritis and osteomyelitis are similar, varying more with the age of the patient than whether one or the other of these infectious problems is present.

In the neonate and infant, signs of systemic illness may not be as evident as in the older child. A septic infant may appear irritable and not feed well, but often does not have a high fever. The parents usually note that the baby does not move the affected extremity, refusing to kick one of the legs or refusing to use an arm to help hold a bottle or other object. If limited movement of an extremity has been present for more than a few days, significant swelling of the extremity is generally seen.

In a child who is over the age of 1 to 1½ years, systemic symptoms and signs are generally more obvious. The child will look very ill and have a high fever, often in the range of 103° to 104°F. The other common finding noted by the parents is the development of a limp or refusal to walk.

Physical examination cannot clearly differentiate osteomyelitis from septic arthritis, except in the unusual instances in which the infection involves the long bone shaft rather than the metaphyseal region. Soft-tissue swelling is always present in an infection of the bone or joint. There is increased warmth over the area and there is striking tenderness to palpation of the involved region. In a neonate or infant, passive movement of the involved extremity will evoke crying. In the older child, splinting of the extremity to prevent movement is commonly used to avoid pain that is present with motion of the extremity.

Of particular note should be evaluation of the child for an infection of the hip. The hip joint is less easy to palpate, and the diagnosis and treatment of hip infections may be delayed, with a disastrous functional result. An infant or child with swelling in the thigh and refusal to move the lower extremity should be suspected of having septic arthritis of the hip. In the older child, limitation of internal rotation of the hip associated with a fever and refusal to walk should evoke an emergency workup for septic arthritis of the hip or proximal femoral osteomyelitis. In any joint, but particularly the hip or shoulder, delay in diagnosis of septic arthritis is common and results in rapid and extensive destruction of the articular cartilage and the physis.

Laboratory Studies

Laboratory studies that are used to diagnose infection of the bone or joint at an early stage are the white blood cell count and differential and the erythrocyte sedimentation rate. The white blood cell count is elevated with a predominance of polymorphonuclear leukocytes and the presence of band forms. The sedimentation rate, normally below 10 to 15 mm/hr, is significantly elevated.

In a child with suspected infection, early efforts should be made to identify the specific causative bacteria prior to the initiation of antibiotic therapy. Blood cultures should be obtained at initial presentation. When there is no obvious joint effusion, direct aseptic needle aspiration of the tender and swollen area, with the needle proceeding down to bone, may provide a drop or two of blood or purulent fluid that will identify the causative organism. In a febrile child with a joint that is swollen and tender, aspiration of the joint fluid for culture is routine. Cultures for both aerobic and anaerobic bacteria should be obtained as well as a white blood cell count and a Gram stain of the aspirated joint fluid.

Imaging examinations are useful for identification of the site and the extent of infection. In the early stages of osteomyelitis a radiograph will demonstrate normal bone. Soft-tissue swelling is present in the first days of infection; however, radiographic changes in the bone do not occur for 7 to 10 days after the onset of infection. The earliest change seen is periosteal new bone formation resulting from periosteal elevation by a subperiosteal abscess. Periosteal new bone formation takes 1 to 2 weeks to become dense enough to be visualized on radiographs (Fig. 16.4). In cases of septic arthritis, particularly of the hip, lateral displacement of the femoral head from the acetabulum may occur as a result of increased fluid volume within the hip joint. In advanced cases, the femoral head may slip off the metaphysis from damage to the physis. Ultrasonography is very sensitive in the detection of fluid within a joint and serves as a guide as to whether enough fluid is present within the hip joint to attempt needle aspiration.

Radioisotope studies are sensitive and specific in the workup of possible bone and

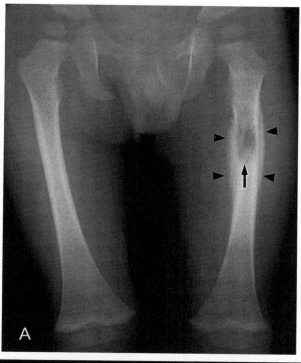

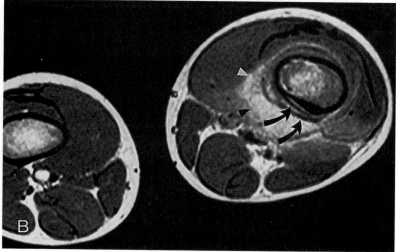

Figure 16.4.   A, This 2-year-old child had been limping for 4 weeks. Radiograph shows chronic medullary osteo-myelitis (*arrow*) and dense periosteal new bone (*arrowheads*) surrounding the area of infection. **B,** Magnetic resonance scan, with a T1-weighted sequence, of chronic osteomyelitis shows medullary destruction of the femur and layered periosteal new bone (*arrows*) around the outside of the femur. Note edema of soft tissues (*arrowheads*).

joint infections. The three-phase technetium bone scan is helpful in diagnosing inflammation or infection in the joint capsule by demonstrating increased uptake during the initial postinjection vascular flow phase and will diagnose early osteomyelitis by showing increased radioisotope uptake in the affected bone in delayed images. Abnormalities are noted on bone scans several days before the changes are visible on radiographs. A gallium scan requires 48 hours for determination of a site of infection but is useful if the technetium scan does not specifically demonstrate an infection in a child in whom a bone or joint infection is considered likely. Scans with indium-labeled white blood cells can localize white blood cell aggregation at the site of localized infection.

Organisms versus Age

Though it is preferable to obtain positive cultures for specific identification of the bacteria causing septic arthritis or osteomyelitis, a calculated guess can be made as to which organisms will produce infection based on the age of the child. In general, treatment with a broad-spectrum antibiotic is optimal until specific culture results are available.

Staphylococcus aureus is the most common causative agent for bone and joint infection. In the neonate and infant, *S. aureus* is the most common infecting organism, but in the neonatal age group Gram-negative bacterial sepsis is frequently the source of these infections. In neonates, septicemia often leads to multifocal metaphyseal infections, a condition uncommon in other age groups. In children between 6 months and 3 years of age, upper respiratory infection or otitis media is a common precursor to osteomyelitis. Since *Haemophilus influenzae* infection is frequently a cause of ear and upper respiratory infections, bacteremia can lead to *H. influenzae* infection of the bones and joints of this age group. *S. aureus*

remains very common in this toddler age group. Above the age of 3 years, *S. aureus* is by far the most common causative organism for septic arthritis and osteomyelitis. Special circumstances occur in certain patients, including children with sickle cell anemia who also develop *Salmonella* infections. Children with underlying immune compromise are more likely to develop infections with opportunistic organisms.

Treatment of Septic Arthritis

The treatment of septic arthritis begins with the early recognition of the condition. Aspiration of the involved joint should be performed whenever this diagnosis is entertained. Most joints are very accessible for aspiration, although the hip and the shoulder joints are somewhat more difficult to tap.

Aseptic techniques should be used when aspirating joints. The physician should use sterile gloves, and an aseptic prep solution should be employed. Each joint has an avenue of needle placement that allows ready access to the joint. The knee is generally easiest to aspirate with the needle inserted below the patella on the lateral side. The preferred direction for ankle aspiration is from the anterolateral side of the ankle, just anterior to the fibula with the foot in the neutral position. The elbow should be aspirated from the lateral aspect superior to the radial head to avoid the risk of neurovascular involvement. The wrist is generally aspirated from the direct dorsal approach between the radius and ulna.

The hip may be aspirated by medial, anterior, or lateral routes (see Fig. 12.25, p. 156). The authors' preferred method is anterior. The femoral artery is palpated and the needle entry point generally is approximately 1 cm lateral to the neurovascular bundle and 1 to 2 finger breadths inferior to the inguinal ligament with the hip in neutral position. As with the medial and lateral approaches, aspiration is best carried out under fluoroscopy. The medial approach employs placement of the needle just anterior to the adductor longus muscle, palpable in the groin with the hip abducted. The lateral approach involves needle placement just anterior to the greater trochanter as pictured in Figure 12.25. When fluid is obtained by aspiration, cultures, a white blood cell count, and Gram stain of this fluid should be obtained. If no fluid is obtained on the attempted aspiration, 2 or 3 ml of contrast medium is injected into the hip to confirm that the needle is appropriately located in the hip joint. Ultrasonography is useful before attempted aspiration to determine the presence or absence of an effusion, particularly in proximal joints such as the hip and shoulder. The usual aspiration direction for the shoulder is from a direct anterior approach.

The purpose of treatment of septic arthritis is to allow antibiotics to enter the joint cavity in sufficient concentration to eradicate the infection. While antibiotics are always used, surgery is usually needed for joint irrigation and drainage, though in some selected circumstances surgery may not be needed. Surgical incision and drainage are *always* urgently necessary in children with septic arthritis of the hip and shoulder. For more peripheral joints, in addition to appropriate antibiotics, treatment may include open irrigation and drainage of the joint, arthroscopic irrigation, or daily joint needle aspirations. If the infection has been present a very short time and there is not a large amount of purulent effusion within the joint, a trial of antibiotics for 24 to 48 hours can be considered, provided the child is not systemically ill. While in early infection the use of antibiotics alone may be successful, in more established infections surgical treatment of the joint is indicated, both to prevent articular cartilage damage from bacterial products and breakdown products of white blood cells and to enable the antibiotics to be delivered to the entire joint surface to eradicate the infection.

There is some controversy regarding whether the joint should be splinted or mobilized when infection is present. Traditionally a splint has been applied to limit joint motion, with the idea that this immobility decreases the child's pain and allows for a quicker resolution of the infection. Immobilization should not be used for prolonged periods of time, however, since children with septic arthritis can develop joint stiffness. Once an initial improvement in the infection has been obtained, a therapy program to reestablish joint motion should be utilized in children with any signs of stiffness.

Treatment of Osteomyelitis

Effective treatment of osteomyelitis in children, as with septic arthritis, begins with an early diagnosis of the condition. Any child with a sudden change in walking status without a history of recent trauma or with unexplained swelling of the extremity should be considered to be at risk for osteomyelitis. In children, these symptoms are usually accompanied by an elevation in temperature, but in the neonatal age group limb swelling or failure to move an extremity is considered presumptive evidence that an infection is present. Although certain bacteria are most commonly identified with certain age groups, it is useful to try to obtain a culture of the specific organism involved by aspiration of the region of maximum tenderness. This should be done aseptically, and if no fluid can be obtained by direct aspiration, 1 ml of saline solution can sometimes be injected and then re-aspirated to be used for culture material.

The diagnosis of acute osteomyelitis should be suspected by physical examination. With fever, tenderness and swelling of an extremity, limp, or refusal to walk or stand, the presumptive diagnosis of osteomyelitis should be made and antibiotics begun. A bone scan is used to confirm the clinical impression, but treatment need not be delayed until the radioisotope study has been completed. Aspiration of a joint or of a location of suspected osteomyelitis will not influence the bone scan within the first 24 to 48 hours after aspiration.

If the child has had signs or symptoms of infection for only a few days, intravenous antibiotics are given for 24 to 48 hours and the response monitored. If the patient remains systemically ill and no local improvement is noted, surgical drainage is often necessary. If the child responds to antibiotic treatment alone within the first 2 to 3 days, parenteral antibiotics are continued for a minimum of 3 weeks, usually in an outpatient setting. Once a local response has occurred and swelling and pain are absent, ambulation can be begun.

If the child has had signs and symptoms for more than 2 or 3 days, surgical treatment is usually needed to augment the appropriate antibiotics. Consider drainage of an acute osteomyelitis as similar to drainage of a soft-tissue abscess. The incision into bone is accomplished by removing a window of bone and allowing the purulent material inside the bone to be adequately drained. Since the involved bone is hyperemic, drainage of the bone abscess allows antibiotics to reach the infected area and effectively eradicate the infection. Intravenous antibiotics are used in this setting for at least 3 weeks and may be used longer if the infection is more widespread or if there is a significant delay in response of the erythrocyte sedimentation rate. If a hole in the bone has been created, the bone is initially splinted and, once the local infection has been controlled, a cast is applied. It takes approximately 4 to 6 weeks for the bone to regain its strength following this type of surgical procedure.

If signs and symptoms of an infection have been present for a few weeks to a few months, extensive surgical debridement is necessary to remove dead bone and to ensure that adequate drainage is obtained. In acute osteomyelitis of only a few days' du-

ration, the skin can generally be closed over the drainage area; however, if the infection has been present for several weeks or months, the wound is left open and allowed to granulate slowly, and skin grafting is sometimes necessary. In more extensive infections, antibiotics need to be given intravenously for a 6-week period, and oral antibiotics may be needed thereafter.

Although intravenous administration of antibiotics is generally the preferred treatment for osteomyelitis, oral antibiotics may be used provided a bactericidal blood level of an appropriate antibiotic is obtained. If it is elected not to administer intravenous antibiotics for 3 weeks, but to switch to oral antibiotics earlier, it is mandatory that appropriate peak and trough levels of antibiotics be obtained on a daily basis initially to ensure that appropriate bacterial inhibition is present. Failure to treat an infection appropriately for a minimum of 3 weeks will increase the child's risk of developing chronic osteomyelitis.

Sequelae of Bone/Joint Infections

Septic arthritis and acute osteomyelitis that has not been treated as an emergency or that has not been diagnosed promptly will often lead to permanent damage to the joint, growth plate, or long bone.

GROWTH DISTURBANCE

A feared complication of acute osteomyelitis is damage to the growth plate. Although acute osteomyelitis begins in the metaphyseal area near the zone of provisional calcification of the growth plate, if the infection is inadequately treated, is ignored, or advances rapidly, the infection will spread across the growth plate, destroying the replicating and germinating cells at the growth plate. Additionally, the infection may spread to the epiphysis adjacent to the growth plate. If these cells are damaged, focal growth disturbance occurs. Growth plate disturbances can also occur in purpura fulminans associated with meningococcemia, in which multiple growth plates are injured as a result of septic emboli to the metaphyseal and physeal regions.

If growth plate injury occurs as a result of infection, surgical attempts to re-establish growth in these regions are less successful than if the partial growth plate disturbance resulted from a fracture. Although the entire growth plate can be involved, osteomyelitis usually causes only partial destruction of the growth plate, leading to an angular deformity rather than limb length inequality.

JOINT DESTRUCTION OR ARTHRITIS

If pus has been left in a joint for several days, the lysosomes and proteases produced by the white blood cells and bacteria lead to permanent damage to the articular cartilage of the joint. Thinning of the articular cartilage is seen on radiographs. This loss of articular cartilage followed by bone destruction will lead to decreased movement in the affected joint and, in some cases, fibrous ankylosis or fusion when sufficient articular cartilage damage has occurred.

CHRONIC OSTEOMYELITIS

If adequate antibiotic treatment has not been provided, chronic osteomyelitis may result and last a lifetime. Inadequate antibiotic treatment may result from either too low a dose of antibiotics, the wrong antibiotics, too short a treatment with antibiotics, or inadequate surgical drainage. Chronic osteomyelitis is extremely difficult to eradicate fully. While children and adults may have several months or even years of quiescent periods in which no drainage is present, the usual course of chronic osteomyelitis is one of periodic flare-ups requiring antibiotics and surgical drainage. Adults who have had chronic infection drainage for decades are at risk for developing squamous cell carcinoma at the sinus tract.

PATHOLOGIC FRACTURE OR NONUNION

A fracture may occur either at the site of chronic infection or at the site of a bone window that has been used to drain an osteomyelitis. Fractures heal slowly or not at all in the face of active local infection. If a nonunion develops at the fracture site, extensive surgical treatment, including vascularized bone or soft-tissue transfers may be needed to allow healing to occur once the infection has been eradicated.

Suggested Readings

Choi, I.H., Pizzutillo, P.D., Bowen, J.R., et al.: Sequelae and reconstruction after septic arthritis of the hip in infants. J. Bone Joint Surg. 72A:1150–1165, 1990.

Cole, W.G.: The management of chronic osteomyelitis. Clin. Orthop. 264:84–89, 1991.

Fink, C.W. and Nelson, J.D.: Septic arthritis and osteomyelitis in children. Clin. Rheum. Dis. 12: 423–435, 1986.

Green, N.E. and Edwards, K.: Bone and joint infections in children. Orthop. Clin. North Am. 18: 555–576, 1987.

Gustilo, R.B., Gruninger, R.P., and Tsukayama, D.T. (eds.): Orthopaedic Infection: Diagnosis and Treatment. Philadelphia, W.B. Saunders, 1989.

Jacobs, R.F., McCarthy, R.E., and Elser, J.M.: *Pseudomonas* osteochondritis complicating puncture wounds of the foot in children: A 10-year evaluation. J. Infect. Dis. 160:657–661, 1989.

Morrissy, R. and Haynes, D.W.: Acute hematogenous osteomyelitis: A model with trauma as an etiology. J. Pediatr. Orthop. 9:447–456, 1989.

Sundberg, S.B., Savage, J.P., and Foster, B.K.: Technetium phosphate bone scan in the diagnosis of septic arthritis in childhood. J. Pediatr. Orthop. 9: 579–585, 1989.

Wopperer, J.M., White, J.J., Gillespie, R., et al.: Long-term follow-up of infantile hip sepsis. J. Pediatr. Orthop. 8:322–325, 1988.

17

Torsional and Angular Conditions in the Lower Extremity

Parental concern over possible rotational or angular abnormalities of the lower extremity in their children, particularly the first born, is widespread. While active treatment is occasionally needed, many of these conditions correct by themselves with growth alone. The primary care physician must be able to evaluate these various conditions and establish the appropriate diagnosis, offering reassurance to the parents in instances when self-correction is expected and offering orthopaedic referral when progressive conditions are present.

Torsional or Rotational Conditions

There are four torsional problems that may be present in the lower extremity. Even though these problems occur in the tibia or the femur, the concerns generally expressed by the parents are of the child's in-toeing or out-toeing when walking. In-toeing results from internal tibial torsion and/or internal femoral torsion, also known as increased femoral anteversion. (Metatarsus adductus may also cause an in-toeing gait but is not a rotational problem and is discussed in Chapter 15.) Out-toeing is seen in children with external tibial torsion and/or external femoral torsion, also called femoral retroversion.

While imaging studies, such as computed tomographic (CT) and magnetic resonance (MR) scans, are available to help quantitate the amount of rotational deformity that may

be present, the diagnosis of torsional problems is essentially a clinical one, made on the basis of physical examination and the observation of the child's gait.

The child should be observed walking both toward and away from the examiner. When the child is walking toward the physician, the position of the patella should be noted: does it point medially or straight ahead when the foot is on the ground? The *foot progression angle* is estimated for both feet: if a line were to be drawn in the direction the child is walking, do the feet point in, out, or straight ahead? (Fig. 17.1) Limping and pain are generally absent with torsional conditions, so the child should spend equal time on each foot as walking proceeds.

Three different positions are used to fully examine the child for torsional deformity while on the examining table. Because toddlers and young children often fear shots and become upset when placed in a lying position, the initial examination is performed with the child sitting on the edge of the table, with the knees and hips flexed. In this position, the tibial tubercle is palpated and the tibia is placed so the tubercle is directed straight forward. The medial and lateral malleoli at the ankle are then palpated with the other hand, with the thumb usually placed on the lateral malleolus and the index finger placed medially (Fig. 17.2). Normally, the lateral malleolus lies 20° to 30° posterior to the medial malleolus, and this

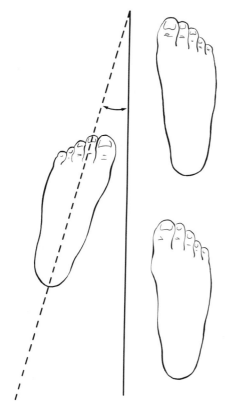

Figure 17.1. Evaluation of the foot position during walking will allow estimation of a foot-progression angle. Normally, the foot should be pointed straight forward, as shown on the right side of this diagram. The left foot in this example is internally rotated, due to internal torsion of either the tibia or the femur.

be obtained with the child supine, but these motions are more accurately measured with the child prone.

With the child in the prone position, the hips are extended, a position that better simulates the hip position when the child is standing and walking. The knee is flexed to 90° and the internal and external rotation of the hip is measured. Normally, a child has a combined rotation of approximately 90°, with 45° each of external and internal rotation. Internal rotation is assessed by allowing the flexed leg to rotate laterally. External rotation of the hip is measured by medial rotation of the flexed leg, while the examiner's hand steadies the buttock area to prevent rocking of the pelvis (see Chapter 12, p. 138). If excessive internal rotation is noted, the child has increased femoral anteversion, while excessive external hip rotation connotes femoral retroversion.

With the child still in the prone position and the knee flexed, the examiner notes the *thigh-foot angle* (the position of the foot relative to the long axis of the thigh) to estimate the amount of tibial torsion present (Fig. 17.3). Normally, a line drawn through the long axis of the foot should demonstrate slight external rotation compared to the long axis of the thigh. If the foot is in an internally rotated position, internal tibial torsion is present. In this same position, the plantar aspect and lateral margin of the foot can be assessed for a possible metatarsus adductus component to the in-toeing.

While all of these torsional positions can be measured by goniometers, in clinical practice the magnitude of the torsion positions are generally estimated to the nearest 5° or 10°. Though this may seem to be relatively inaccurate, estimates can become quite reproducible with a little practice and are adequate for appropriate assessment of possible torsional problems. If surgical correction of these torsional conditions is contemplated, CT scans can be used preoperatively to provide more accurate quantitation of rotation.

position is designated as neutral torsion. If the lateral malleolus is at the same level as the medial malleolus, 20° to 30° of internal tibial torsion exists. If the lateral malleolus is more than 30° posterior to the medial malleolus, external tibial torsion is present.

After estimating the degree of tibial torsion in this manner, the child is placed supine and the range of motion of the hip, knee, and ankle is noted. This is done to rule out the possibility that the rotational deformity has resulted from the child holding the limb in this position to minimize pain due to a joint abnormality. An estimate of internal and external rotation of the hip can

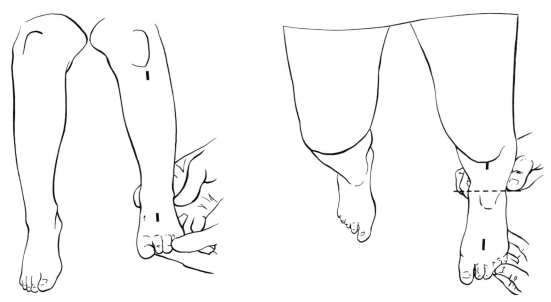

Figure 17.2.   The amount of tibial torsion present is estimated by evaluating the intermalleolar axis at the ankle relative to the position of the tibial tubercle. Normally, with the tibial tubercle facing forward, the lateral malleolus is 20° to 30° posterior to the medial malleolus, a position defined as neutral torsion. The illustration on the right side demonstrates an intermalleolar angle of 0°, or 20° to 30° of internal tibial torsion.

INTERNAL TIBIAL TORSION

Most commonly diagnosed between the ages of 6 months and 2 years, internal tibial torsion is generally thought to be secondary to molding due to the intrauterine position of the legs during later fetal development. In this position, the legs are crossed and the foot is rotated inward, the medial side of the foot being in contact with the front of the opposite tibial region. Internal tibial torsion is not seen in a stillborn fetus born several weeks preterm.

Although internal tibial torsion may not be diagnosed until later, it has been present since birth. Internal tibial torsion does not develop after delivery and is not a progressive deformity. At birth and for the first year of life, many infants have external rotation soft-tissue contractures at the hips, also related to the intrauterine position. With the hips externally rotated and the tibia internally rotated, the feet will appear to point straight forward. As internal rotation movement of the hip increases during the first year of life, the internal tibial torsion becomes more obvious, and the foot appears to begin pointing more inward. When the child begins to stand, the internal rotation becomes even more exaggerated in appearance, and the parents might seek the advice of a physician. The presence of internal tibial torsion will not delay motor milestone development.

Evaluation of the thigh-foot angle will demonstrate medial deviation of the foot. Assessment of the malleolar position will confirm that the lateral malleolus is parallel with the medial malleolus. With walking, the foot progression angle will be pointed inward.

Radiographs of the tibia are normal, unless the rotation is marked, in which case the knee will be seen in an anteroposterior view and the ankle will be viewed obliquely. A CT scan with a single cut of the proximal

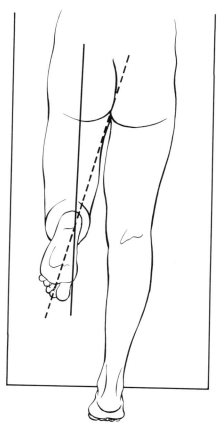

Figure 17.3. An easier method to determine the amount of tibial torsion is the evaluation of the thigh-foot angle. As shown in this diagram, a line along the long axis of the foot should point slightly externally to a line along the long axis of the thigh. If the foot points internally, internal tibial torsion is present.

tibia and a single cut of the distal tibia, with the leg held in the same position, can be used to quantitate the amount of torsion present, but this is unnecessary for usual clinical assessment.

No treatment is needed in the large majority of children with internal tibial torsion, as there will be gradual resolution of this internal torsion by 2 or 3 years of age. Improvement in the internal torsion is slower in children who sleep on their stomachs, because the feet are held internally rotated during sleep.

Generally, children should be observed for at least 6 months after walking begins before active treatment is even considered. If improvement is occurring, no treatment is offered. If moderate to marked internal tibial torsion persists after 18 months of age, the use of a Denis-Browne bar and shoes can be discussed with the parents. No scientific evidence exists to indicate that this treatment is better than simple observation. However, if this treatment is used, high-top shoes are positioned on the Denis-Browne bar in an externally rotated position of 30° to 45° and the bar and shoes are worn when the child sleeps. The length of the bar should be the same as the width of the child's pelvis or shoulders; if the bar is too long, excessive stress is placed on the child's knees and knock-knee deformity may be produced. Generally, this type of bar and shoes can be used up to age 3 years but is poorly tolerated thereafter.

If internal tibial torsion persists into later childhood or into adult life, this is primarily a cosmetic problem, not a functional one. In fact, many excellent athletes have some mild residual internal tibial torsion. There is no evidence that internal tibial torsion will lead to early degenerative arthritis of the knee or ankle in adult life. If the internal tibial torsion is asymmetrical or interferes with walking or running, surgical treatment with derotational tibial osteotomy can realign the lower leg, though surgical treatment of this condition should be delayed until at least 4 years of age to allow the normal expected improvement to occur.

EXTERNAL TIBIAL TORSION

Infants or toddlers with out-toeing of the feet generally have relative external rotation of the tibia. This is most likely caused by the intrauterine position of the legs, causing the foot to dorsiflex to such a degree that the dorsum of the foot abuts the anterior tibial region of the same leg. When the foot is in this position of excessive dorsiflexion, the tibia assumes an externally rotated position. When combined with the external rotation soft-tissue contractures of the hips (again from the intrauterine position) the infant with these rotational conditions will appear to have marked external rotation of the foot.

The normal position of the lateral malleolus is approximately 20° or 30° posterior to the medial malleolus. If the lateral malleolus is further posterior so a larger intermalleolar angle is seen, external tibial torsion is present. If this angle measures 20° or 30° with tibial rotation normal, the foot still may be out-turned due to the hip position. Careful attention to the level of the rotational condition is important for appropriate management and advice to parents.

On examination, infants or toddlers with external tibial torsion will have an intermalleolar angle greater than 30°. During walking, the foot-progression angle will be in an external rotation position. The thigh-foot angle check will reveal the foot to be externally rotated in relation to the long axis of the thigh.

In the standing position, the child may markedly rotate the foot externally, even up to 90°, depending on the degree of external rotation at the hip level. In this position, the supple foot will often appear to be a marked flatfoot, but since the line of body weight passes medially to the foot in this condition, no specific foot treatment is needed as long as the foot appears normal when not bearing weight. As the external rotation contractures at the hip level improve, the foot will assume a less out-turned position. While the "external" tibial torsion does not change with growth, the improvement of hip internal rotation with time will be sufficient to allow the older child to place the foot straight forward when walking.

As a rule, no treatment is needed for this condition. The relative external tibial torsion should improve by itself. The supple flatfoot condition will improve as the external rotation position of the foot improves, and special shoes are *not* needed. The use of a Denis-Browne bar is virtually never

necessary. Long-term sequelae are essentially nonexistent. Surgical treatment of external tibial torsion is indicated only in the unusual circumstance of persistent symptomatic or asymmetrical external tibial torsion after the age of 4 years.

INTERNAL FEMORAL TORSION OR EXCESSIVE FEMORAL ANTEVERSION

While internal tibial torsion is the most common cause of in-toeing in the early walking years, internal femoral torsion is the usual cause of in-toeing after the age of 3 years.

The magnitude of the internal femoral torsion, also called femoral anteversion, is measured by an angle formed by the intersection of a line drawn through the bicondylar axis of the distal femur and an anteriorly directed line drawn up the axis of the femoral neck and head. The physician needs to recall that only a portion of the femoral head is in contact with the acetabulum in the normal standing position, with the anterior and lateral portions of the femoral head cartilage partially outside the acetabulum, in this way allowing for more movement at the hip joint. Quantitation of the amount of femoral anteversion is possible by measuring the rotation on limited-segment CT scans at the proximal and distal femur. However, the amount of anteversion is generally determined clinically, by estimating the degree by which internal hip rotation exceeds external hip rotation with the child in a prone position.

At the time of birth, 30° to 40° of femoral anteversion is normally present, although in infants this cannot be detected on examination because of the external rotation contractures present as a result of the intrauterine fetal position. As the child grows, however, the amount of femoral anteversion normally decreases slightly each year, with the skeletally mature teenager or adult having about 10° to 15° of femoral anteversion. The majority of this remodeling with growth takes place prior to the age of 8 years.

In children with excessive femoral anteversion, observation of the gait will demonstrate an internally directed foot-progression angle. The anterior aspect of the patellae will be directed medially, a feature that helps differentiate this condition from tibial torsion. With the child prone, the thigh-foot angle will be normal, with a slightly external position of the foot relative to the thigh, since this internal rotation is not in the tibia. In the prone position, internal rotation of the hip will be greater than external rotation. Because of this ease of internal rotation of the hip, the child will prefer to sit with the lower extremities in the "W" position rather than in the crossed-leg position.

Radiographs of the femur are generally interpreted as normal. However, if the femoral anteversion is quite marked, apparent coxa valga will be noted. Generally, the femur radiograph is obtained with the patella directed anteriorly; in children with marked femoral anteversion, this position will also cause the femoral neck and head to be directed more anteriorly, resulting in the appearance of increased valgus of the femoral neck. In these cases, the true neck-shaft angle of the proximal femur can be determined by a pelvis radiograph with the hips internally rotated. With the leg held in one position, a limited CT scan of the proximal and distal femoral areas will allow for quantitation of the amount of internal femoral torsion present.

Treatment of increased femoral anteversion generally consists of parental reassurance that gradual improvement will occur by the time the child is about 8 years old. There is no evidence that any of a wide variety of nighttime or daytime braces or special shoes will lead to a more rapid improvement in this internal femoral rotation. Although many physicians recommend having the child sit in the tailor or crossed-leg position to increase the amount of external rotation

at the hips, it is unclear whether this is efficacious. This crossed-leg position has no effect on the bone rotation but may stretch hip muscles to allow slightly more external rotation.

From a practical standpoint, if a child has at least 10° or 15° of external hip rotation with the child in the prone position, no treatment will be needed. As peer pressure builds during the elementary school years to walk with the feet directed forward, children will usually correct the walking position of the feet by themselves. If no external hip rotation is present and in-toeing persists past the age of 8 years, derotational osteotomy of the femur can be performed if functional or cosmetic concerns warrant this surgery.

Longer-term effects of persistent internal femoral torsion vary with the patient. Most are asymptomatic, with only a mild cosmetic problem from the in-toeing. There is no evidence that persistent excessive femoral anteversion will lead to earlier degenerative arthritis of the hip or knee. In teenagers with increased femoral anteversion and mild knock-knees, patellar region pain may occur from lateral subluxation of the patella in the patellofemoral groove of the distal femur. Children with Legg-Perthes disease of the hip characteristically have more femoral anteversion than normal.

EXTERNAL FEMORAL TORSION OR FEMORAL RETROVERSION

The presence of true external femoral torsion is less common than internal femoral torsion, though some children and teenagers who walk with their feet in a significant out-toeing position, in the "Charlie Chaplin" position, will be found to have this condition.

At the time of delivery, the infant will generally have about 90° of external rotation at the hip and essentially no internal rotation. This is *not* external femoral torsion or retroversion. Even though the child generally has 30° or 40° of femoral anteversion or internal femoral torsion at the time of birth, this bony internal torsion cannot be detected clinically because of the presence of soft-tissue (muscles, hip capsule, ligaments, etc.) contractures in the hip area as a result of the fetal position in the uterus. These soft-tissue "contractures" will resolve within the first year of life, at which point the evaluation of the internal and external rotation of the hip can be a reasonable clinical tool for estimating the amount of femoral anteversion or retroversion that is present.

In the child or adolescent, the physical examination for evaluating a child with out-toeing is the same as for in-toeing. With the child walking, the foot-progression angle is noted; check for symmetry here too, as excessive external rotation of only one foot may be a sign of unilateral hip disease. Any type of limp is noted and the Trendelenburg test is performed. On the examining table, the child's hip is examined with the child in both the supine and prone positions. In the supine position, the amounts of external and internal rotation are assessed. As the hip is flexed, if the thigh is pushed into further external rotation, consider that a slipped capital femoral epiphysis may be present. With the child prone, there is significantly more external hip rotation than internal rotation in children with femoral retroversion.

Radiographs of the hips and femurs of children with femoral retroversion alone appear normal. Quantitation of retroversion is possible with limited CT scans, as described under femoral anteversion.

It appears that increased femoral retroversion may predispose the child to a more serious hip disorder, particularly slipped capital femoral epiphysis. The "classic" clinical appearance of a child with slipped capital femoral epiphysis is an obese teenager who walks with both feet externally rotated, but with the affected leg further outturned. CT or MR studies of these children will often demonstrate either a relative or absolute amount of femoral retroversion.

Why femoral retroversion seems to produce these hip problems is not well defined.

Treatment of external femoral torsion by itself is not necessary. No splints, orthotics, or special shoes will affect the rotation, and corrective osteotomy is rarely indicated.

Angular Deformity

In addition to rotational variations in the lower extremity, the child may exhibit angular abnormalities such that the standing child will have either excessive bowlegs (genu varum) (Fig. 17.4) or knock-knees (genu valgum) (Fig. 17.5). Although mild bowlegs or knock-knees are often normal at some stages of growth, severe angular deformity or asymmetrical angular position of the lower extremities should alert the examiner to try to identify growth plate disorders that may have caused these abnormalities.

When the normal adult stands with the legs together, the medial aspects of the knees are just touching and the ankles are separated by a few centimeters. In this position of mild knock-knees there is approximately 5° to 7° of genu valgum. This lower-extremity position of mild valgus is normal after the age of 6 years.

From the time the child begins to walk until about 6 years of age, there are normal changes in the angular alignment of the lower extremities that occur as growth proceeds. When the child begins to stand, mild bowlegs are commonly present. In addition to the physiologic bowing at this age, children often have some internal tibial torsion, the combination of which will give the appearance of more bowing than is actually present. Between the ages of 2 and 3 years, this physiologic bowing gradually changes to a mild knock-knee or physiologic valgus position. Between the ages of 3 and 5 years, there is often more valgus or knock-knee present than after age 6 years, by which time the "adult" angular configuration is present (Fig. 17.6).

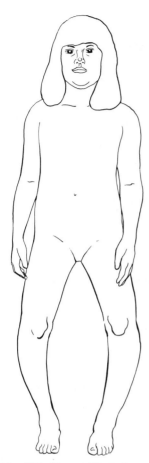

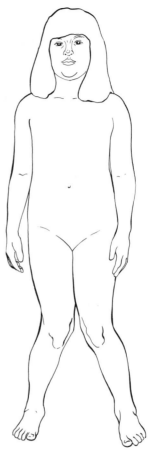

Figure 17.4. This diagram illustrates a girl with genu varum or bowed legs. Varus (inward) angulation is generally defined by the bone distal to the reference joint pointing toward the midline. Here the tibia distal to the knee (genu) is pointing toward the midline, and genu varum is diagnosed.

Figure 17.5. The girl illustrated has genu valgum or knock-knees. Valgus (outward) angulation is present when the bone distal to the reference joint points away from the midline. After the age of 6 years, genu valgum of about 5° is normal.

This dynamic pattern of growth of the lower extremity between the ages of 1 and 6 years will explain many of the concerns parents might have over the position of their child's legs when standing. It should be remembered, though, that these physiologic conditions, which are expected to improve with time, should be symmetrical and should be matched with the age and stage of growth noted above. Growth plate or metabolic disorders should be suspected if the angular condition involves one leg only or occurs at the wrong age, such as bowing past the age of 3 years.

BOWLEGS OR GENU VARUM

In a child with bowleg deformity, four possible diagnoses should come to mind: (*a*) physiologic bowing, (*b*) Blount's disease, (*c*) rickets, and (*d*) growth plate injury from trauma or infection. A careful history will be helpful in establishing the correct diagnosis. The time when the bowing was first

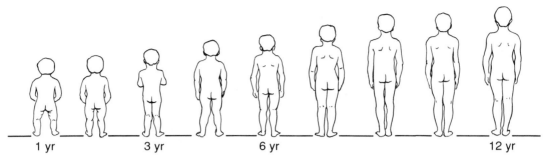

Figure 17.6.   As a child ages, the angular position of the lower extremities commonly changes. When the child is first beginning to walk, bowlegs are common. By age 3, most children develop knock-knees, which resolves by age 5 or 6. After the age of 6, the normal "adult" angular alignment should be present and should remain unchanged after this age.

noted is important, as is the parents' impression as to whether the bowing is improving or worsening. The child's nutrition history, especially the intake of vitamin D-fortified milk or vitamin supplements, is determined, as well as whether the child was obese at early walking age. A history of significant limb trauma or infection is usually readily obtained from parental questioning, though some babies requiring intensive care as neonates may have had an undiagnosed osteomyelitis as a part of generalized neonatal sepsis. A family history of bowing should also be sought.

Physical examination for bowlegs concentrates on the observation of the child standing and walking, in addition to measurement of the angular alignment of the lower extremities, though the entire lower-extremity examination needs to be noted. With the child standing, the legs are placed so the patellae are directed straight forward, to decrease the effect of rotational conditions on the angular position of the legs. In this standing position with the medial sides of the ankles touching, the femorotibial angle formed by lines along the long axes of the thigh and lower leg is noted, as well as the distance between the knees. Tape measurement of the distance between the knees in this position will provide a simple method of serial clinical assessment in the office to help decide whether the bowing is improv-

ing or worsening on subsequent examinations. In this same standing position, the examiner should determine whether the bowing involves both the femur and the tibia or only the tibia. With the child walking, the examiner should look specifically for any lateral thrust of the knee area as the foot is placed on the floor.

On the examining table, the femorotibial angle is measured again, preferably with the use of a goniometer for better accuracy. The laxity of the knee joint collateral ligaments is tested. Femoral and tibial rotation is noted. If rickets is suspected to be the cause of the bowing, the upper extremity and thoracic cage are also evaluated.

Not all children with bowing require radiographic evaluation. However, those with severe or progressive bowing and those with asymmetrical bowing should have a standing anteroposterior radiograph of the lower extremities, preferably on a film that includes the hip, knee, and ankle on a single radiograph. Unless it is being used to further investigate an abnormality seen on the standing radiograph, a supine radiograph of the knee is not routinely needed when evaluating a child for bowlegs. Other special imaging studies are reserved for those with an abnormality seen on the standing radiograph.

Serum investigations for calcium, phosphorus, and alkaline phosphatase are indicated in children suspected of having rickets by either physical findings or radiographic changes.

PHYSIOLOGIC BOWING

Far and away the most common type of bowing seen, physiologic bowing is present primarily between the ages of 1 and 2 years, with gradual improvement noted by age 2 or 3 years. The bowing is seen to involve both the femoral and tibial areas. No lateral thrust of the knee is seen when walking. No ligament instability is found at the knee. The remainder of the lower extremity examination is normal. Serum studies are normal.

If radiographs are obtained, the bowing is seen to involve both the distal femur and the proximal tibia. In more marked cases, there may be some delay in the ossification of the medial epiphyses of the distal femur and the proximal tibia. If serial radiographs are evaluated, this delay in medial epiphyseal ossification improves as the physiologic bowing improves (Fig. 17.7).

No treatment is needed for physiologic bowing, as improvement occurs over a period of several months. Physiologic bowing should not be diagnosed after the age of 3 years. This diagnosis should be used sparingly between the ages of 2 and 3 years and should not be used for bowing that worsens after the age of 2 years.

BLOUNT'S DISEASE OR TIBIA VARA

Blount's disease, called tibia vara because the bowing occurs in the proximal tibia only, is the most common nonphysiologic cause of bowing in the young child. This condition is found primarily in obese or large children who have begun walking at 9 or 10 months of age. It is more common in black children than in other racial groups. The diagnosis of Blount's disease should be suspected in all children with progressive bowing, asymmetrical bowing, or significant bowing that persists after the age of 2 years.

Abnormal function of the medial portion of the proximal tibial growth plate is the cause of the bowing in Blount's disease. It is generally accepted that the forces on the medial part of this physis exceed physiologic limits when a large or obese child walks early on a leg with normal physiologic bowing. This excessive force on the medial physis inhibits normal growth in this segment, leading to progressive bowing of the proximal tibia as the lateral portion of this physis continues to grow normally. If these abnormal medial forces persist with continued growth, the bowing continues to worsen, and if it remains untreated, permanent damage to the medial portion of the growth plate will occur. Microscopic evaluation of the medial physis in Blount's disease demonstrates disordered growth in the physeal cell columns, a change that becomes less reversible the longer this condition is present.

In a child with Blount's disease, the physical examination will clearly demonstrate bowing of the lower extremity. The thigh is not bowed, and the bowing is seen to begin at or just below the knee level. Bowing may be unilateral or bilateral. Persistent internal tibial torsion remains in the affected tibia. With walking, a lateral thrust of the knee may be noted during the early stance phase of gait as each step is taken. Pain and tenderness are absent in the young child, but may be present in the adolescent.

The diagnosis of Blount's disease is confirmed by a standing anteroposterior radiograph of both lower extremities after the age of 2 years. Prior to this age, generally insufficient changes have occurred to clearly establish this diagnosis radiographically. The femur is usually normal. The medial aspect of the proximal tibial metaphysis may demonstrate a "beak" with some delay in ossification at this site (Fig. 17.8). The longer Blount's disease remains untreated, the more physeal and metaphyseal changes are seen on the medial aspect of the proximal tibia. As described by Langenskiold, six radiographic stages can be noted; the assign-

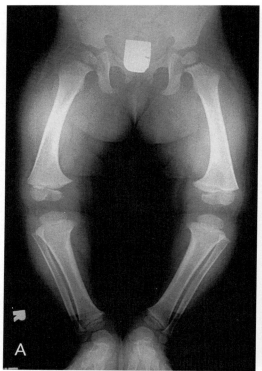

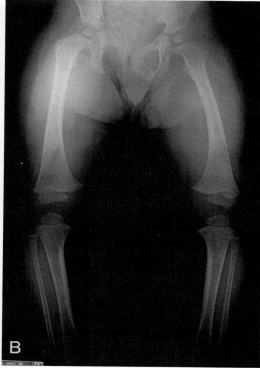

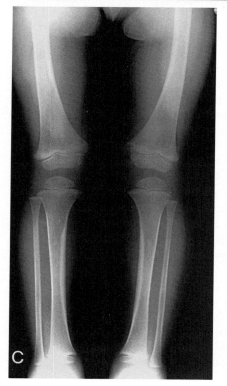

Figure 17.7. **A,** Standing anteroposterior radiograph of a 15-month-old child shows symmetrical bowing of femurs and tibiae characteristic of physiologic bowing. The medial aspect of the distal femoral and proximal tibial epiphyses commonly have a delay in ossification in association with this normal bowing. **B,** Standing radiograph of the same child at 2½ years of age shows significant improvement of the physiologic bowing. There is still some delay in ossification of the medial distal femoral epiphysis. **C,** Standing radiograph at 4 years of age demonstrates resolution of the bowing and evolution into a normal mild valgus position of the lower extremities without any active treatment.

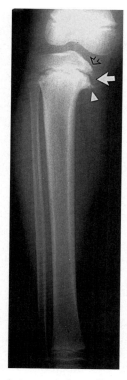

Figure 17.8. Anteroposterior radiograph of the tibia in a child nearly 3 years old shows widening of the medial growth plate (*white arrow*) and flattening of the medial aspect of the proximal tibial epiphysis (*open arrow*), characteristic of Blount's disease or tibia vara. A medial metaphyseal beak is also seen (*arrowhead*).

ment of a specific radiographic stage to a child will guide the treatment recommendations that are subsequently made (Fig. 17.9). The lateral knee radiograph will often reveal a posteriorly directed bony prominence at the metaphyseal level.

Two measurements are useful in evaluating a child for Blount's disease. On a standing anteroposterior radiograph of the lower extremities, the femorotibial angle is formed by the intersection of a line drawn up the femoral shaft and a line drawn up the tibial shaft. This angle is used to assess progression or improvement in bowing on consecutive radiographs. The metaphyseal-diaphyseal angle appears to be more useful than the femorotibial angle to make the initial diagnosis of Blount's disease. This angle is formed by a line drawn transversely from the medial metaphyseal beak to the proximal lateral metaphysis at the growth plate as it intersects with a line drawn perpendicular to the long axis of the tibial shaft. Virtually all children with a metaphyseal-diaphyseal angle greater than 11° have been shown to require treatment for Blount's disease.

The treatment used for Blount's disease depends on the stage of the disease and the age of the child, but all children with the diagnosis of Blount's disease should have some type of orthopaedic treatment.

The two general forms of orthopaedic

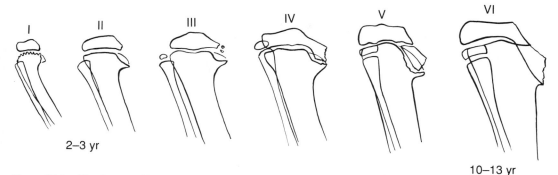

Figure 17.9. The Langenskiold classification of tibia vara or Blount's disease includes six groups. Stage I and II findings are reversible by treatment with either bracing or surgery, while stage III and greater usually cannot be fully reversed to normal. The earlier the diagnosis is made and treatment instituted, the better the result. Redrawn from Langenskiold, A.: Tibia vara: A critical review. Clin. Orthop. 246:195–207, 1989.

care are brace treatment and surgical management. Brace treatment is useful only in the early stages of Blount's disease and is best used in children between the ages of 2 and 3 years. A long leg brace is used, either without a knee joint or with the knee joint locked in full extension, since valgus-producing forces are less effective in correcting bowlegs if the knee is allowed to flex. This brace should be worn full-time during the hours the child is awake, so the legs are held in the supported position during weight bearing. The braces can also be worn at night during sleep. Brace wear is generally needed for at least 9 to 12 months to obtain a discernible effect. Standing anteroposterior radiographs (with the brace off) are obtained at 4- to 6-month intervals to assess the effect of the brace treatment. If improvement occurs, the brace is continued until the radiographs are essentially normal. If improvement does not occur within a year of the initiation of treatment, the brace treatment is terminated and surgical treatment is needed.

The most common type of realignment surgical treatment used for Blount's disease is a valgus-producing osteotomy of the affected tibia and fibula. For children below the age of 5 years, a single osteotomy will be successful over 75% of the time in obtaining a permanent correction of the bowing. In older children or in those with recurrent bowing, more extensive realignment surgery is used, but the best results with surgery are obtained if this condition is diagnosed and treated at a relatively early age and stage.

Although Blount's disease occurs most often in early childhood, *adolescent tibia vara* can be discovered in a teenager not previously noted to have bowlegs. There is a predilection for black teenagers. It is most likely that the teenager did have a mild form of bowing as a young child that did not fully resolve. Clinically, the bowing in this condition is more subtle to diagnose, measuring only 10° to 15°, and is most readily diag-

nosed when the bowing is unilateral. Medial knee pain with activity may be present. A standing anteroposterior radiograph of the lower extremities will demonstrate a varus deformity of the proximal tibia, with the height of the epiphysis less on the medial side than laterally. Proximal tibial osteotomy to realign the leg is needed to relieve the medial knee joint stress or else degenerative arthritis of the medial compartment of the knee will develop in early adult life.

RICKETS

Bowlegs may be caused by a variety of types of rickets, the most common being vitamin D-resistant rickets, nutritional rickets, and renal rickets. Regardless of the cause of the rickets, the result is similar: a buildup of unossified cartilage at the growth plate. Histologically, this produces widening of the physis, since the zone of hypertrophic cells becomes wider and the zone of provisional calcification is essentially absent, due to the metabolic imbalance of serum calcium and phosphate (Fig. 17.10). Radiographically, the most obvious sign of rickets is a widened physis, particularly at the knee and the wrist, where the bones are most rapidly growing.

As a result of the widened physis, mechanical stresses across the affected bones may cause either a varus or a valgus deformity. Bowing is the most common result of nutritional rickets and vitamin D-resistant rickets, though renal rickets seems to lead more often to valgus.

In a child with bowlegs, the diagnosis of rickets is initially suspected by a standing anteroposterior radiograph, which shows the bowing as well as widening of the distal femoral physis. If a wide physis is noted on radiographs, serum calcium, phosphate, alkaline phosphatase, and urea nitrogen measurements should be ordered to confirm the diagnosis of rickets and to determine which type of rickets is present. In nutritional rickets, the serum calcium and phosphate will be low. With vitamin D-resistant rickets,

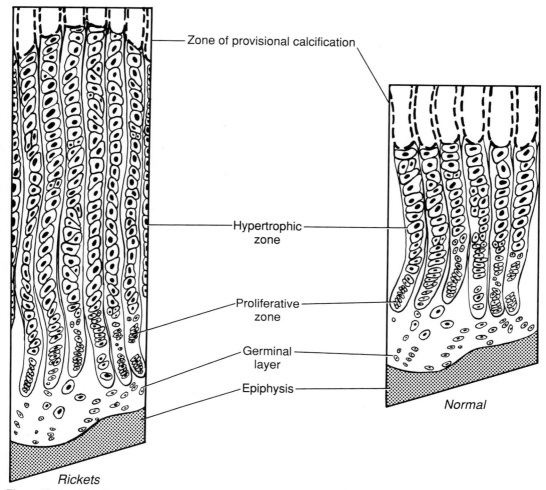

Zone of provisional calcification

Hypertrophic zone

Proliferative zone

Germinal layer

Epiphysis

Normal

Rickets

Figure 17.10.   This illustration portrays the changes seen in the rachitic physis compared to the normal physis. In rickets, the hypertrophic zone is widened, as is the zone of provisional calcification, since the new osteoid formed cannot be calcified. This lack of calcification of the osteoid produces a palpable enlargement of the physis on examination and a visible widening of the physis on radiographic evaluation.

also known as hypophosphatemic rickets, the serum calcium is either normal or low and the serum phosphate is very low. Children with renal rickets will generally have low calcium and normal phosphate values, with elevated urea nitrogen and creatinine. Calcium and phosphate determinations on a 24-hour urine collection may be useful if the serum studies are inconclusive in determining the type of rickets present.

If the bowlegs are due to rickets, the initial treatment is medical, to reverse the ab-

normal calcium-phosphate balance present. If nutritional rickets is the cause, vitamin D supplements will correct the rickets, and remodeling of the bowed legs may occur over a period of several months without the need for surgical treatment. In renal rickets, the underlying renal problem is addressed first. In hypophosphatemic rickets, vitamin D and phosphate supplements may correct the metabolic imbalance, but improvement of the bowing without surgery is rarely seen.

Braces are relatively ineffective in correcting bowing due to rickets. Once the metabolic imbalance is satisfactorily corrected, proximal tibial osteotomy can be done to correct the bowlegs. If surgical correction is attempted prior to the improvement in the metabolic status of the child, recurrence of deformity is common, since the osteoid that forms at the osteotomy will not calcify sufficiently to allow healing of the osteotomy. Children who receive supplemental phosphates or vitamin D preoperatively need to be observed closely for hypercalcemia during the period of bed rest after surgical treatment.

Unfortunately, children with bowing due to rickets often need to undergo more than one osteotomy to maintain alignment of the lower extremity. Even if metabolic control is well maintained for several years, there are often enough periods of poor control to lead to the reappearance of bowing with continued growth.

Knock-Knees or Genu Valgum

Physiologic valgus of the knees is present between the ages of 3 and 5 years, with a gradual return to "adult" values by age 6. If the valgus is asymmetrical or if it persists past the age of 5 years, rickets should be suspected. Renal rickets and hypophosphatemic rickets are the most common types that may lead to an increased knock-knee deformity.

In children with increased genu valgum, the standing anteroposterior radiograph of the lower extremities will allow quantitation of the amount of valgus. If rickets is present, the physes at the distal femur and the proximal tibia will be wider than normal.

If the diagnosis of rickets is made, metabolic control is the first step of treatment, as discussed under Bowlegs above. After metabolic control has been achieved, proximal tibial osteotomy will correct the excessive valgus. Appropriate metabolic management of the rickets must be consistently continued to avoid recurrence of angular deformity.

Angular Deformity due to Growth Plate Damage

Partial damage to the growth plate may occur after fracture or bone infection. Generally, if the cause is a prior injury, the history will help determine this. Children who have been in the hospital for a month or two as neonates may have had an unsuspected infection of the metaphysis of the involved bone, leading to partial permanent injury to the physis. Children with prior episodes of meningococcemia also have a high rate of physeal injury, often in multiple sites.

If the physeal cartilage has been sufficiently damaged, growth in that portion will stop. The remainder of the physis will continue to grow. If the damage is to the medial physis, bowing will occur, while if lateral physeal injury has occurred, a progressive knock-knee deformity will be seen.

If less than half of the physis has been injured, surgical resection of the injured portion and replacement with an inert spacer will often allow for restitution of normal longitudinal growth of the involved long bone. If over half of the physis has been damaged, as is common after an adjacent infection, realignment osteotomy and surgical closure of the remainder of the damaged physis is recommended to prevent further deformity, with the possible need for later leg lengthening if the leg length difference caused by this growth arrest is great enough.

Suggested Readings

Carter, J.R., Leeson, M.C., Thompson, G.H., et al.: Late-onset tibia vara: A histopathologic analysis: A comparative evaluation with infantile tibia vara and slipped capital femoral epiphysis. J. Pediatr. Orthop. 8:187–195, 1988.

Cook, S.D., Lavernia, C.J., Burke, S.W., et al.: A biomechanical analysis of the etiology of tibia vara. J. Pediatr. Orthop. 3:449–454, 1983.

Engel, G.M. and Staheli, L.T.: The natural history of torsion and other factors influencing gait in childhood: A study of the angle of gait, tibial torsion, knee angle, hip rotation, and the development of the arch in normal children. Clin. Orthop. 99:12–17, 1974.

Foreman, K.A. and Robertson. W.W., Jr.: Radiographic measurement of infantile tibia vara. J. Pediatr. Orthop. 5:452–455, 1985.

Henderson, R.C., Lechner, C.T., DeMasi, R.A., and Greene, W.B.: Variability in radiographic measurement of bowleg deformity in children. J. Pediatr. Orthop. 10:491–494, 1990.

Kling, T.F., Jr.: Angular deformities of the lower limbs in children. Orthop. Clin. North Am. 18:513–527, 1987.

Kling, T.F., Jr. and Hensinger, R.N.: Angular and torsional deformities of the lower limbs in children. Clin. Orthop. 176:136–147, 1983.

Langenskiold, A.: Tibia vara: A critical review. Clin. Orthop. 246:195–207, 1989.

Mankin, H.J.: Rickets, osteomalacia, and renal osteodystrophy: An update. Orthop. Clin. North Am. 21:81–96, 1990.

Salenius, P. and Vankka, E.: The development of the tibiofemoral angle in children. J. Bone Joint Surg. 57A:259–261, 1975.

Staheli, L.T., Corbett, M., Wyss, C., et al.: Lower-extremity rotational problems in children: Normal values to guide management. J. Bone Joint Surg. 67A:39–47, 1985.

Svenningsen, S., Apalset, K., Terjesen, T., et al.: Regression of femoral anteversion: A prospective study of intoeing children. Acta Orthop. Scand. 60:170–173, 1989.

Wolfson, B.J. and Capitanio, M.A.: The wide spectrum of renal osteodystrophy in children. CRC Crit. Rev. Diagn. Imaging 27:297–319, 1987.

18

Orthopaedic Concerns in Neuromuscular Disease

Since the skeletal system depends on muscles and nerves for normal function, neuromuscular diseases have a prominent effect on extremity function, primarily through weakness or contractures produced by these disorders. Any child with a delay in developmental motor milestones or with an unexplained deterioration of extremity function needs an evaluation for neurologic or muscle disease.

The diagnosis of neuromuscular disease can be made at different ages throughout childhood and adolescence, so the clinician must stay alert to these possible diagnoses. Spina bifida or myelomeningocele is diagnosed prenatally or at birth. In severe cases, cerebral palsy is diagnosed in infancy, but a mild case of cerebral palsy may escape detection until toddler age. Most children with muscular dystrophy seem normal in infancy and early childhood, and the diagnosis is often not made until 5 or 6 years of age. Some of the peripheral neuropathies and less severe muscle disorders cannot be recognized until the teenage years.

As a general rule, certain orthopaedic findings point toward an underlying neurologic or muscular problem. Foot deformities that develop during childhood or adolescence (such as a cavus foot or claw toes), asymmetrical foot size, leg length discrepancy that is associated with muscle atrophy, congenital joint contractures, and spotty extremity muscle weakness may each be the first indication that a neuromuscular disor-

der is present. If a child is seen with any of these findings, do not ignore them or pass them off as normal. Referral to an orthopaedist and a neurologist at an early stage is preferable. Muscle or nerve biopsy may be needed to establish the correct diagnosis.

It is impossible to discuss here all the neuromuscular disorders that may have orthopaedic implications. Several of the more common problems have been chosen as representative of this large group. Though less common muscle and neurologic diseases are not included, *all* neuromuscular diseases have the potential for developing problems of an orthopaedic nature and require periodic orthopaedic assessment as growth proceeds.

Spina Bifida

Myelomeningocele, the most common form of spina bifida, is readily diagnosed at the time of delivery in the newborn infant with a large dorsal sac filled with cerebrospinal fluid and vestigial neural structures in the lower back. This condition is commonly diagnosed in the prenatal period by α-fetoprotein assays or by ultrasonography.

Normally, the cells from each side of the neural crest join in the midline of the embryo to form the spinal cord (neural canal). In association with spinal cord development, the spinous process of each vertebra is formed by the union of half of the spinous process from each side in the fetal spine with these bony elements closing over the spinal cord and joining in the midline to encircle the neural canal. In children with spina bifida, normal formation of the dorsal spinal cord and spinous process region does not occur. When a myelomeningocele forms in the developing fetus, the result is a dural sac filled with cerebrospinal fluid and vestigial neural elements in the portion of the spine involved. If the meninges alone are involved and the spinal cord is not, a meningocele develops and the neurologic deficit is less severe or minimal. If only the bony spinous processes fail to unite at more than one level and the neural elements form normally, a spina bifida occulta occurs and is usually of little clinical consequence.

In a child with a myelomeningocele, the functional deficit of the lower extremities is linked to the level of the neuroanatomic defect. The level of motor function may be slightly different in each extremity, although both extremities are nearly always involved. The sensory level may also vary between the two extremities.

The level of neurologic function can be closely approximated by performing a physical examination of the child's muscle function in the newborn nursery. This is best done by spending some time in simple observation of the child to see what parts of each lower extremity are actively moving and which are not. Care must be taken not to confuse reflex movements with usable motor function. If the baby's leg flexes when withdrawing from the stimulation of the foot only, with no other unprovoked movement of the leg seen, this motion is likely mediated by a single arc reflex below the level of useful spinal cord function.

If no active lower-extremity movement is seen in the newborn, a low thoracic level of spina bifida is present. Infants with defects at the high lumbar level have hip flexion and adduction. Those with mid-lumbar–level defects have knee extension and flexion. Children with low lumbar-level lesions have dorsiflexion of the ankle, while those with defects at the sacral neurologic level have foot inversion and some eversion as well. Correlation of observed physical findings with the anteroposterior spine radiograph, noting the levels where the spinous processes are unfused and the pedicles flared and rotated, will allow accurate identification of the neurologic level (Figs. 18.1 to 18.3). Based on this information, it is possible to discuss with the parents the expected extremity function, the child's walking potential, and potential orthopaedic problems that lie ahead.

Neurosurgical closure of the myelomeningocele is urgently needed shortly after birth to prevent infection with meningitis. Hydrocephalus may also require early placement of a ventriculoperitoneal shunt. On the other hand, orthopaedic care is seldom essential at birth but is needed throughout the child's life, as the majority of orthopaedic problems arise as a result of muscle imbalance or weakness leading to joint contractures or walking difficulty. Because of the associated multiple neurologic and urologic problems as well as other medical and social concerns, these children are best managed through multidisciplinary clinics.

ESTIMATION OF WALKING ABILITY

Characteristically, orthopaedists divide ambulation into four main categories: community, household, exercise, and wheelchair. A community ambulator may require braces or crutches for assistance but can walk virtually everywhere; a household ambulator uses a wheelchair outside the house or school; an exercise ambulator walks only at physical therapy sessions; a wheelchair ambulator uses a wheelchair nearly full time but may take a few steps with much support.

In general, a child with a low thoracic or high lumbar spina bifida will be a wheelchair or exercise ambulator, although household ambulation is feasible for a child in a very motivated family. Children with mid-lumbar–level spina bifida are household and

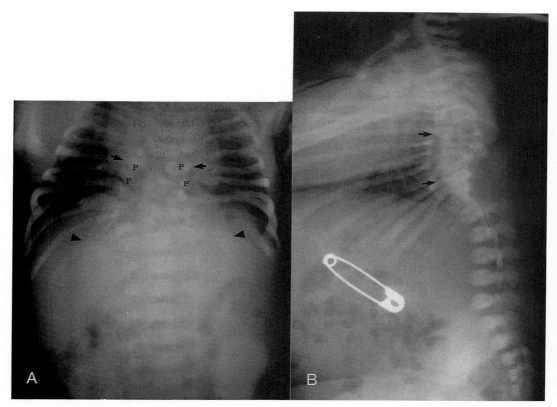

Figure 18.1. **A,** Frontal view of the spine of an infant shows a meningomyelocele starting in the mid-thoracic spine (*arrows*) with flaring of the pedicles (*P*) from T7 caudally. The soft tissue mass of the meningomyelocele is noted overlying the midline (*arrowheads*). **B,** Lateral spine radiograph of the same infant shows tethering and focal lordosis (*arrows*) in the thoracic region and lumbar kyphosis.

sometimes community ambulators. Children with low lumbar and sacral-level spina bifida are often community ambulators. If hydrocephalus is a persistent problem, ambulation at these predictive levels is less likely.

As some community-ambulator children become teenagers, many will find that use of a wheelchair will allow for less energy expenditure and more ease of movement in school and in the community than walking using braces and crutches. This is particularly true in teenagers who become obese, a common problem in older children with myelomeningocele.

SPECIFIC ORTHOPAEDIC PROBLEMS

Kyphosis

A rigid kyphosis is seen at birth in some children with thoracic-level spina bifida. During embryonic development, failure of posterior closure of the spine leads to marked flexion of the lumbar spine, which becomes fixed. This immobile kyphosis makes sitting difficult, and skin breakdown over the apex of the insensate kyphosis is troublesome. Bracing is ineffective due to the rigid nature of the kyphosis, and surgical resection of the kyphosis may be the recommended treatment.

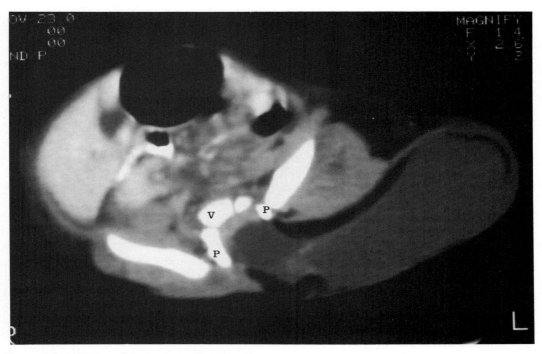

Figure 18.2. CT scan of the lumbosacral lipomeningocele shows widespread pedicles (*P*), S1 vertebra (*V*), and a large posterior defect with a mass of meningomyelocele.

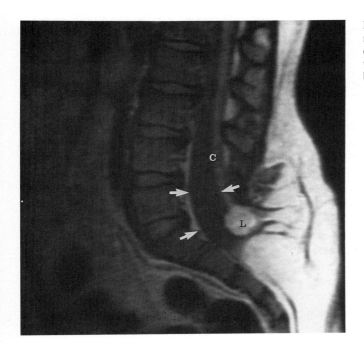

Figure 18.3. Sagittal MR scan of a lipo-meningocele shows a tethered spinal cord (*C*), a lipomatous mass (*L*), and a widened spinal canal (*arrows*) in the lum-bosacral region.

Scoliosis

Unlike the kyphosis that is present at the time of birth, scoliosis develops in later childhood or during adolescence. It is most common in children with thoracic or high lumbar-level involvement. Unilateral hip dislocation and pelvic obliquity may further predispose to the development of scoliosis.

During the early stages of scoliosis, a thoracolumbar-sacral orthosis (TLSO) can often prevent further progression of the spinal curvature. Spinal instrumentation and fusion are indicated if the scoliosis is severe enough to interfere with sitting or walking function.

Whenever the progression of scoliosis is rapid or is associated with further impairment of lower-extremity function, the cause of the rapid change may be from a tethered cord or lipoma at the base of the spinal cord, both of which often coexist with spina bifida. If these neurologic problems are suspected, a magnetic resonance study of the thoracic or lumbar spine is needed. If either a lipoma or a tethered cord is present, it should be treated surgically prior to treatment for the scoliosis.

Hip Instability

Hip instability is a common occurrence in children with spina bifida who have innervation of the hip flexor and adductor muscles but have no function in the hip extensor or abductor muscles. Hip dislocation most commonly occurs in children with a neurologic functional level that stops at the third or fourth lumbar level. Hip dislocation is rare in children with spina bifida who have innervation to the sacral level.

The need for and extent of treatment of hip dislocation in children with myelomeningocele is somewhat controversial. Pain is rarely present, and passive hip movement is usually well maintained, even in those with unstable hips. It has been well demonstrated that ambulatory children with spina bifida and bilateral dislocated hips are able to walk as well as those with located hips, provided the dislocation has not caused significant pelvic obliquity. Bracing is not very effective in preventing dislocation, since the instability is related to muscle imbalance. If the dislocation is bilateral, no treatment may be needed. If there is a unilateral dislocation, surgical relocation of the hip, combined with a muscle transfer (such as the external oblique muscle of the abdominal wall) to maintain the reduction, is generally recommended, especially if pelvic obliquity begins to develop.

Foot Deformity

Foot deformities are very common in children with myelomeningocele. At birth, the most common foot problems are rigid clubfoot deformity and congenital vertical talus (see Chapter 15). Although serial casting is helpful to allow partial correction, surgical treatment is inevitably needed to correct the deformity and place the feet in a plantigrade position for standing and walking. Because these feet are often insensate, it is important to provide the child with a foot that bears weight relatively evenly, avoiding bone prominences that can lead to pressure sores with weight bearing, especially if braces are worn to facilitate walking. The parents of walking children who have poor or absent sensation in the foot must check for skin pressure areas at least daily, a chore that older children and teenagers should assume for themselves.

Foot deformity that arises during childhood results from asymmetrical muscle action on the foot or a progressive neurologic loss. An example of asymmetrical muscle pull is the development of a calcaneus foot deformity. In children with L4-level innervation, the anterior tibialis muscle will provide unopposed foot dorsiflexion at the ankle. Since no plantarflexion muscles are working, the foot remains dorsiflexed, placing all weight with standing or walking on the heel, at times resulting in skin breakdown there. Surgical treatment, consisting of either a tendon transfer or a tendon release, will permit the foot to return to a position that allows distribution of weight over the entire foot.

No matter what the specific foot deformity that results from uneven muscle pull, a surgical procedure to better balance the muscle pull can be devised to allow improved standing or walking.

Joint Contractures

Flexion contractures at the hip in children with a low thoracic or an upper lumbar myelomeningocele result from intact psoas muscle function, which may produce hip instability. Even if the hips are stable, stretching exercises and periods of prone lying can minimize these contractures. If a hip flexion contracture develops, surgical tendon lengthening may be needed to allow the use of a reciprocating gait orthosis that can be employed at an early age to allow ambulation.

Knee flexion contractures are a result of intact medial hamstring muscle function with little or no quadriceps muscle power. In the younger child, daily stretching exercises can often prevent contractures. The primary reason for considering surgical treatment in these cases is to facilitate the use of braces for standing or walking.

Stretching exercises at home can be very useful to prevent significant contractures at the hip and knee. If surgical correction is needed, bracing and continued home exercise postoperatively can prevent the recurrence of contractures.

Cerebral Palsy

Cerebral palsy is a nonprogressive neurologic disorder that results from significant ischemia of the central nervous system deep white matter in a neonate or young infant. Cerebral palsy occurs most commonly after intraventricular hemorrhage and periventricular leukomalacia in preterm infants. Similar clinical patterns of spastic cerebral palsy are seen in children with meningitis and cerebritis in infancy and in those with anoxic brain injury as a result of near-drowning. Cerebral palsy is a constellation of neurologic findings that results from significant injury to the brain.

Several manifestations of cerebral palsy occur, and one child may exhibit characteristics of more than one type. Most common is the spastic type, recognizable by the presence of increased muscle tone in the involved extremities. Within this group, the term *spastic diplegia* indicates involvement of the lower extremities only, *spastic hemiplegia* describes involvement of both the upper and the lower extremity on one side of the body, and *spastic quadriplegia* describes a child with total body involvement.

Most common is the spastic type of cerebral palsy, in which the spasticity results from aberrant function of the stretch receptors in the involved muscles. Normally, when a muscle is stretched, the stretch receptors signal the muscle to elongate to allow the stretching to occur. In spastic cerebral palsy, the attempted stretching of a muscle results instead in contraction of the muscle. For example, in a child with spastic cerebral palsy, a sudden movement of the foot into a dorsiflexed position will begin to stretch the calf muscles, leading to a sudden contraction of the gastrocnemius and resultant plantarflexion of the foot. In the lower extremity, the muscles most commonly affected are the hip flexors and adductors, the hamstrings, and the gastrocnemius, while in the upper extremity this spasticity primarily involves the finger and wrist flexor muscles and the biceps muscle.

The second most common form of cerebral palsy is the athetoid type, which is seen primarily in children with kernicterus during the neonatal period. It has become less common, as neonatal hyperbilirubinemia is now more effectively treated. Involuntary extremity and head movements are the hallmark features of this type of cerebral palsy. Although contractures of the extremity occur, they are less common than in the spastic type. Limited ambulation is difficult or impossible due to the involuntary movements and problems with balance. However, many of these children can learn to control and drive a powered wheelchair for improved independence. The use of communication boards should be evaluated for most of the children with the athetoid form of cerebral palsy, since speech is often significantly impaired even though intelligence is often normal.

Other forms of cerebral palsy are the rigid type, choreoathetoid type, and a variety of mixed types. The remainder of the discussion in this chapter addresses the spastic type only, since this is the form of cerebral palsy that most often results in orthopaedic problems.

DIAGNOSIS

In some very premature infants with generalized body involvement, the diagnosis of spastic cerebral palsy can be made early. However, in a larger number of cases, the manifestations are more subtle and the diagnosis may not be established for months or even until toddler age. Certain aspects of the medical history and physical examination should suggest to the primary care physician that cerebral palsy may be present.

Any child with a delay in developmental motor milestones should be considered to possibly have cerebral palsy. Normally a child should be sitting by 6 months of age and walking at about 1 year. Although there is normal variation in development, a child who is not walking by 15 months of age has a delay in motor milestones. If a child was premature, sustained a significant anoxic episode perinatally, or had low Apgar scores, the diagnosis of cerebral palsy should be strongly considered.

The primary physical finding is the presence of increased muscle tone or spasticity in the extremities, most easily detected in the lower extremities, at the hips and ankles. Rapid passive abduction of the hips

is used to detect spasticity in the adductor muscles. If the hips "catch" when passively abducted, increased tone is present. In the ankle, sudden dorsiflexion of the foot will detect spasticity in the gastrocnemius muscle of the calf.

To differentiate the limitation of joint movement due to fixed contracture from that due to spasticity ("dynamic contracture"), the examiner should provide firm, continued pressure to stretch the involved muscle, thus overcoming the aberrant stretch response and allowing muscle elongation and joint movement to occur. In the ankle, for example, if sudden dorsiflexion meets resistance due to spasticity of the gastrocnemius muscle, continued dorsiflexion pressure will "overpower" the spasticity, allowing the foot to be brought into a dorsiflexed position. In a static or fixed contracture, it is impossible to place the foot into the dorsiflexed position. It is important to differentiate between dynamic and fixed contractures, since fixed contractures usually need surgical treatment, while dynamic contractures usually do not.

Although a magnetic resonance (MR) scan may detect brain abnormalities in some children, there is no specific laboratory test to confirm the diagnosis of cerebral palsy. The diagnosis is made by the combination of medical history, delayed motor milestones, and the physical examination finding of increased motor tone.

GENERAL ORTHOPAEDIC CONSIDERATIONS

Even though the neurologic lesion in spastic cerebral palsy is not progressive, the orthopaedic problems that result from this neurologic lesion are commonly progressive. At birth, even in infants with marked spasticity, fixed contractures of the extremities are unusual. These contractures result from asymmetrical muscle pull over time as the more spastic muscles overpower those with less spasticity.

The more spastic the child, the harder it

is to control the extremity muscles individually. This lack of control leads to either flexion or extension patterns linking the action of several muscles together and causing functional problems. In the lower extremity, hip adduction and extension, knee extension, and foot plantarflexion are characteristic of an extensor pattern; with a flexion pattern in the upper extremity, shoulder internal rotation, elbow flexion, and wrist flexion commonly exist together. Knowledge of these mass action patterns helps to understand why a child with spasticity has problems with extremity function and helps guide treatment to improve this function.

The goal of orthopaedic treatment of children with spastic cerebral palsy is to maximize function by controlling the adverse effects of spasticity through physical therapy, use of braces, and/or surgical treatment. Temporary or permanent reduction of spasticity can be effected by selective dorsal lumbar rhizotomy, but the role of this operative procedure in the overall management of spastic cerebral palsy is not fully defined.

Stretching exercises, to prevent or delay the appearance of contractures, are instituted once the diagnosis of spastic cerebral palsy is made. Effective use of stretching exercises requires parental interest and cooperation, as these exercises must be performed at least daily and preferably several times a day. A physical therapist instructs the parents in the proper method of passive stretching and checks the child periodically to monitor progress. When the child is young, stretching exercises are more effective than when the child is older, larger, and stronger.

The optimal amount of time spent in physical therapy varies. The long-term effect of physical therapy is difficult to assess accurately, but in the short term the pediatric physical therapist is very helpful in supervising the program of stretching exercises and in providing information and support to the parents. As the child becomes older, the decision must be made as to whether the child is better served by spending time with peers or by spending time in formal physical therapy sessions. The availability of a parent to take the child to physical therapy may also become an issue in making this decision.

Orthotics are used for two primary purposes: to facilitate walking and standing and to prevent contractures. Orthotics are named according to the joints crossed by the brace. A short leg brace is called an ankle-foot orthosis (AFO), while a long leg brace is termed a knee-ankle-foot orthosis (KAFO). The orthosis most commonly used is the AFO, which functions in several ways. The AFO holds the foot flat when walking or standing, may prevent progressive equinus or plantarflexion contractures, and may improve sitting ability by "breaking up" the extensor mass action pattern and facilitating hip and knee flexion. Orthotics are commonly used for several months following surgical treatment to prevent the recurrence of contractures. Since orthotics are meant to facilitate function, children who walk should be assessed periodically with and without braces to ensure that the child functions better with the orthotic than without it.

Children with spastic cerebral palsy should have regular orthopaedic evaluations. If a child is primarily being observed, an annual evaluation may suffice. However, if orthotics are being used or if a physical therapy program has been prescribed, the child should be evaluated by the orthopaedist for progress or new problems every 3 to 6 months.

Surgical treatment is recommended to treat joint contractures that interfere with function and are too fixed to be treated with stretching or orthotics. In a child who is walking, thorough evaluation prior to surgical treatment is often facilitated by computerized gait analysis studies. Using this objective information on muscle activity, joint motion, and rotational position of the lower extremities during walking, the orthopaedic surgeon can carefully construct a surgical plan to treat all orthopaedic problems of the extremities that interfere with walking. Since it takes several months after operative procedures for an ambulatory spastic child to regain good walking ability, it is important to avoid annual surgery by planning surgery no more than once or twice during childhood. Intensive physical therapy postoperatively will speed the return of the child to walking, and the use of postoperative orthoses to prevent recurrence of contractures will help preserve the surgical gains.

"TOE-WALKING"

In a child with mild involvement from spastic cerebral palsy, toe-walking may be the problem for which the parents bring the child to the physician. Toe-walking can be normal for many children beginning to walk and may even be considered normal in some children up to age 3 years. In some normal children there may be a family history of toe-walking. However, any child with toe-walking needs to be evaluated with the passive dorsiflexion stretch test to see if increased tone is present in the calf muscles. If no increased tone is noted and the child can stand flat-footed when not walking, simple follow-up will usually demonstrate the development of a normal heel-toe walking pattern. However, if increased calf muscle tone is present or if the child was premature, had an anoxic episode as an infant, or had delayed motor milestones, the toe-walking should be considered a manifestation of spastic cerebral palsy (albeit mild if this is the only extremity finding present). Parents should be informed of this diagnosis, and other testing (for example for learning disorders) should be considered.

If toe-walking is due to spastic calf muscles, a stretching program should be instituted for use at home by the parents. An AFO will generally improve the child's walking and will help prevent a fixed equinus or plantarflexion contracture. If the foot cannot be dorsiflexed past a neutral position at the ankle, surgical lengthening of the Achilles tendon is indicated. Extreme care must be taken not to over-lengthen this tendon. Over-lengthening the Achilles tendon will lead to a crouch-type gait that will require the use of an orthotic for life, so having to re-lengthen the Achilles tendon at a later age is preferable to the initial over-lengthening of the tendon.

KNEE FLEXION CONTRACTURES

Flexion contracture of the knee secondary to increased spasticity of the medial and lateral hamstring muscles is common in spastic cerebral palsy. The medial hamstring muscles are the gracilis, semitendinosus, and semimembranosus. The biceps femoris is the lateral hamstring muscle. These muscles cross both the hip and the knee joints, arising from the ischial region of the pelvis and inserting onto the proximal tibia and fibula, thereby acting as hip extensors and knee flexors.

The two major effects of hamstring contractures are inability to straighten the knee when walking and difficulty sitting. If a knee flexion contracture is present, energy requirements when walking are increased since much more muscle activity is required from the quadriceps muscle to stand and walk. In fact, the farther the child walks with bent knees, the more likely the child will have a progressive increase in knee flexion as the quadriceps muscle tires. Even if a child with spastic cerebral palsy does not walk, hamstring contractures can affect the way he or she sits in the wheelchair or a seat. Tight hamstrings extend the hip, tending to throw the trunk posteriorly. This either leads to a total kyphosis position of the spine or causes the child to lose sitting balance and fall backward.

In the young child, hamstring stretching by extending the knee with the hip flexed can help prevent progressive hamstring contractures. However, once these contractures are present and interfere with the child's function, partial surgical lengthening of the hamstring muscles is needed. Hamstring lengthening is often combined with other procedures, such as hip flexor lengthening and Achilles tendon lengthening, to better prevent a recurrence of a crouched gait. Over-lengthening of the hamstring muscles, which will lead to a recurvatum deformity of the knee, must be avoided in a child who is walking.

HIP CONTRACTURES AND HIP INSTABILITY

Spasticity of the psoas and adductor muscles produces flexion and adduction contractures of the hip in a child with spastic cerebral palsy. The adduction contractures can interfere with function at various stages, making sitting difficult, causing "scissoring" when attempting to walk, and potentially causing hip dislocation. Flexion contracture may also lead to hip dislocation and cause a crouched gait. If the adductor and flexion contractures interfere with func-

tion, surgical lengthening of these spastic muscles is indicated and useful.

In children with limited abduction due to adductor spasticity, periodic anteroposterior radiographs of the pelvis should be obtained to monitor the development of the hips (Fig. 18.4). If hip subluxation is detected early, surgical lengthening of the hip adductors (and possibly the psoas) can allow the hip to develop well, provided hip abduction is preserved postoperatively. At a later age, hip subluxation or hip dislocation requires a proximal femoral osteotomy and possibly a pelvic osteotomy to maintain hip stability.

In all children with spastic cerebral palsy and hip instability, even children who are totally dependent, the author recommends surgical treatment to maintain hip stability. In ambulatory children, walking ability will be preserved. In nonwalking children, sitting ability and perineal hygiene will be enhanced compared with a child with pelvic

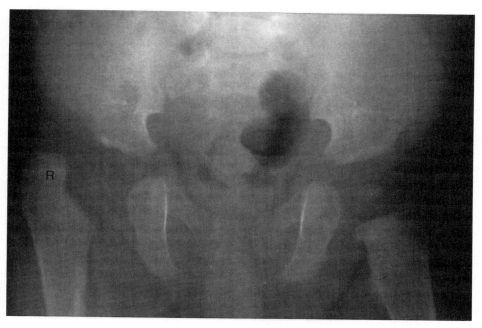

Figure 18.4. Anteroposterior pelvic radiograph in a young child with spastic cerebral palsy demonstrates a right hip dislocation and apparent bilateral coxa valga.

obliquity from a unilateral hip dislocation. In some older spastic children, hip dislocations will become painful with attempted leg movement and may precipitate progressive scoliosis.

SCOLIOSIS

Progressive scoliosis occurs most often in children with cerebral palsy who have total body involvement and who are unable to walk. Many of these children develop scoliosis in mid- to late childhood, and it progresses rapidly in the teenage years. It is uncommon for children with spastic diplegia or spastic hemiplegia to require treatment for scoliosis.

Reasons for the development of scoliosis are unclear. At times, asymmetrical hip contractures or even a unilateral hip dislocation may lead to pelvic obliquity, which in turn leads to a progressive long C-shaped thoracolumbar scoliosis, but this is not always the case. Once scoliosis develops, worsening can be expected. Since the scoliosis is in the lumbar and thoracolumbar regions, pulmonary function is less affected than with thoracic curves.

Treatment of scoliosis in children who have spastic quadriplegia cerebral palsy is difficult. When it is detected early, wearing of an orthosis is recommended to prevent progression, but children are seldom able to wear the brace as prescribed due to feeding problems, seizures, skin breakdown, and other coexisting health concerns. As a result, bracing is seldom fully successful.

As the scoliosis worsens, it needs to be decided whether or not surgical treatment is warranted. If the child has useful hand function, surgical treatment—usually an anterior and posterior spinal fusion with spinal instrumentation—is indicated and will stabilize the spine and allow stable sitting without the need for the child to use one hand or arm for support. However, if no useful upper-extremity function is present, the primary gains from spinal surgery will be to improve the sitting position and facilitate attendant care. In instances when the parents

and the physician conclude that extensive spinal surgery for scoliosis may not provide enough gain to warrant the risks and expense of surgery, a seating support system can be built into the wheelchair to facilitate care.

UPPER-EXTREMITY CONTRACTURES

A flexion pattern develops in the upper extremity as a result of spasticity, causing the shoulder to rotate internally, the elbow to flex, and the wrist and fingers to flex. Primary attention is given to the wrist and finger flexion resulting from this spasticity.

Normally, the hand has the strongest grip when the wrist is in an extended position, thus allowing the finger flexors to generate the most power. If the wrist is flexed (try it out for yourself!), the finger flexor muscles are effectively lengthened and provide only weak grasp. One of the goals in treating spastic cerebral palsy is to position the wrist in a neutral or extended position.

The hand, likewise, cannot function well if the fingers cannot be extended out of the palm to allow the hand to grasp an object. Because of the spasticity in the finger flexor muscles, including those of the thumb, voluntary finger extension may be difficult or impossible, inhibiting the grasping of objects. If this spastic involvement is only in one arm, as in spastic hemiplegia, the involved arm is often used little.

Hand splints can be used in most children with spastic upper extremities to improve wrist extension and to keep the thumb out of the palm. However, if the child is markedly retarded or has no active volitional movement of the hand, passive splinting may be all that is needed. In selected children, when they have reached an age to cooperate postoperatively with occupational therapy, surgical tendon lengthening or tendon transfer can improve function.

Muscular Dystrophy

Several forms of muscle disease first appear during childhood. Although some myopathies are diagnosed during infancy, most muscle disorders appear later in childhood, with the child having normal motor milestones initially only to lose function with increasing age. When presented with this clinical picture, the physician must strongly consider the possibility of muscle disease.

The large number of muscle disorders that exist cannot be fully covered here. The primary focus is on Duchenne's muscular dystrophy, but physical findings of increasing weakness and decreasing motor function are similar for many other muscle diseases.

Duchenne's muscular dystrophy occurs only in boys, but other muscle disorders occur in children of both sexes. Because of the delay in onset of this muscle weakness, other children may be born into the affected family before the diagnosis of the muscle disease has been made in the older boy.

Boys affected with Duchenne's muscular dystrophy appear normal at birth and have normal motor development milestones. At about 3 years, the parents note some increased clumsiness and a tendency to fall. Over the next year, there is a decrease in the child's stamina and he tires easily. The parents' concern over the boy's declining motor abilities usually prompts them to seek the advice of a physician when the child is about 5 years of age. Physical examination at that time allows the diagnosis to be made clinically, with confirmation by appropriate laboratory studies. The most striking physical finding in Duchenne's muscular dystrophy may be the pseudohypertrophy or disproportionate enlargement of the calf muscles. These calf muscles appear large but weakness is present as a result of fatty replacement of muscle. A positive Gowers' sign, in which the child must use his hands to ''climb up'' the legs when getting up from the floor into a standing position, is present due to more pronounced weakness in the hip area than more distally in the lower extremity.

As the boy with Duchenne's muscular dystrophy becomes older, other physical findings characteristically occur. Lumbar lordosis increases during standing, a result of hip extensor weakness and hip flexion contractures. Toe-walking, due to an equinus contracture of the calf muscles, becomes common. Weakness continues to progress, and the affected boy usually stops walking by around age 12. If hip flexion and ankle equinus contractures progress untreated, loss of walking ability occurs earlier. Once the child becomes nonambulatory, scoliosis appears and generally continues to worsen during teenage years. Pulmonary function deteriorates relentlessly as the result of the muscle disease, and the presence of a progressive scoliosis accelerates this loss of pulmonary function. Eventual death in the late teens or early twenties is due to respiratory compromise.

Laboratory studies will confirm the clinical diagnosis of Duchenne's muscular dystrophy. Serum creatinine phosphokinase will be strikingly elevated. A muscle biopsy will demonstrate characteristic histopathologic changes. The most specific test for Duchenne's muscular dystrophy is genetic analysis for the presence of dystrophin.

Once the diagnosis is established, other male siblings should be screened for possible Duchenne's muscular dystrophy and the parents should be counseled about the 50% risk of future male offspring having this disorder. The family should be referred to a Muscular Dystrophy Association center for continuing care and family support. To date, no cure is known for Duchenne's muscular dystrophy.

The initial orthopaedic care for these boys involves the use of passive stretching exercises by the parents and therapists to prevent or delay the appearance of hip flexion and ankle equinus contractures, since both these contractures lead to early cessation of walking. If these contractures appear, tendon lengthening of the hip flexor muscles and the heel cord can prolong walking ability for 1 to 2 years, but long leg braces are required for walking following this surgery. Once the older child is nonambulatory, these contractures usually do not need surgical treatment.

When a child with Duchenne's muscular dystrophy becomes wheelchair bound, scoliosis begins. Bracing is not effective in preventing the progression of scoliosis. If the scoliosis exceeds 30° when the child is sitting, spinal instrumentation and fusion surgery is indicated to improve sitting balance and to delay the impairment of pulmonary function seen in boys with progressive scoliotic deformity. This surgical treatment should be completed while the child still has reasonable pulmonary function, or prolonged respirator support following surgery may be needed.

Arthrogryposis Multiplex Congenita

Confusion over the exact meaning is commonplace when one encounters the term arthrogryposis in the medical literature or in clinical practice. Literally meaning bent or crooked joints, the word *arthrogryposis* is used by some (including most orthopaedists) to describe a specific condition involving all four extremities and resulting in multiple orthopaedic problems. However, for others this term is more appropriately used to denote a condition of limited joint motion, present at birth and resulting from soft-tissue contractures. Using this latter sense, over 100 different syndromes have been described that include arthrogryposis as one part of a more generalized syndrome. This section focuses on the use of the term *arthrogryposis* as synonymous with the conditions described variously as arthrogryposis multiplex congenita or, more recently, amyoplasia.

Typically, a child with this condition is born with contractures of essentially all joints in all four extremities. Breech presentation is common and delivery may be difficult, leading to the relatively common appearance of one or more fractures at birth. Most often, these contractures produce po-

sitions of internal rotation and adduction at the shoulder, extension at the elbow, flexion at the wrist and fingers, adduction and flexion at the hips, and flexion at the knees. Foot deformity, either a clubfoot or a congenital vertical talus, is present in the majority of infants. There is usually a striking lack of normal skin creases at the joints. The long, slender fingers have been described as having a wax-like appearance. The face is round at birth, and a capillary hemangioma on the face is common.

Other features differentiate this condition from others that include congenital joint contractures. In arthrogryposis multiplex congenita, there are no abnormalities of the viscera and intelligence is normal. The occurrence of this condition appears to be sporadic, and there is no evidence that it is a genetic disorder.

The deformities seen in this condition seem to be the result of diminished intrauterine fetal movement. These infants have a decrease in the number of anterior horn cells in the spinal cord, but whether this neurologic abnormality is due to an unrecognized teratogen, a maternal viral infection, or some other cause is unknown. This lack of fetal movement, commonly noted by the mother during the pregnancy, leads to abnormal amniotic fluid circulation and to oligohydramnios, which in turn may produce abnormal fetal position. The lack of fetal movement produces soft-tissue contractures that lead to the joint contractures seen at birth, even though the joints have been formed normally in an embryologic sense. (A condition similar to that of human arthrogryposis has been produced in chicks by injection of a fertilized egg with a paralyzing agent.)

The diagnosis of arthrogryposis multiplex congenita is made by history (lack of fetal movements and negative family history of a similar condition) and by physical examination of the infant. Muscle biopsy will demonstrate fibrofatty replacement of muscle tissue, but a muscle biopsy is not usually needed. Radiographs will demonstrate the joint contractures and a lack of muscle mass around the normal long bones. Hip dislocation is common but not specific for this condition.

Early treatment of these contractures is often helpful. Passive motion exercises should be started in the newborn period and continued regularly by the parents under the guidance of a physical or occupational therapist. Splints can be effectively used in conjunction with a passive exercise program to maintain gains in joint movement. The majority of the multiple soft-tissue contractures will improve, at least partially, with this program of passive exercise and splinting.

Surgical treatment is beneficial in managing several of the associated orthopaedic abnormalities. The foot deformity, be it a clubfoot or a congenital vertical talus, is treated surgically during the first year of life, with the goal of producing a plantigrade foot to facilitate standing and walking development. Unilateral hip dislocation is surgically reduced to decrease the later development of pelvic obliquity and progressive scoliosis. However, bilateral hip dislocation is often left untreated, as walking potential is essentially the same for those with bilateral hip dislocations as for those children with reduced hips. Persistent knee flexion contractures that interfere with walking can be corrected by soft-tissue release and extension osteotomy of the femur. Progressive scoliosis in the older child is initially managed with bracing but requires surgical treatment if worsening of the spinal deformity continues.

The intellectual and cognitive development of these children is normal. With appropriate orthopaedic care, about 75% of the children with this condition will be able to walk, though rarely in a normal manner. However, difficulty with mobility, lack of full independence in activities of daily living, and absence of normal social and sexual relationships often combine to markedly delay psychosocial development in children and adolescents with this condition.

Charcot-Marie-Tooth Disease

Charcot-Marie-Tooth disease is the most common peripheral neuropathy that results in significant orthopaedic problems. In most peripheral neuropathies that involve the growing extremity asymmetrically, a deformity of the hand or foot will result. This is also true of conditions involving the central nervous system, and a thorough workup is needed to clearly define the exact cause of the extremity dysfunction or deformity.

Charcot-Marie-Tooth disease is a familial disorder, inherited as an autosomal recessive trait. This condition primarily affects the peroneal nerve in the lower extremity and, later, the ulnar nerve in the upper extremity. Involvement is bilateral, although one side may be affected slightly more than the other. The severity of this condition can be judged to some degree by the age of onset, and children diagnosed before 10 years of age have the most extensive involvement.

The presenting complaint usually involves parental concern over deformity of the child's foot. This deformity may be a cavus or high-arched deformity or an inturned position of the foot. The foot problem, not noted in early childhood, becomes progressively worse as the child grows. Activity levels are not usually affected early in the course of the disease.

Physical examination will confirm the presence of foot deformity. Weakness of the peroneal muscles will be noted and ankle deep tendon reflexes will be diminished. When walking, the child will often recruit the use of the long toe extensors to help try to dorsiflex the foot during the swing phase of gait. When this physical finding is noted, weakness of the dorsiflexor muscles of the foot and ankle is usually present. Atrophy of the intrinsic muscles of the hand, specifically those innervated by the ulnar nerve, is generally seen later than the changes due to peroneal nerve involvement.

Confirmation of the diagnosis of Charcot-Marie-Tooth disease is made by electrodiagnostic studies. Nerve conduction is delayed along the peroneal nerve between the knee and the ankle and along the ulnar nerve in the upper extremity. Electromyographic changes of denervation are present in the peroneal muscles of the legs. Nerve or muscle biopsy is not needed to establish this diagnosis.

In the lower extremity, the asymmetrical muscle weakness that results leads to a progressive cavus deformity of the foot, often associated with clawing of the toes. The result is excessive weight-bearing pressure placed on the heads of the metatarsals, and painful callosities often occur at this site. Shoe modification may be effective in children who are less involved, but surgical correction of the cavus and claw-toe deformity is generally the best treatment to preserve function. It is not unusual for the child to require more than one operative procedure during the years of growth. While foot deformity is by far the most common orthopaedic problem seen in children with this disease, observation and examination for hip disorders and spinal deformity are also needed.

Poliomyelitis

Although poliomyelitis rarely occurs in the United States since the introduction of polio vaccine, this disorder still strikes children in Third World countries. In regions with a large immigrant population from these countries, the primary care physician may encounter children with the sequelae of this disease.

Poliomyelitis is a viral infection that affects the anterior horn cells of the spinal cord. The usual history is that the child was normal until the occurrence of muscle weakness following a febrile illness. The effect of this infection on walking and general motor function depends on the muscles affected and the severity of involvement.

In general, a child who has strong calf muscles for plantarflexion and a strong gluteus maximus muscle for hip extension can walk if no knee flexion contracture is present, even if the strength of several other muscles in the leg is weak or absent. A thorough lower-extremity muscle strength examination should be completed at the initial evaluation to determine what function is present and what potentially could be improved with orthotic or surgical treatment. For example, a child with good hip extension strength but no muscle power below the knee should walk well with an ankle-foot orthosis (AFO) that compensates for the lack of plantarflexion.

Unlike a condition such as cerebral palsy in which selective muscle control is often difficult or impossible, poliomyelitis often spares muscles with selective control, and these may be surgically transferred to substitute for absent muscle function. Avoidance of joint contractures through passive exercises and/or braces should be a major goal as the child grows, since these contractures make orthotic or surgical treatment more difficult. No two children with muscle weakness from poliomyelitis are the same, so it is essential to assess potential treatment options individually, based on a thorough extremity muscle examination.

Persons who have had poliomyelitis in childhood may note an increase in weakness during middle age, a condition aptly called "post-polio syndrome." This weakness is not due to a recurrence of the spinal cord infection but is related to an increased tendency of the weaker muscles to fatigue with activity or exercise.

Suggested Readings

Bleck, E.E.: Locomotor Prognosis in Cerebral Palsy. Dev. Med. Child Neurol. 17:18–25, 1975.
Bleck, E.E.: Orthopedic Management of Cerebral Palsy. J.B. Lippincott, Philadelphia, 1987.

Brooke, M.H.: A Clinician's View of Neuromuscular Disease, 2nd ed. Williams & Wilkins, Baltimore, 1986.

Duval-Beaupere, G., Kaci, M., Lougovoy, J., et al.: Growth of trunk and legs of children with myelomeningocele. Dev. Med. Child Neurol. 29:225–231, 1987.

Goldberg, M.J.: The Dysmorphic Child: An Orthopedic Perspective. Raven Press, New York, 1987.

Green, N.E.: The orthopaedic care of children with muscular dystrophy. Instr. Course Lect. 36: 267–274, 1987.

Jones, E.T. and Knapp, D.R.: Assessment and management of the lower extremity in cerebral palsy. Orthop. Clin. North Am. 18:725–738, 1987.

Mazur, J.M. and Menelaus, M.B.: Neurologic status of spina bifida patients and the orthopedic surgeon. Clin. Orthop. 264:54–64, 1991.

McDonald, C.M., Jaffe, K.M., Mosca, V.S., and Shurtleff, D.B.: Ambulatory outcome of children with myelomeningocele: effect of lower-extremity muscle strength. Dev. Med. Child Neurol. 33:482–490, 1991.

McLaughlin, J.F., Shurtleff, D.B., Lamers, J.Y., et al.: Influence of prognosis on decisions regarding the care of newborns with myelodysplasia. N. Engl. J. Med. 312:1589–1594, 1985.

Nelson, K.B. and Ellenberg, J.H.: Antecedents of cerebral palsy: multivariate analysis of risk. N. Engl. J. Med. 315:81–86, 1986.

Miller, G. and Vannucci, R.C.: Hereditary motor and sensory neuropathies. Pediatr. Ann. 18:428–431, 1989.

Palmer, F.B., Shapiro, B.K., Wachtel, R.C., et al.: The effects of physical therapy on cerebral palsy: a controlled trial in infants with spastic diplegia. N. Engl. J. Med. 318:803–808, 1988.

Sarwark, J.F., MacEwen, G.D., and Scott, C.I., Jr.: Current concepts review: amyoplasia (a common form of arthrogryposis). J. Bone Joint Surg. 72A: 465–469, 1990.

Sutherland, D.H.: Gait Disorders in Childhood and Adolescence. Williams & Wilkins, Baltimore, 1984.

Thompson, C.E.: Raising a Handicapped Child: A Helpful Guide for Parents of the Physically Disabled. Ballantine Books, New York, 1991.

19
The Limping Child

The ability to walk without pain or disability is an essential part of normal everyday life. Normal walking is characterized by symmetrical movement of both lower extremities in a regular pattern called the gait cycle. Simply stated, the gait cycle for each leg consists of a stance phase and a swing phase, with a short period when both feet are in contact with the ground. The stance phase begins with heel strike, then proceeds to a flat foot position, and ends with toe off, as the foot pushes off from the ground. The swing phase begins with toe off, proceeds through mid-swing, to end with the next heel strike. Both feet are on the ground for about 20% of the gait cycle, with stance and swing phases each accounting for approximately 40% of this gait cycle (Fig. 19.1).

An aberration of this normal gait cycle, be it due to deformity or pain, will result in a limp. In attempting to determine the cause of a limp in a child, the first step is to assess what type of limp is present. The three primary types of limp are antalgic type, abductor lurch or Trendelenburg type, and short-leg type.

An *antalgic gait* is a limp caused by pain in one of the extremities and is sometimes called a "quick step" gait. This type of limp is easily detected since the child will have a shorter stance phase on the affected leg, manifested by a quick step on to and then off the painful leg. The stance phase of the gait cycle will be lengthened on the normal leg, though a quicker swing phase is present on the normal side.

The *abductor lurch or Trendelenburg gait* is characteristic of children with a chronic problem involving the hip. This manner of walking is manifested by the trunk swinging over the affected leg that is on the ground during stance phase. If both hips are involved, the trunk will swing from one side to the other as walking proceeds. This type of walking results from weakness of the primary hip abductor muscle, the gluteus medius muscle. The time spent standing on each foot is the same for both legs.

Normally, the gluteus medius muscle is strong enough to keep the pelvis level when the opposite leg is off the ground during the swing phase of gait, with the trunk remaining in the midline. If the gluteus medius muscle is weak, as is the case with virtually all conditions affecting the hip for more than a few weeks, the opposite side of the pelvis drops down when the leg on that side is lifted off the ground. The child compensates for this hip abductor weakness by leaning the trunk over the weak side, resulting in the trunk sway characteristic of this type of abnormal gait.

If hip abductor weakness is suspected, a Trendelenburg test should be performed. When one leg is lifted off the ground, that side of the pelvis should become somewhat elevated as the opposite gluteus muscle contracts (see Fig. 12.4). However, if the pelvis drops down, a positive Trendelenburg test is present, demonstrating gluteus medius weakness on the side that is standing on the ground (see Fig. 12.5).

A *short-leg gait* results from either a true or an apparent leg length discrepancy. The

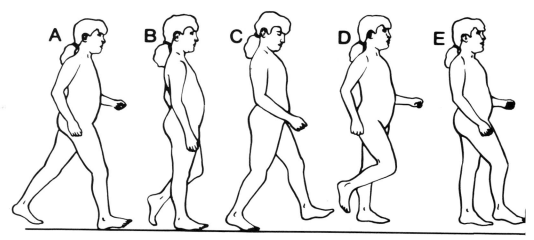

Figure 19.1. Sagittal-plane angular movement of the lower extremities during walking changes little after early childhood. This normal manner of walking, termed the *gait cycle*, is divided into different phases. Each leg normally has a stance and swing phase, with about 20% of the gait cycle consisting of both feet on the ground. In this illustration, the right leg positions are described. In **A**, "heel strike" begins the stance phase. In **B**, the right foot is in mid-stance, while in **C**, terminal stance or toe-off is present. In **D**, the right leg is in swing phase, with all the body weight supported on the left side. In **E**, the right foot is in terminal swing phase, just prior to the next heel strike as seen in **A**. This cycle is repeated for each leg continually as walking takes place. Determination of which phase of the gait cycle is affected when a child limps will be helpful in determining the cause of the limp.

long leg will either demonstrate some persistence of knee flexion when the child is standing or the child will walk on the toes of the shorter leg. In such a child, the pelvis will move up and down more than normal during walking. Since there is no pain with this gait, an equal amount of time is spent on each leg.

A true leg length discrepancy can be determined by measuring the distance from the anterior superior iliac spine to the medial malleolus or by assessing the height of each side of the pelvis with the child standing. An apparent leg length discrepancy is due to contractures of one or more muscles around the hip. If there is an adduction contracture, the affected lower extremity will seem to be shorter than it actually is, while abduction contractures lead to apparent lengthening of the extremity when walking. Apparent leg lengths can be quantitated by measuring from the umbilicus to the medial malleolus of each leg. If a co-existent foot deformity is present, the tape measure-

ments should be made to the bottom of the heel to include possible heel height discrepancy.

Clinical evaluation of a child with a limp should include evaluation of the following items:

- Careful history from parents or child
- Vital signs, especially temperature check
- Assessment of forward spine flexion
- Straight leg raising test for hamstring tightness or sciatic nerve irritation
- Assessment of the hip range of motion, especially internal rotation, abduction, and extension
- Palpation of the sacroiliac joints
- Evaluation of the thigh and calf for bruises and tenderness
- Tape measurement of thigh and calf circumference to assess for muscle atrophy
- Tape measurement of leg length
- Thorough knee evaluation
- Comparison of ankle range of motion with the normal side

- Visual and palpation examination of the foot
- Neurologic evaluation of the lower extremities, including reflexes, sensation, and motor strength

Determining the type of limp will narrow the differential diagnosis significantly. If there is no pain with the limp, the examiner should concentrate on possible hip or spine problems and on assessing the leg lengths. If pain is present, a careful examination of the entire affected lower extremity is in order, as noted above.

Since children, especially young children, often cannot accurately communicate the location of the pain that may be causing the limp, imaging studies are extremely useful in this situation to determine the cause of the pain. Radiographs from the hip to the foot, and sometimes including the spine, are used initially. If these appear normal, a bone scan is an excellent screening test to localize problems that are causing the pain, including fractures, infection, or tumors. Computed tomographic and magnetic resonance studies can be used to further delineate the disorder if there is an area of increased isotope uptake noted on the bone scan.

The differential diagnosis of a child with a limp contains many potential disorders of the lower extremity and spine (Table 19.1). Brief notes on many of these possible disorders are presented below, but most are discussed in more detail in the chapter on the particular anatomical section, elsewhere in this book.

Spine

The primary spinal conditions that may cause a child to limp are discitis, spinal or spinal cord tumors, tethered cord, and spondylolysis/spondylolisthesis. The main physical findings are limitation of forward bending of the spine and hamstring spasm with attempted straight leg raising. Specific neurologic findings in the lower extremity serve to further localize the spinal disorder.

Table 19.1.
Differential Diagnosis of the Limping Child

Spine	Discitis or disc space infection
	Spine or spinal cord tumor
	Tethered cord
	Spondylolysis/spondylolisthesis
Pelvis	Sacroiliac joint septic arthritis
	Ankylosing spondylitis
	Pelvic osteomyelitis
	Benign or malignant bone tumor
	Avulsion fracture of apophysis of iliac spine or ischium
Hip	
1–3 years	Septic arthritis or osteomyelitis
	Developmental dysplasia of the hip (DDH)
	Congenital short femur
	Congenital coxa vara
3–10 years	Transient synovitis (up to age 6)
	Legg-Perthes disease
	Septic arthritis or osteomyelitis
	Bilateral hip dysplasia
10–16 years	Slipped capital femoral epiphysis
	Avascular necrosis of the femoral head
	Osteomyelitis
	Bone tumor
	Idiopathic chondrolysis
	Effects of childhood hip dysplasia
Femur and thigh	Referred pain from hip disorder
	Bone tumors, especially osteosarcoma
	Myositis ossificans in quadriceps muscle
Knee	Meniscal or ligament injury
	Osgood-Schlatter disease
	Patello-femoral malalignment
	Osteochondritis dissecans
	Juvenile rheumatoid arthritis
Leg	Stress fracture of upper third of tibia
	Toddler's fracture (up to age 3)
	Shin splints
	Flat feet
	Bone tumor
	Osteomyelitis
Ankle	Sprain
	Growth plate fracture of distal tibia or fibula
	Osteochondritis dissecans of the talus
Foot	Calcaneal apophysitis (ages 9–12)
	Köhler's disease (ages 5–7)
	Avulsion fracture of the fifth metatarsal
	Tarsal coalition
	Cavus foot deformity
	Congenital foot anomaly
Miscellaneous	Congenital limb length discrepancy
	Acquired limb length discrepancy
	Brain injury causing hemiplegia
	Poorly fitting shoes

Besides plain radiography, the imaging studies most useful in delineating the underlying cause are bone scans and magnetic resonance scans.

Pelvis

Lesions in the pelvic area cause pain with weight bearing or as a result of pressure on the femoral or sciatic nerve, causing pain to radiate into the lower extremity. The most common conditions to consider are sacroiliac joint infection or inflammation, benign or malignant bone tumors, and an avulsion fracture of a secondary ossification center of the iliac spine or ischium.

Infection of the sacroiliac joint may be difficult to diagnose. However, if hyperextension of the hip causes pain at the sacroiliac joint, this diagnosis should be suspected. Whereas septic arthritis of the hip produces pain on internal rotation of the hip, sacroiliac septic arthritis produces pain on external rotation of the hip. If sacroiliac joint infection is strongly suspected, a bone scan should be obtained. In some cases of pelvic or sacroiliac infection, the standard Tc-99 bone scan may appear normal, while the gallium scan will demonstrate the site of infection.

Hip

Disorders in the hip region should be strongly considered whenever there is a limp. A Trendelenburg gait is caused nearly exclusively by a hip disorder, while an antalgic gait may also emanate from the hip.

While a full check of hip range of motion is preferable, the two primary planes of motion to check are internal rotation and abduction. Because of the anatomic features of the hip capsule, its volume capacity is the least with the hip extended and internally rotated. Therefore, fluid in the joint, be it blood, pus, or other effusion, will cause the hip to assume a position of external rotation and flexion. Testing of internal rotation of the hip in extension (with the child lying prone) is *the* most sensitive indicator of early or subtle abnormality of the hip (see Fig. 12.2). Any asymmetrical limitation of hip abduction requires further evaluation.

The most common reason for a limp in a child just beginning to walk is a congenital or developmental hip dislocation, though a congenital short femur or coxa vara will present with a painless limp as well. In a toddler who suddenly refuses to walk, osteomyelitis or septic arthritis needs to be seriously considered.

Transient synovitis of the hip is a common cause of an antalgic limp in children between the ages of 3 and 6 years, while Legg-Perthes disease occurs primarily between 4 and 10 years of age. It may be difficult to differentiate these painful conditions from septic arthritis of the hip, but this evaluation should be done urgently and expeditiously. Ultrasound evaluation can be useful in identifying a hip effusion. If any question of hip septic arthritis exists, an aspiration of the hip and fluid evaluation is needed. Failure to treat hip septic arthritis in an emergent manner will lead to permanent hip disability. While failure to treat transient synovitis or Legg-Perthes disease as an emergency is less important, infection must be ruled out quickly. Juvenile rheumatoid arthritis rarely presents as hip pain; it is commonly first seen at the knee or ankle. In the age range from 3 to 10 years old, the most common cause of a painless limp is either hip dysplasia or a leg length discrepancy.

Over the age of 10 years, the most common condition producing a painful limp is a slipped capital femoral epiphysis. Though usually found in obese pre-adolescents, individuals with a more slender body habitus can also be affected. With chronic slips, pain may be mild, though a Trendelenburg gait is always present and the child will walk with the foot and leg more externally rotated than on the normal side. On physical examination, the hip will go into an externally rotated position as hip flexion is attempted in this condition. Idiopathic chondrolysis and avascular necrosis of the femoral head occur less commonly, but both will demonstrate diminished internal rotation of the hip on examination. A painless limp in teenagers is usually due to a leg length discrepancy.

Femur and Thigh

Thigh pain is most commonly due to radiating pain from the affected hip. Continuing thigh pain, particularly in the lower thigh, should lead to evaluation for a possible tumor, since the midshaft and distal femur region is the most common site of malignant bone tumors. Persistent pain in the quadriceps after direct trauma may signal the onset of myositis ossificans at the site of a prior hematoma.

Knee

A knee disorder will generally cause an antalgic limp unless a fixed contracture of the knee is present, in which case the affected leg will appear shorter than the normal leg. If a knee is painful and swollen, it will usually be held in a flexed position. Inability to fully extend the knee makes pushing off difficult during walking, resulting in a shorter step with that leg.

The causes of knee pain are multiple, but most knee conditions that cause pain will also have an associated effusion of the knee. Being in a subcutaneous position, the knee joint can be palpated easily to determine the site of maximal tenderness. Meniscal and ligament injuries, as well as patellar problems and Osgood-Schlatter's disease, can be diagnosed quite often by simple physical examination. If there is increased warmth over the knee and an effusion is present without a history of traumatic injury, it should be remembered that one of the most common regions for presentation of juvenile rheumatoid arthritis is at the knee.

Leg

The primary tibial problems causing a limp are fracture, infection, and tumor. In the toddler age group, refusal to walk is fre-

quently associated with the so-called "toddler's fracture," an often unwitnessed spiral fracture of the mid-tibia that is either nondisplaced or minimally displaced. Swelling may be minimal but tenderness is present over the mid-tibia. Osteomyelitis in this age group will demonstrate tenderness over the metaphyseal area. Since the radiographs of early osteomyelitis are essentially normal for several days, tenderness at the ends of the bones, particularly without specific injury to this area, is enough to suspect osteomyelitis in a young child. Stress fractures may occur in the proximal mid-tibia in teenagers during the early days of running long distances to get in condition for a varsity sport. A stress fracture should not be confused with shin splints; bone tenderness is present with a stress fracture, while tenderness over the anterior muscle compartment of the leg may be seen with shin splints. A bone scan will be abnormal with all three of these conditions, even if the radiographs are normal.

If pain is present mainly on the medial aspect of the calf, the child should be evaluated for possible symptomatic flat feet. With marked flat feet, the posterior tibialis tendon becomes overactive in an attempt to provide medial arch support, and pain may develop along the posterior tibialis muscle belly in the calf, producing a limp.

Ankle

Ankle swelling and pain are generally due to a ligament sprain, a growth plate fracture, arthritis, or infection. Ligament sprains and physeal fractures can usually be differentiated by localizing the anatomic site of maximal tenderness to palpation. The ankle is one of the two most common sites for the presentation of juvenile rheumatoid arthritis, with limitation of ankle motion being common at the time of the first office visit. Passive ankle dorsiflexion and plantarflexion should be compared with the normal ankle to detect small differences and to measure the amount of motion limitation that is present.

Foot

Because the foot provides the only contact between the body and the ground, any painful condition or anatomic deformity in the foot will usually result in a limp. Visualization of the foot will diagnose congenital anomalies, while careful palpation will localize points of maximal tenderness or pain. Heel pain in children between the ages of 9 and 12 years usually means calcaneal apophysitis is present. Midfoot pain and tenderness in children 5 to 7 years old may indicate Köhler's disease of the tarsal navicular. A marked flatfoot with limited subtalar motion usually indicates that a tarsal coalition is present between two of the hindfoot bones. Tenderness at the base of the fifth metatarsal generally indicates an avulsion fracture at that site. A high-arch or cavus foot deformity, whether unilateral or bilateral, should always lead to a further search for an underlying neurologic cause; while the cavus foot deformity might cause a limp, the limp in this condition may be from muscle weakness elsewhere in the affected leg.

SUMMARY

A child with a limp should be approached in much the same way a detective may approach a crime. Even though the young child will not be able to give many details, evidence can be gathered by physical examination and careful observation of the child. Based on the positive physical findings present, the laboratory studies expected to provide the most information in that child should be judiciously ordered. If a diagnosis can be reached after the examination and laboratory data have been collated, specific treatment should be administered. If no cause of the limp or extremity pain can be determined, even after the imaging studies have been completed, re-examination at regular intervals may allow discovery of a physical finding previously not apparent. Above all, a limp in a child should not be dismissed as being "growing pains."

Suggested Readings

Sutherland, D.H.: Gait Disorders in Childhood and Adolescence. Baltimore, Williams & Wilkins, 1984.

Sutherland, D.H., Olshen, R., Cooper, L., et al.: The development of mature gait. J. Bone Joint Surg. 62A: 336–353, 1980.

Todd, F.M., Lamoreux, L.W., Skinner, S.R., et al.: Variations in the gait of normal children: A graph applicable to the documentation of abnormalities. J. Bone Joint Surg. 71A:196–204, 1989.

20
Arthritis of Childhood

Joint inflammation in children can result from a great number of potential causes. While joint pain or arthralgia is common, only a small percentage of children with joint pain have clinical findings of arthritis, which include pain, restriction of joint movement, and joint effusion.

Of all arthritides in childhood, the type that must be diagnosed and treated as an emergency is septic arthritis, which is discussed fully in Chapter 16. With all other types of arthritis, the initial step is to rule out septic arthritis before continuing the diagnostic workup. Failure to accurately diagnose and treat joint infection in a timely manner leads to permanent damage of articular cartilage and often growth cartilage as well. Needle aspiration of joint effusions, using aseptic technique, should be freely used to establish or eliminate the possible diagnosis of septic arthritis. Once the diagnosis of septic arthritis has been eliminated, the other diagnoses discussed in this chapter can be considered.

Juvenile Rheumatoid Arthritis

Although its etiology remains unknown, juvenile rheumatoid arthritis (JRA) is the most common connective tissue disorder in children and accounts for 75 to 80% of pediatric connective tissue disease. Girls are affected more often than boys. The initial joint signs and symptoms present between 1 and 4 years of age, although JRA may appear at any time during childhood and early adolescence.

Since JRA usually presents after walking is begun, a child limping or refusing to walk may be the first sign noted by the parents. There may be a history of increased fatigue, fever, weight loss, and irritability associated with this abnormal gait.

Physical examination will demonstrate pain and limitation of motion in one or more joints. A palpable effusion may also be present. The onset of JRA usually occurs at the knees, ankles, wrists, or elbows. Initial involvement of the hip is uncommon with JRA. Joints of the hand and feet may be involved either early or late. The polyarticular form of JRA is diagnosed if five or more joints are involved with arthritis, while in the pauciarticular form four or fewer joints are involved.

Serum laboratory studies may or may not be able to specifically confirm the diagnosis of JRA. The erythrocyte sedimentation rate is elevated and, in more severely involved children, anemia and leukocytosis are common. Among children with JRA, rheumatoid arthritis factor testing is positive only 20% of the time or less, but a positive antinuclear antibody test may be present more often. The white blood cell count of the joint fluid is commonly elevated to 10,000 to 30,000/mm^3, but this count may be higher than 50,000/mm^3, in which case JRA is often confused with septic arthritis in children with only one joint involved.

The early radiographic findings are soft-tissue swelling and joint effusions (Fig. 20.1). If synovitis has been present for some time, epiphyseal enlargement or accelera-

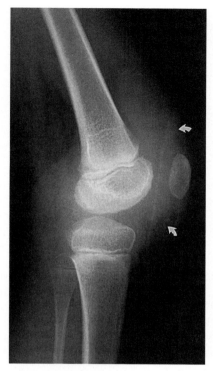

Figure 20.1. Lateral knee radiograph of a child who presented with early JRA demonstrates a large effusion (*arrows*) in the knee.

tion of epiphyseal ossification relative to the uninvolved extremity may be seen. A characteristic feature is periarticular osteoporosis around the involved joint(s).

As the disease progresses, synovial hypertrophy occurs and is identified within the joint capsule by magnetic resonance (MR) scanning. There is progressive erosion, first of articular cartilage, then eventually of the bony articular surfaces. Radiographically the changes are manifested as narrowing of joint spaces, erosion of the neighboring surfaces of bones, and eventual fusion of bones (Fig. 20.2). MR studies will demonstrate more abnormalities than are seen on plain radiographs. Sometimes the synovium causes cysts within the bone. The cysts are produced by gradual protrusion of the proliferating synovial pannus into the adjacent bone. Most commonly involved with these changes are the knees and ankles. The hips demonstrate cartilage erosion and protrusion of the femoral heads into the acetabula, the wrists show carpal fusion (Fig. 20.3), and the facets of the cervical spine commonly fuse (Fig. 20.4).

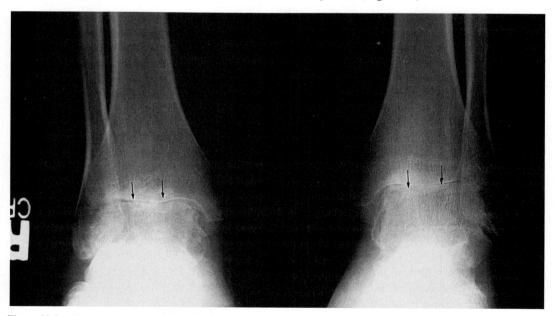

Figure 20.2. Anteroposterior radiograph of both ankles in a teenager with JRA shows extreme narrowing of joint spaces (*arrows*).

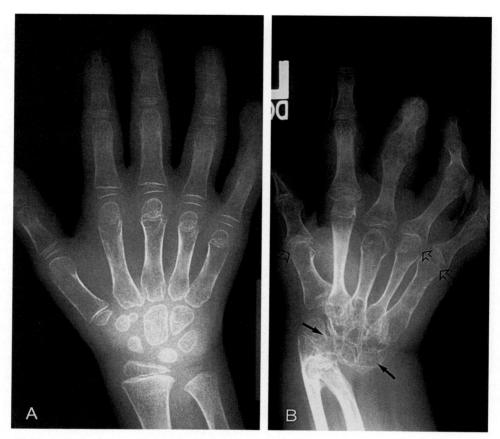

Figure 20.3. **A,** Early changes of JRA are osteoporosis and carpal irregularity. Note the soft-tissue swelling of the proximal interphalangeal joints in this anteroposterior hand radiograph. **B,** Late hand changes in JRA are fusion at the radial-ulnar joint and destruction and fusion of the carpal bones (*solid arrows*). Marked erosions involve most of the joints of the fingers (*open arrows*).

Since the serum studies specific for the diagnosis of JRA are inconclusive about 80% of the time, JRA often becomes a diagnosis of exclusion. If other causes of juvenile arthritis have been excluded and the joint(s) have been symptomatic for 2 or 3 months, the diagnosis of JRA can be made in young patients under the age of 16 years.

Aside from the orthopaedic manifestations of this disease, JRA is a leading cause of blindness in children, the blindness caused by chronic uveitis. Once the diagnosis of JRA has been established, repeated slit-lamp eye examination is important to ensure the prevention of permanent visual changes, particularly in young girls with pauciarticular disease.

The initial treatment for JRA is medical. Salicylates or nonsteroidal anti-inflammatory medication is administered under the supervision of a pediatric rheumatologist as initial treatment, but more potent anti-inflammatory agents may be needed if the disease cannot be controlled.

The initial orthopaedic care rendered to children with JRA consists of physical and occupational therapy to preserve a functional range of joint motion and to prevent joint contractures. Periodic splinting of the inflamed joints is useful. The therapy pro-

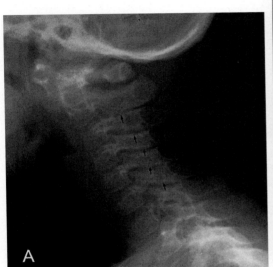

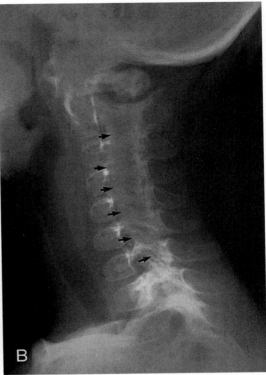

Figure 20.4. A, Early lateral radiograph of the cervical spine shows irregularity of the surfaces of the facets (*arrows*). **B,** One year later, facets C2 to C7 (*arrows*) have fused.

gram needs to be performed daily at home as well as in professional therapy sessions (Fig. 20.5).

Over half of the children with the diagnosis of JRA recover without continued progressive arthritis into adulthood. However, if systemic or polyarticular arthritis does persist, orthopaedic surgical care is needed to relieve pain and restore extremity function. Synovectomy may be needed and is used primarily if one specific joint has been resistant to medical control, though in some series synovectomy has not significantly changed the course of the disease. In more advanced stages, total hip or total knee arthroplasties are effective in relieving pain and improving extremity function. However, total joint arthroplasties in a teenager are apt to require one or more replacements during the patient's lifetime, and this surgi-

cal treatment is usually delayed until function significantly deteriorates and pain is severe.

Lyme Disease

First described in the 1970s, Lyme disease has become a common cause of childhood joint pain, producing recurrent asymmetrical arthritis. The larger joints are predominantly involved. Girls and boys are involved in approximately equal numbers. This condition can easily be confused with JRA unless the diagnosis of Lyme disease is kept in mind.

Lyme disease is caused by a spirochete, *Borrelia burgdorferi,* which is transmitted to the human via a tick bite, though a history of a tick bite is commonly absent. While this disease was originally described in the

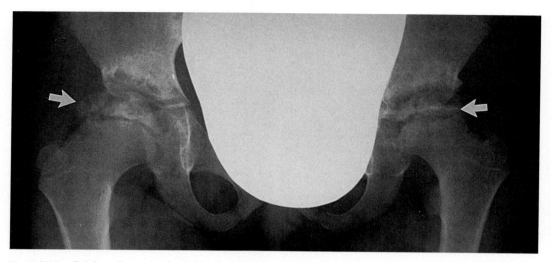

Figure 20.5.   Pelvic radiograph of a child with JRA. Destruction of articular surfaces of both femoral heads has occurred, the left more severe than the right. Initial orthopaedic care is nonoperative and is directed toward relieving inflammation and improving hip motion.

Lyme, Connecticut, area, Lyme disease occurs throughout the United States. A characteristic annular skin lesion appears within several days after the tick bite, and is followed by the appearance of arthritis weeks or months later. If not diagnosed early, central nervous system and cardiac signs and symptoms may appear.

Typically, joint pain is the first musculoskeletal manifestation seen in Lyme disease. The knee is commonly involved, often developing an effusion with associated painful movement. Although each arthritis episode may last only a few weeks, recurrent attacks of arthritis may continue for several months or even years.

It is important to differentiate Lyme disease from JRA in children. A careful history of recent outdoor activity or tick bites needs to be sought. While the erythrocyte sedimentation rate is elevated, as with JRA, serum muscle enzymes may also be elevated and urine examination may show proteinuria and hematuria in Lyme disease. Specific antibody titers are most useful to confirm the diagnosis of Lyme disease.

Since Lyme disease is caused by a spirochete, the treatment consists of administra-

tion of appropriate antibiotics. Tetracycline is used in older children with mature teeth, but penicillin or erythromycin will eradicate this disease as effectively in younger children. Joint symptoms generally resolve after antibiotic treatment, but in a small percentage of children, permanent articular cartilage damage occurs, necessitating ongoing orthopaedic care.

Juvenile Ankylosing Spondylitis

Pain in the lower back and sacroiliac region may result from a number of conditions referred to as seronegative spondyloarthropathies. This group includes Reiter's disease, inflammatory bowel disease, and psoriasis, but the most common condition in this group is juvenile ankylosing spondylitis.

Ankylosing spondylitis affects boys 90% of the time, with the first symptoms usually appearing in the mid-teen years. A family history of ankylosing spondylitis may be elicited. The initial complaints are usually of low back pain and increasing stiffness, worse in the morning.

Physical examination will localize the

back pain to the sacroiliac joints and to the low lumbar region. Limitation of forward flexion of the lumbar spine is common. Pain may be produced by hip movement, and limitation of internal rotation of the hips may be noted. The neurologic examination is normal.

Radiographs of the painful region should be obtained. Usually a lumbar spine series is performed. On the anteroposterior view, the sacroiliac joints should be assessed, as well as the lumbar spine. If the sacroiliac joint is poorly defined, oblique projections of the sacroiliac joints should be obtained to assess for joint space narrowing, bone erosions, or sclerosis at this site.

Serum laboratory studies are helpful to confirm the diagnosis of ankylosing spondylitis. The erythrocyte sedimentation rate is elevated, but identification of the HLA-B27 antigen is the most specific serum test for this disorder.

Nonsteroidal anti-inflammatory medication is the initial treatment for ankylosing spondylitis, and this generally relieves the pain. Orthopaedic care is initially directed toward physical therapy to prevent spine deformity or hip contractures. As the disease progresses, there is progressive ossification of the anterior and posterior longitudinal ligaments of the spine, producing marked restriction of spine motion and leading to a kyphotic deformity of the entire spine. If the thoracic spine ligaments also ossify, chest movements are restricted and respiratory restriction may occur. The arthritis in ankylosing spondylitis mainly affects proximal joints (hip and shoulder). Progressive destructive arthritis of the hips may eventually require total hip arthroplasty.

Traumatic Synovitis and Arthritis

Inflammation of joints may be noted as a consequence of a sports injury or as a result of excessive athletic activity. If a joint effusion is present in children or teenagers, sports or playground activity should be stopped until the cause of the effusion has been determined.

If joint pain and swelling have a gradual onset and occur primarily after extensive exercise, the most common cause is an intra-articular abnormality leading to synovial and articular cartilage inflammation with joint movement. Examples include osteochondritis dissecans of the knee, ankle, or elbow, chondromalacia of the inferior surface of the patella, or a chronic tear of one of the menisci in the knee. Typically, the child or teenager notes increased swelling of the joint with stiffness or limitation of motion several hours after sports activity, although pain during exercise may have been minimal.

With synovitis of this type, aspiration of the joint fluid yields a clear, yellowish fluid with a low white blood cell count and normal viscosity. The erythrocyte sedimentation rate is usually normal. Radiographs of the joint may demonstrate bony change, such as osteochondritis dissecans, and magnetic resonance imaging is sensitive to delineate meniscal, ligamentous, or articular cartilage damage.

In activity-related synovitis treatment consists of limiting the activity that caused the synovitis and treatment of the underlying intra-articular condition. Long-term use of nonsteroidal anti-inflammatory medication for this condition is not advocated by the author, nor is any intra-articular corticosteroid injection. If an intra-articular abnormality is amenable to surgery, either arthroscopic or open surgical procedures should be completed before the child or teenager returns to normal sports activity.

When acute swelling of a joint occurs as a result of an injury, bloody fluid is obtained if joint aspiration is attempted. If radiographs of the injured joint appear normal, joint aspiration can be helpful in diagnosing a chondral fracture (such as in the knee after patellar dislocation) from the presence of bone marrow fat in the bloody joint aspirate.

Most skeletally mature teenagers with an acute hemarthrosis of the knee should be evaluated either by MR imaging or by arthroscopic examination because of the high incidence of anterior cruciate ligament and meniscal injury with this clinical presentation.

Chronic knee effusion from traumatic arthritis is rarely seen in children or teenagers. If seen, this is usually due to an intra-articular fracture that has been inadequately treated at the time of injury. Intra-articular fractures and joint injury from sports activity more often produce chronic joint pain and swelling during middle age. Because of the degenerative arthritis seen in middle-aged adults who have had a complete medial meniscectomy in their youth, treatment of meniscal tears has been changed so that meniscal injuries in teenage athletes are repaired arthroscopically or the torn segment of the meniscus is only partially excised.

Other Arthritides

There are long lists of reported causes of joint inflammation, swelling, and restriction of motion that are not included in this text. Arthritis may result from hematologic disorders, including sickle cell disease; from acute rheumatic fever; from neoplastic disorders; and from inherited disorders.

The most important thing to remember in evaluating a child with joint pain and limitation of joint motion is first to exclude the diagnosis of septic arthritis. Septic arthritis demands emergency treatment for the best outcome, while a more leisurely approach to the evaluation and treatment of the other arthritides can be accepted.

In children and teenagers engaged in sports activity, if the joint is swollen and painful, sports activity should be curtailed until joint symptoms resolve. The presence of these joint signs and symptoms should be a signal to the physician that a problem exists and continued sports activity with limited joint motion predisposes the young athlete to further—and potentially more permanent—injury.

Suggested Readings

Cristofaro, R.L., Appel, M.H., Gelb, R.I., and Williams, C.L.: Musculoskeletal manifestations of Lyme disease in children. J. Pediatr. Orthop. 7: 527–530, 1987.

Culp, R. W., Eichenfield, A.H., Davidson, R.S., et al.: Lyme arthritis in children: an orthopaedic perspective. J. Bone Joint Surg. 69A:96–99, 1987.

Hensinger, R.N., DeVito, P.D., and Ragsdale, C.G.: Changes in the cervical spine in juvenile rheumatoid arthritis. J. Bone Joint Surg. 68A:189–198, 1986.

Miller, J.J., III, and White, P.H. (eds): Arthritis in childhood [Symposium]. Clin. Orthop. 259:1–91, 1990.

Senac, M.O., Jr., Deutsch, D., Bernstein, B.H., et al.: MR imaging in juvenile rheumatoid arthritis. Am. J. Roentgenol. 150:873–878, 1988.

Sheerin, K.A., et al.: HLA-B27-associated arthropathy in childhood: long-term clinical and diagnostic outcome. Arthritis Rheum. 31:230–232, 1988.

21

Musculoskeletal Tumors of Childhood

Both benign and malignant tumors of muscle or bone occur in children of all ages. Many of these are asymptomatic and are discovered in an incidental manner, for example when examining an extremity following trauma. Others are painful as a result of a small fracture in the area of the bone involved with the tumor. Still other tumors present as a mass that impedes joint movement.

While tumors of the musculoskeletal system can be present at any age, those discussed in this chapter are primarily found during childhood and adolescence. Knowledge of the location of a bone lesion—whether it is epiphyseal, metaphyseal, or diaphyseal—is very useful in establishing a differential diagnosis (Fig. 21.1). While physical examination is important, imaging studies and histologic evaluation are the keys to establishing the final diagnosis. Metastasis of other tumors to bone, the most common type of bone lesion found in the adult population, is uncommon in children.

Benign Bone and Cartilage Tumors

OSTEOCHONDROMA

A common benign tumor seen in the extremities, an osteochondroma (or osteocartilaginous exostosis) generally is a solitary lesion. When multiple osteochondromas are present, the child likely has the autosomal-dominant genetic condition of multiple hereditary exostoses.

The location of an osteochondroma within a long bone is identical whether one or multiple tumors are present. These tumors arise in the metaphyseal region of the long bones and, as they grow, are directed toward the diaphysis, away from the adjacent joint. The spine, pelvis, scapula, ribs, and clavicle are less frequently involved than the bones of the extremities.

An osteochondroma is thought to be caused by separation of cartilaginous tissue from the margin of the normal growth plate. This cartilaginous tissue functions as an isolated growth plate, producing a bony prominence as growth occurs in this aberrant cartilage. At the tip of this bony projection is a mushroom-shaped cartilage cap. If multiple osteochondromas are present, genetic factors allow these bony projections to arise at the growth regions of virtually all bones.

An osteochondroma is noted either because of focal pain or through the incidental discovery of a lump in the arm or leg. The pain is generally caused by impingement on muscles, tendons, or nerves by the osteochondroma, though a fracture of an osteochondroma may be present when acute pain follows limb trauma. When a large osteochondroma is located deep to a tendon, such as in the proximal medial tibia, local tendon inflammation may occur with repeated joint movement. If nerve compression is present,

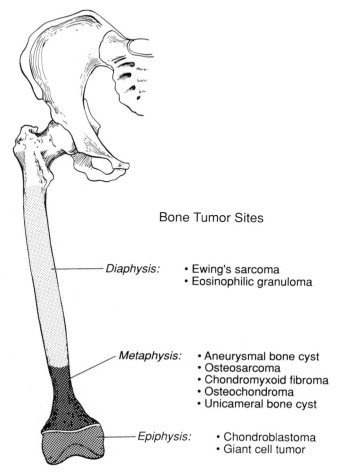

Bone Tumor Sites

Diaphysis: • Ewing's sarcoma
                  • Eosinophilic granuloma

Metaphysis: • Aneurysmal bone cyst
                  • Osteosarcoma
                  • Chondromyxoid fibroma
                  • Osteochondroma
                  • Unicameral bone cyst

Epiphysis: • Chondroblastoma
                  • Giant cell tumor

Figure 21.1.   Each bone tumor has a characteristic location in the long bone, where occurrence is most common. The tumor conditions located primarily in the diaphysis, metaphysis, and epiphysis in all long bones (not only in the femur illustrated), are shown in this diagram.

the hand or foot distal to the osteochondroma may demonstrate motor or sensory abnormalities.

A bony prominence in the region of the pain is palpable. If an osteochondroma is identified in the metaphyseal region of one bone, the metaphyses of all other extremity bones, as well as the pelvis and shoulder girdle, should be carefully examined for other unsuspected lesions. Any limitation of joint motion should be noted and a neurologic examination distal to the osteochondroma should be completed. If multiple le-

sions are present, angular deformity of the long bones requires evaluation, especially in the lower leg and in the phalanges of the hand.

Anteroposterior and lateral radiographs of the affected bone will confirm the diagnosis of an osteochondroma (Fig. 21.2). The lesion appears smaller than palpated, because the tip of the osteochondroma is cartilaginous and is not seen on radiographs. If the osteochondroma is small, a tangential radiograph, obtained at a right angle to the base of the osteochondroma, will best dem-

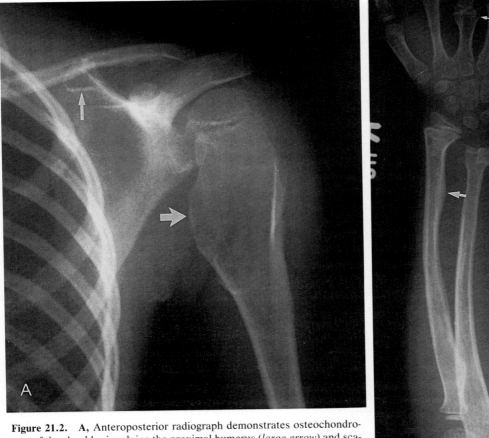
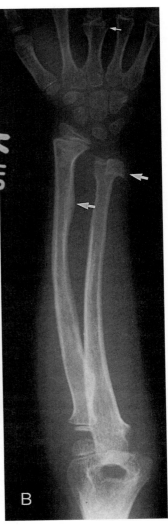

Figure 21.2. **A,** Anteroposterior radiograph demonstrates osteochondromas of the shoulder involving the proximal humerus (*large arrow*) and scapula (*small arrow*). **B,** Osteochondromas of the distal radius, ulna, and metacarpals (*arrows*) may lead to accompanying growth disturbance with bowing and shortening of the involved bones. This child has multiple hereditary exostoses.

onstrate the tumor. Although it is not indicated in cases of a solitary osteochondroma, a baseline skeletal survey should be obtained when multiple lesions are noted on physical examination. The use of special imaging studies such as computed tomography (CT) or magnetic resonance (MR) is reserved for osteochondromas that are very large or cases in which malignant transformation is suspected (Fig. 21.3).

Treatment of a solitary osteochondroma consists of either observation or surgical ex-

cision. If a solitary osteochondroma is painless and is not interfering with extremity growth or function, observation is appropriate. The radiographic appearance is characteristic enough that an excisional biopsy is not needed to confirm this diagnosis if no symptoms are present. Malignant degeneration of a solitary osteochondroma occurs well below 1% of the time and, when present, is accompanied by a sudden increase in tumor size and pain. Surgical removal is indicated if the osteochondroma is painful

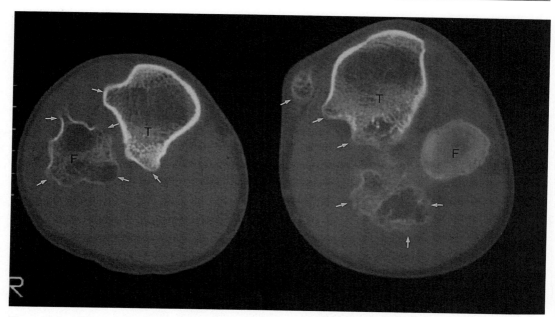

Figure 21.3.   CT scan of the tibiae (*T*) and fibulae (*F*) near the knee of a child with multiple hereditary exostoses shows extensive osteochondromas (*arrows*), resulting in distortion of the normal oval cross-sectional appearance. Nerve or artery compression may result from these large lesions.

or interferes with extremity function. If surgical excision is chosen for a solitary lesion, local recurrences are uncommon.

Treatment of a child with multiple osteochondromas differs somewhat from the management of a solitary lesion. Once baseline radiographs are obtained to evaluate all the involved bones, annual physical examinations to check for pain, joint motion limitation, or angular deformity are used, with subsequent radiographs reserved for areas noted to have a change in physical findings. If pain is present or growth disturbances are apparent, surgical excision of the responsible lesion(s) is needed. If the proximity of the osteochondroma to the physis has resulted in significant angular deformity, an osteotomy is needed to straighten the bone at the same time the osteochondroma is excised. Because of the large number of osteochondromas present in this condition, the likelihood of malignant degeneration into a chondrosarcoma is higher than with a solitary lesion, though still quite small. Rapid

enlargement of one of the multiple lesions should raise the suspicion that malignant change is occurring, and surgical excision should be performed.

UNICAMERAL BONE CYST

A condition that is uncommon in skeletally mature patients, a unicameral (simple) bone cyst is often present for several years prior to its discovery in a child. These cysts arise in the metaphysis adjacent to the growth plate and enlarge by affecting the bone formed in the distal zone of the physis as growth proceeds. A unicameral bone cyst does not involve multiple bones in the same child.

Why a unicameral bone cyst forms is unclear. These cysts are filled with a thin serous or serosanguineous fluid that has been demonstrated to have a high level of prostaglandin E activity. At biopsy, a thin cellular lining is molded around the periphery of this fluid-filled cyst.

Unicameral bone cysts are discovered

either when pain results from a fracture of the cyst wall or when seen incidental to obtaining a radiograph for other reasons. If a stress fracture of the cyst wall is present, localized tenderness is noted. If a displaced fracture has occurred through the weakened bone replaced by the cyst, the physical examination is no different than for a routine fracture in that bone. Without an overt or stress fracture, pain and tenderness are usually absent.

Anteroposterior and lateral radiographs will demonstrate a radiolucent lesion in the medullary bone with smooth thinning of the cortex of the bone at this location. Expansion or widening of the shaft at the affected region, usually near the end of the bone, is common. A cyst that abuts the physis is termed "active," while an inactive cyst has normal-appearing bone between the physis and the cyst. A fracture line may be noted in the cortex. If a portion of the cyst cortical wall has fractured and fallen into the cyst,

this bone piece may be lying at the distal extent of the cyst and produce the "fallen leaf sign" nearly pathognomonic for unicameral bone cysts (Fig. 21.4). Aneurysmal bone cyst is the primary disorder to be included in the radiographic differential diagnosis for this lesion.

The goal of treatment is to prevent further enlargement of the cyst and restore bone to the cystic region. Several methods have been attempted and all have failure rates of approximately 10% to 20%, with cyst recurrence despite the treatment.

If a displaced fracture occurs through the cystic region and the radiographic appearance is characteristic for a unicameral bone cyst, the fracture is treated the same way a fracture of the involved bone would be treated without the presence of a cyst, usually with cast immobilization. Fracture healing is not delayed in this condition, and the fracture sometimes produces enough new bone to partially obliterate the cyst and

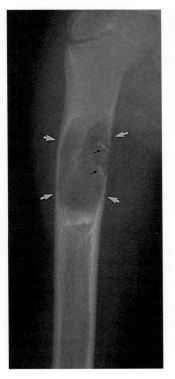

Figure 21.4. Unicameral or simple bone cyst of the inactive type is noted in this proximal humerus radiograph (*white arrows*). At the site of the cyst fracture, the cortical fracture fragments producing the "fallen leaf sign" (*black arrows*) are noted. This cyst is "inactive," since normal bone has formed between the physis and the cyst.

increase bone strength without the need for other treatment (Fig. 21.5). If open reduction is needed to treat the fracture appropriately, biopsy and bone grafting of the cyst region should be performed at the same time as the fracture surgery. If a fracture in the cyst wall is nondisplaced, the cyst cannot be expected to resolve as a result of this injury.

The most commonly used method to treat unicameral bone cysts today is intralesional injection with corticosteroids. This technique involves anesthetizing the child and inserting two needles into the cystic lesion. If the aspirated fluid is yellow or yellowish-red, no biopsy is needed and a unicameral bone cyst is assumed to be present. Since other lesions, in particular aneurysmal bone cysts, may have similar radiographic appearances to a unicameral bone cyst, a biopsy is considered if bloody fluid is aspirated. After thorough cyst irrigation through the two needles, the corticosteroid

suspension is injected into the cyst. Frequently, two or three corticosteroid injections at 6- to 8-week intervals may be needed to produce sufficient response to obliterate the cyst at least partially. Prostaglandin E activity within the cyst has been shown to decrease progressively with each injection. Although after injection the cyst is usually still visible on radiographs, the cyst walls become thicker, trabeculae of bone form within the cyst, and fracture becomes unlikely. Complete resolution of the cyst generally occurs by the time of full skeletal maturity.

While cyst injection can be done easily in an outpatient surgery facility, other treatment methods involve more extensive surgery. The most commonly employed open surgical method consists of removing a part of the cyst wall, curetting the entire cyst wall to remove the cyst lining, and filling the entire cyst with either autogenous or allograft bone graft. Cast immobilization is

Figure 21.5.   This humeral radiograph shows a unicameral bone cyst (*arrows*) in a 6-year-old boy with a fracture after falling. Early healing is seen (*open arrows*). This type of fracture within a unicameral bone cyst may lead to cyst closure without injection or surgery.

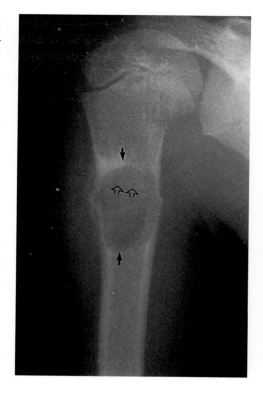

needed postoperatively, and several weeks are needed for bone graft healing. Since this open surgical procedure is unsuccessful with approximately the same frequency as the corticosteroid injection method, cyst injection should usually be the first therapy used for a unicameral bone cyst, with the possible exception of a cyst in the femoral neck.

OSTEOID OSTEOMA

This fascinating bone lesion may occur in any bone, though is most common in the femur, tibia, and spine. The diagnosis of osteoid osteoma is commonly delayed for several weeks or months due to the small size of this lesion. Because of the vague and poorly localized pain complaints associated with this condition, psychological disorders or "growing pains" are diagnoses that have often been given prior to reaching the correct diagnosis.

The history can be very important in this condition. Pain is typically present at night and is often absent during the day. Pain relief is excellent with aspirin or other nonsteroidal anti-inflammatory agents, while even codeine or other more potent analgesics are ineffective. If back pain is present from an osteoid osteoma, the child usually notes stiffness of movement and may develop scoliosis.

The source of this pain is a nidus of inflammatory tissue found within the cortex of the involved bone. This benign tumor incites the local region to increase bone production, leading to a marked thickening of the bone cortex adjacent to the nidus location. The histologic appearances of osteoid osteoma and osteoblastoma are similar, and these two lesions are differentiated by lesion size and bone location.

Physical findings are often minimal. In fact, pain may be absent at the time of the examination. If the complaint is back pain, the patient should be checked for back stiffness, scoliosis, and hamstring tightness. If the pain is in the leg, all joints should be checked for range of motion and a careful neurologic examination should be performed. Tape measurements of the thigh and calf may reveal muscle atrophy in one location. When no specific physical findings are found, pain has been present for several weeks, there is no history of trauma, and the pain is characteristically present at night more than during the day, an osteoid osteoma should be suspected.

Initial evaluation of the spine or extremity for an osteoid osteoma requires anteroposterior and lateral radiographs. If this lesion has been present for some time, thickening of one cortex in the involved bone will be seen (Fig. 21.6A). A small radiolucent region, representing the nidus, may be visible in the central region of this hyperostotic area (Fig. 21.6B). In the long bones, a CT scan of the involved area will clearly demonstrate the exact location and extent of the nidus region—information important for surgical planning. In a long bone, the radiographic differential diagnosis should include sclerosing osteomyelitis, stress fracture, and intracortical abscess.

An osteoid osteoma of the spine is more difficult to diagnose than when this lesion involves a long bone. In children with scoliosis and back pain, particularly if little vertebral rotation is noted in conjunction with the scoliosis, a spinal osteoid osteoma should be considered. Since this lesion is frequently too small to be noted on radiographs, a technetium-99 bone scan is valuable to localize an osteoid osteoma, which characteristically demonstrates an intense increase in isotope uptake in the involved region. After the region of the spine with the increased isotope uptake has been defined with the bone scan, a CT scan is used to delineate the anatomic location of the osteoid osteoma.

Surgical resection of the nidus is the preferred treatment for osteoid osteoma, even though use of anti-inflammatory agents may relieve the pain. It is not necessary to resect all the new bone that has formed in response

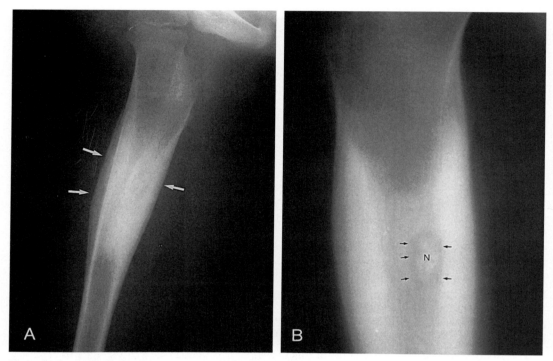

Figure 21.6. **A,** Radiograph of an osteoid osteoma in a 5-year-old boy shows the marked hyperostosis present with cortical thickening (*arrows*) and sclerosis of the proximal femur. **B,** This linear tomogram of an osteoid osteoma shows the radiolucent ring (*arrows*) around a small, dense central nidus (*N*).

to the presence of this osteoid osteoma nidus. If histologic confirmation of the nidus is present in the resected specimen, the lesion should not recur, and pain relief should be noted almost immediately postoperatively. If painful scoliosis has resulted from an osteoid osteoma, removal of this lesion will allow at least partial improvement of the scoliosis to occur spontaneously.

HISTIOCYTOSIS X OR LANGERHANS' CELL HISTIOCYTOSIS

The clinical manifestations of the three primary forms of histiocytosis X or Langerhans' cell histiocytosis (LCH) vary greatly, but one or more bones are virtually always involved in all forms. Letterer-Siwe disease is a life-threatening form that affects the youngest children, usually by age 3, and involves multiple viscera in addition to multiple bones. Hand-Schüller-Christian dis-

ease is a chronic disseminated form that usually occurs between the ages of 3 and 5 and, though multiple organs can be involved, is less severe than Letterer-Siwe disease. The most benign condition, a solitary eosinophilic granuloma of bone, is the most common as well, and has a peak incidence between 5 and 10 years of age.

Eosinophilic granuloma of bone involves the skull and the flat bones of the trunk most commonly (Fig. 21.7A). In the long bones, this lesion may occur either in the diaphysis or the metaphysis, with a predilection for the femur and humerus (Fig. 21.7B). Boys are affected twice as often as girls. The histologic appearance of affected regions in histiocytosis X consists of histiocytes mixed with cells characteristic of both acute and chronic inflammation, primarily eosinophils. It is unknown why one child develops a solitary lesion and another has multiple

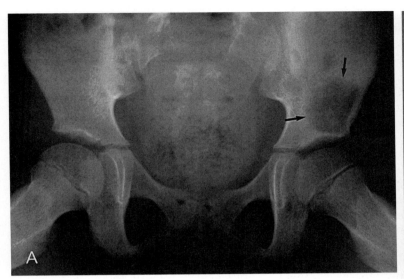

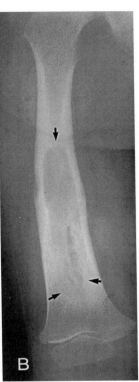

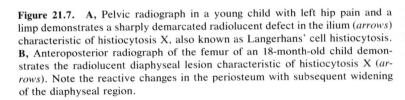

Figure 21.7. **A,** Pelvic radiograph in a young child with left hip pain and a limp demonstrates a sharply demarcated radiolucent defect in the ilium (*arrows*) characteristic of histiocytosis X, also known as Langerhans' cell histiocytosis. **B,** Anteroposterior radiograph of the femur of an 18-month-old child demonstrates the radiolucent diaphyseal lesion characteristic of histiocytosis X (*arrows*). Note the reactive changes in the periosteum with subsequent widening of the diaphyseal region.

sites of involvement, though age appears to be a factor.

Pain is the usual presenting complaint, with the pain sometimes resulting from a fracture through the lesion. Tenderness is present over the lesion site. With a solitary eosinophilic granuloma of bone, the skin lesions and hepatosplenomegaly found in the disseminated forms are absent.

Radiographs of the painful region demonstrate a well-defined radiolucent region with loss of bone trabeculae and thinning of the bone cortex from the inner or marrow edge. Some lesions show little periosteal reaction. If the radiolucency is present in the diaphysis of a young child, eosinophilic granuloma is the most likely diagnosis. If eosinophilic granuloma is suspected on the initial radiograph, a complete skeletal survey—including the long bones, spine, and skull—is indicated to look for other sites. The skeletal

survey is probably more accurate than the bone scan in determining multicentric disease, since some histiocytosis X lesions will not demonstrate increased isotope uptake.

The typical radiographic presentation of eosinophilic granuloma in the spine is the appearance of vertebra plana. The vertebral body is flattened into a wafer-thin structure as a result of the eosinophilic granuloma within the vertebral body. Compression is symmetrical and spinal deformity is seldom significant. This radiographic picture is so characteristic of eosinophilic granuloma that no biopsy or surgical treatment is needed except in the rare instance of a coexisting neurologic deficit.

The orthopaedic treatment of a solitary eosinophilic granuloma in a long bone of a child is begun by obtaining an accurate histologic diagnosis by open biopsy. The diagnosis can usually be made intraoperatively by microscopic examination of a frozen tissue sample. Curettage of the yellow-brown tissue from the lesion is sufficient treatment, and the lesion will usually fill in by itself over the ensuing weeks without the need for bone grafting. Corticosteroid injection into an eosinophilic granuloma of bone has also been reported to eradicate this lesion.

If multiple bone lesions are seen on the skeletal survey, an evaluation of abdominal viscera for possible systemic disease is needed. If only multiple skeletal sites are present, systemic chemotherapy with vinblastine or corticosteroids may be added to whatever local surgery may be needed to restore skeletal stability. Low-dose radiotherapy is occasionally used for lesions that have not responded adequately to surgical or chemotherapeutic treatment.

In the case of a solitary eosinophilic granuloma of bone, the prognosis is excellent and recurrence is uncommon. In the chronic disseminated form, skeletal lesions can generally be controlled with chemotherapy, but diabetes insipidus or pulmonary fibrosis can be more serious sequelae. In Letterer-Siwe disease, a fatal outcome is common in the very young, but the prognosis improves if the child survives past the age of 3 years.

CHONDROBLASTOMA

Chondroblastoma is an uncommon benign bone tumor that occurs primarily between the ages of 10 and 20. It is typically present in the epiphysis of a long bone, most commonly the femur or the humerus.

Pain is the primary presenting complaint. Tenderness is noted on physical examination and joint symptoms may be present on attempted movement.

Radiographs of the affected region demonstrate a well-demarcated radiolucent region within the epiphysis (Fig. 21.8). If the lesion has been present for some time, or if the epiphyseal plate is closing, the lesion may include a portion of the metaphysis.

Radiographically, the differential diagnosis includes giant cell tumor of bone.

Thorough curettage of this lesion, with bone grafting as needed, is generally curative. Recurrence rates are below 10%, and if a recurrence is noted it can also usually be treated with local surgical excision.

CHONDROMYXOID FIBROMA

Though rare, this benign bone tumor generally occurs in skeletally immature individuals. Typically, chondromyxoid fibroma is found in the metaphysis, with extension toward the diaphysis. It is almost always found in the lower-extremity bones. Pain or a mass is noted by the patient.

Radiographically, an eccentric radiolucent lesion is noted in the metaphyseal region. Multiple bones are not involved. The histologic picture includes benign fibrous and cartilage cells.

Wide surgical removal is the recommended treatment. Radiotherapy should not be used. Recurrence is uncommon.

FIBROUS DYSPLASIA

Fibrous dysplasia should always be considered in the evaluation of bone lesions involving the metaphyseal and diaphyseal regions of long bones in children and adolescents. A very wide spectrum of clinical and radiographic presentation can be seen in this condition.

The two major groups of fibrous dysplasia are monostotic and polyostotic. The monostotic form, the more common of the two, affects only one bone, most commonly the maxilla, femur, or tibia. The polyostotic form involves multiple bones, though generally one side of the body is more involved than the other. The spine is generally spared.

Pain is the most common presenting complaint, with the pain usually resulting from either a microfracture or a fracture through the involved area of the long bone. At times, the first thing noted by the patient

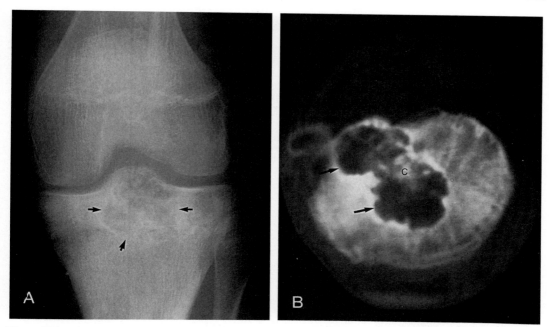

Figure 21.8. **A,** Anteroposterior radiograph of the knee of a 15-year-old male with a limp shows a chondroblastoma. The well-demarcated epiphyseal lesion (*arrows*) contains fine calcifications, indicating its cartilage origin. **B,** CT scan of the epiphysis in this same teenager shows a sharply demarcated destructive lesion (*arrows*) with a calcified central matrix (*C*).

is a hard mass in the leg or face, resulting from bony expansion.

Tenderness is present over the involved region. If prior fractures have occurred, deformity of the limbs may be noted. A specific finding in fibrous dysplasia is the presence of café-au-lait spots on the skin, with an outer border described as the "coast of Maine." Endocrine abnormalities, such as precocious puberty in girls and hyperthyroidism in boys, are sometimes associated with the polyostotic form, and careful assessment for these disorders is needed.

Radiographs of the affected bones demonstrate expansile lesions in the metaphyseal and diaphyseal regions of the long bones. The epiphysis is not involved. The degree of involvement may vary from a localized radiolucent region (Fig. 21.9), similar to that seen with a bone cyst, to involvement of the entire long bone shaft (Fig. 21.10). There is a predilection for the proximal femur, which may develop a progressive varus deformity with time, producing the so-called shepherd's crook deformity of the proximal femur at the hip. The radiographic differential diagnosis should include bone cysts, enchondromas, osteoblastoma, and osteofibrous dysplasia.

If the diagnosis is made by the combination of café-au-lait spots and radiographic appearance of the long bones, observation is the most appropriate treatment course. There is generally little need to take biopsies of these lesions. Corrective osteotomy is appropriate when an angular deformity results from this disorder. However, whether the fibrous dysplasia involves one bone or multiple bones, curettage and bone grafting should be reserved for the adolescent and young adult, if possible. Bone grafts placed in fibrous dysplasia lesions in young children are often resorbed, with recurrence of the underlying bone lesion.

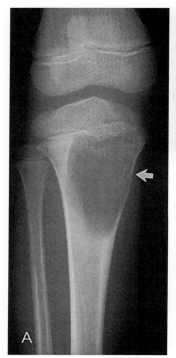

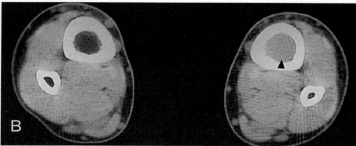

Figure 21.9. **A,** Anteroposterior radiograph of the knee of a child with fibrous dysplasia shows a hazy, well-defined metaphyseal lesion (*arrow*) in the proximal tibia. **B,** CT scan of a child with fibrous dysplasia shows intermediate attenuation of the tibial medullary bone (*arrowhead*) without attenuation of the normal fatty marrow in the other tibia or the ipsilateral fibula.

Figure 21.10. Radiograph of the humerus demonstrates fibrous dysplasia with the typical long segment of expansile medullary lucency and cortical thinning (*arrows*) common with this condition.

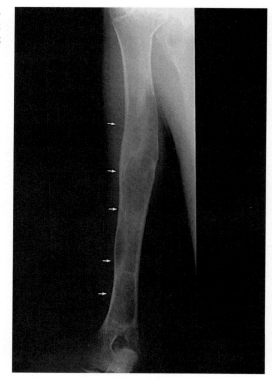

The overall prognosis for this condition is quite good. The activity of these bone lesions seems to diminish at the time of skeletal maturity, so adult problems with this disorder are largely the result of residual deformity from the time of childhood.

Malignant Bone Tumors

OSTEOSARCOMA

Osteosarcoma is the most common malignant bone tumor in the growing child. The incidence of osteosarcoma is approximately 2 to 3 per 1 million people, yet this tumor occurs primarily in the preadolescent and teenage population.

Osteosarcoma occurs primarily in the metaphyseal regions of long bones. The most common sites are the distal femur, the proximal tibia, and the proximal humerus. Approximately 75% of these lesions occur in the knee and shoulder regions, though any bone may be affected.

Pain is the presenting complaint in most of these tumors. The involved area is tender to pressure, and a soft-tissue mass may be palpable on physical examination.

Radiographic studies generally confirm this diagnosis. Radiographs demonstrate a destructive, invasive lesion, usually in the metaphysis of the long bone (Fig. 21.11). The cortex and medullary canal are invaded and formation of new periosteal bone is seen at the margins of the primary lesion. A soft-tissue mass emanating from the bone tumor is commonly present (Fig. 21.12). Radiographically, the differential diagnosis in this age group includes mainly Ewing's sarcoma, which usually occurs more in the diaphysis than in the metaphysis.

To fully evaluate a possible osteosarcoma prior to biopsy, the child should have a bone scan, a CT scan of the chest and lesion area, and an MR study. The bone scan is used to discover other possible sites of tumor. The CT scan of the tumor region will assess bone destruction, but an MR scan will evaluate the extent of cortex and

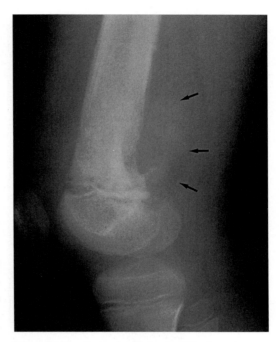

Figure 21.11. Lateral radiograph of the knee demonstrates an osteogenic sarcoma of the distal femur with destruction of the posterior cortex and a partially ossified soft-tissue mass posteriorly (*arrows*).

marrow involvement as well as the size of a soft-tissue tumor mass. The MR image also demonstrates the relationship of the tumor to adjacent arteries, nerves, and muscles. Because of the propensity of osteosarcoma to metastasize to the lungs, a CT evaluation of the lungs is an essential part of the initial work-up as well.

Treatment of osteosarcoma includes both surgical resection and chemotherapy. After a biopsy has established the diagnosis, chemotherapy is used for several weeks, at which point surgical resection is completed. Limb-sparing surgical resection of the tumor is used more often now than amputation, but either surgical procedure can be appropriate. Using current tumor surgery methods, the survival rate and low rate of local recurrence has been shown to be the same for teenagers with osteosarcoma treated with amputation and those treated with limb-sparing procedures. With surgical

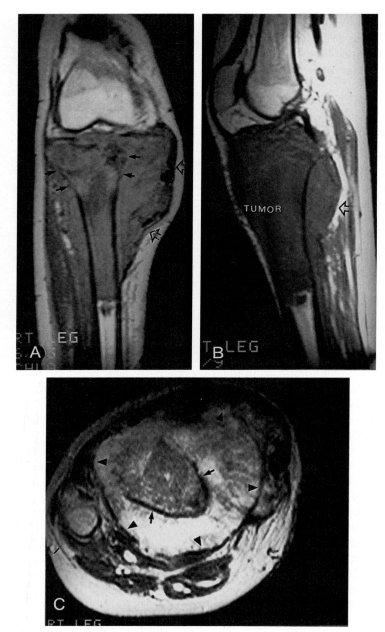

Figure 21.12.   A, The MR scan is extremely useful in the evaluation of the extent of tumor growth, as shown in this osteogenic sarcoma of the proximal tibia in a 12-year-old girl. This coronal T1-weighted MR image shows cortical (*arrows*) and medullary canal destruction by the tumor, with the mass extending into the soft tissues (*open arrows*). **B,** Sagittal MR scan shows the osteosarcoma (*gray area*) extending to the articular surface of the tibia and replacing the marrow of the proximal tibia. Soft-tissue extension (*open arrow*) is well defined posteriorly. **C,** T2-weighted axial MR section of the proximal tibial metaphysis shows the osteosarcoma soft-tissue expansion in white (*arrowheads*) surrounding the ghost of the remaining tibia (*arrows*). Note the distortion and invasion of the soft-tissue structures, including the neurovascular bundle posteriorly and laterally.

resection and pre- and postoperative chemotherapy, the 5-year survival rates for osteosarcoma are approximately 60 to 70%. If metastatic disease occurs, the lungs are primarily affected.

EWING'S SARCOMA

In children and adolescents, Ewing's sarcoma is the second most common malignant tumor of bone. Its peak incidence is between 10 and 20 years of age, being rare before the age of 5 and after the age of 25.

A small round-cell tumor by histologic appearance, Ewing's sarcoma is located most typically in the diaphysis of a long bone. With the exception of osseous lymphoma (rare in children), diaphyseal locations are unusual in bone malignancies. The femur and tibia are most commonly involved, though the pelvis and spine are also relatively common sites of tumor involvement.

Pain is usually the initial symptom with Ewing's sarcoma. A mass may be noted by the patient over the painful area. If the pelvis or spine is involved, neural compression will lead to weakness or sensory change in the lower extremities. Intermittent low-grade fever is not unusual. Weight loss may occur with time.

Tenderness over a palpable mass at the site of the pain is the primary physical finding. A low-grade fever, usually below 38°C, is often noted. With extremity pain, neurologic function should be carefully evaluated. Serum studies will frequently demonstrate elevated erythrocyte sedimentation rate and white blood cell count, but these should not be confused with bone infection.

The radiographic appearance of Ewing's sarcoma is typically a permeative, destructive lesion of the diaphysis, with extension into the metaphyseal region. Erosion of the bony cortex and medulla occurs (Fig. 21.13). An adjacent soft tissue mass is commonly seen. The radiograph may demonstrate multiple layers of periosteal new bone

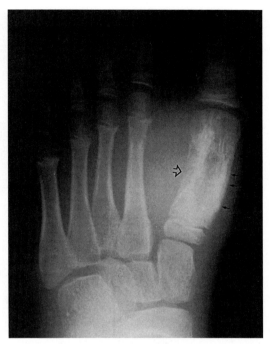

Figure 21.13. Anteroposterior radiograph of the foot demonstrates a Ewing's sarcoma of the first metatarsal in an 8-year-old boy who presented with a puffy, tender foot. There is permeative destruction of the metatarsal with periosteal new bone formation medially (*small arrows*) and cortical destruction laterally (*open arrow*).

formation, the so-called "onion-skin" appearance; however, this radiographic finding is characteristic of, but not pathognomonic for, Ewing's sarcoma (Fig. 21.14). In the growing skeleton, a similar "onion-skin" appearance may be seen in chronic or subacute osteomyelitis, eosinophilic granuloma, lymphoma, leukemia, and osteosarcoma.

As with osteosarcoma, a bone scan and MR scan of the lesion, plus a CT scan of the lungs, should be obtained prior to taking the biopsy if Ewing's sarcoma is strongly suspected. If the frozen section at the time of biopsy confirms the presence of Ewing's sarcoma, an iliac bone marrow aspiration is performed to evaluate for microscopic disseminated disease.

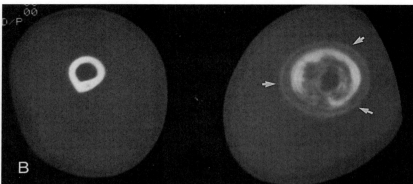

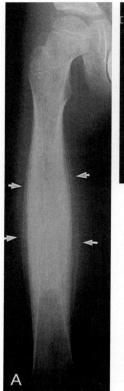

Figure 21.14.   A, Anteroposterior radiograph of a femur with Ewing's sarcoma shows medullary permeative destruction and the "onion-skin" appearance of new bone formation due to the successive elevation of the periosteum by a growing tumor (*arrows*). **B,** CT scan of the same child with Ewing's sarcoma of the femur demonstrates reactive new bone formation around the periphery of the femur (*arrows*). Endosteal destruction by tumor is noted.

The currently advocated treatment for Ewing's sarcoma is surgical resection with chemotherapy before and after surgery. Radiotherapy is added when surgical resection is incomplete or when metastatic lesions occur. Although Ewing's sarcoma is very radiosensitive, tumor recurrence or the appearance of radiation-induced osteosarcoma following radiotherapy has made radiation treatment less desirable as the primary treatment for this malignancy.

The use of chemotherapy and surgical resection for Ewing's sarcoma is very similar to the approach used for osteosarcoma, though the specific chemotherapeutic agents may differ. Chemotherapy is given before and after surgical resection, which generally is performed with a limb-sparing procedure. Five-year survival rates have been impressively improved with this ap-

proach and now approach 50%. Unlike osteosarcoma, which usually recurs early if at all, Ewing's sarcoma may recur at times even after 5 years of apparent disease-free time. When metastases occur, the lungs and other skeletal sites are most commonly affected.

Soft-Tissue Tumors

HEMANGIOMA

A diversity of conditions can be included in this category. From the orthopaedic standpoint, the purely cutaneous hemangiomas do not commonly have an impact on the function of the musculoskeletal system and are not addressed here.

A solitary deep hemangioma is the most common benign tumor involving muscles of the extremities and trunk. Most often found in the lower extremity, a muscle hemangioma is generally confined to one muscle belly, except in the hand or foot. Muscle hemangiomas are rare at birth and usually appear during childhood and adolescence.

A mass in the region of the involved muscle is the usual presenting complaint. Pain may be noted with movement of the adjacent joint, which stretches the muscle containing the hemangioma. With time, a joint contracture may result.

Physical findings include local warmth over a palpable mass in the extremity or trunk muscle affected. Tenderness is commonly absent but may be present. Passive stretching of the involved muscle by passive joint motion can produce pain. Joint motion may be limited, such as limited knee flexion with a quadriceps hemangioma and limited ankle dorsiflexion with a gastrocnemius hemangioma.

Radiographs show a soft-tissue mass that may contain small calcifications. Localized periosteal new bone reaction or cortical erosion is seen infrequently. The lesion is sharply demarcated and the bone may be enlarged (Fig. 21.15A). An MR scan will show the mass and feeding vessels as well as internal vessels and will clearly define the muscle involved, the extent of involvement present, and the degree of vascularity. A specific imaging study to identify a hemangioma is an isotope-labeled red blood cell scan, which localizes these tagged red cells in the soft-tissue tumor in a pattern specific for hemangioma (Fig. 21.15B).

Treatment depends on the extent of the hemangioma and the symptoms produced by this tumor. If pain is absent and no functional limitations are present, periodic physical examination and sequential (perhaps annual) MR studies are used to assess the growth of this tumor. If treatment appears necessary, surgical resection of the entire section of muscle containing the hemangioma is needed. Recurrence after surgery is more common in young children and is more often seen in the hand and foot.

Certain more generalized hemangiomatous conditions, such as the Klippel-Trenaunay-Weber syndrome, may affect multiple muscles and bones, in addition to having extensive skin involvement. Macrodactyly and asymmetrical extremity hypertrophy

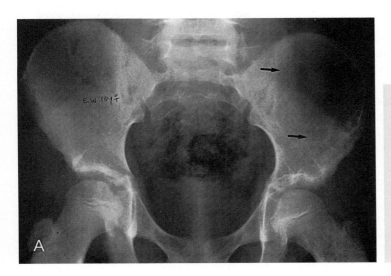
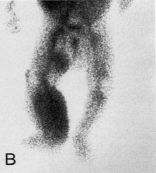

Figure 21.15. **A,** Anteroposterior radiograph of the pelvis shows a hemangioma of the ilium. Note the sharply demarcated replacement of normal bone (*arrows*). **B,** A labeled red blood cell scan demonstrates multiple hemangiomas of the right leg.

generally occurs. Surface bleeding from the hemangiomas with activity may be problematic. Radiographs of the affected limbs should be obtained to determine the degree of bone involvement and resultant skeletal deformity in this condition. Treatment, which usually involves a series of soft-tissue operative procedures to achieve the best functional result, must be individualized.

GANGLION OR MUCOUS CYST

This benign condition, though much more commonly seen in the adult population, can be present in older children and teenagers. The most common locations are at the wrist and the foot, generally on the dorsal aspect of both sites.

A true ganglion does not communicate with the adjacent joint, such as may be seen with a popliteal cyst at the knee. The ganglion arises from mucoid transformation of the connective tissue in the tendon sheath or fascia adjacent to the joint. Enlargement of the ganglion occurs as this mucoid material increases in volume.

The child or parent will note a small mass in the hand or foot region. Pain and tenderness are usually absent. Limitation of adjacent joint movement is rare. Radiographs are normal.

With the usual physical findings of a lump in a typical area for a ganglion, biopsy is not needed. If the ganglion is totally asymptomatic, observation is appropriate. If treatment is indicated, aspiration of the ganglion and corticosteroid injection may lead to resolution. If the ganglion is persistent and symptomatic, surgical excision will effect a cure.

RHABDOMYOSARCOMA

The most common soft-tissue sarcoma in children and teenagers is rhabdomyosarcoma. This sarcoma has a tendency to differentiate into a striated muscle-type cell. Rhabdomyosarcoma may present in the limbs or trunk, in the head and neck region, or in the pelvis or genitourinary system.

Three histologic types of rhabdomyosarcoma are prevalent: embryonal, alveolar, and pleomorphic. The embryonal type is the most common and usually occurs in the young child or pre-adolescent, with a predilection for the head and neck or the genitourinary tract. The alveolar type is found during later childhood and adolescence and is the primary type of rhabdomyosarcoma that occurs in the extremities (Fig. 21.16). The pleomorphic type is found in adults and is rare today.

The discovery of a mass in the extremity is the usual reason the child seeks medical advice. Pain is not common until marked enlargement occurs or a nerve is compressed. Radiographs show a soft-tissue mass, and if the tumor is large, cortical bone erosion may be present. An MR study dem-

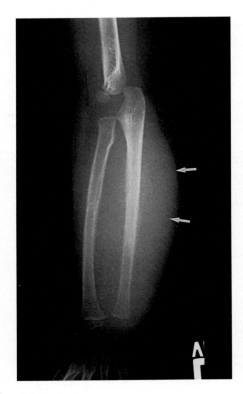

Figure 21.16. This radiograph of the forearm demonstrates a mass in the soft tissues that represents a rhabdomyosarcoma. The regional bones show slight reactive periosteal changes due to this soft-tissue mass.

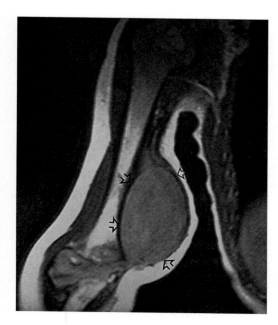

Figure 21.17. This MR study clearly demonstrates the location and anatomical extent of a rhabdomyosarcoma (outlined by *open arrows*).

onstrates the size and anatomical location of this soft-tissue sarcoma well (Fig. 21.17).

Treatment of a rhabdomyosarcoma involves surgical excision with chemotherapy both before and after surgery. Since tumor spread can occur via the lymph system, biopsies should be taken of any enlarged lymph nodes adjacent to the tumor, and lymph node dissection surgery may need to be added to the tumor resection. Although alveolar rhabdomyosarcoma (the type generally found in the extremities) has a worse

prognosis than the embryonal type, 5-year survival for rhabdomyosarcoma in children is now approximately 70 to 80% with surgical resection and chemotherapy.

Suggested Readings

Bohndorf, K., Reiser, M., Lochner, B., et al.: Magnetic resonance imaging of primary tumours and tumour-like lesions of bone. Skeletal Radiol. 15: 511–517, 1986.

Eilber, F.R. and Rosen, G.: Adjuvant chemotherapy for osteosarcoma. Semin. Oncol. 16:312–323, 1989.

Healey, J.H. and Ghelman, B.: Osteoid osteoma and osteoblastoma: Current concepts and recent advances. Clin. Orthop. 204:76–85, 1986.

Makley, J.T. and Joyce, M.T.: Unicameral bone cyst (simple bone cyst). Orthop. Clin. North Am. 20: 407–415, 1989.

Meyers, P.A.: Malignant bone tumor in children: Ewing's sarcoma. Hematol. Oncol. Clin. North Am. 1: 667–673, 1987.

Mickelson, M.R. and Bonfiglio, M.: Eosinophilic granuloma and its variations. Orthop. Clin. North Am. 8:933–945, 1977.

Milgram, J.W.: The origins of osteochondromas and endochondromas: A histopathologic study. Clin. Orthop. 174:264–284, 1983.

Ruymann, F.B.: Rhabdomyosarcoma in children and adolescents: A review. Hematol. Oncol. Clin. North Am. 1:621–654, 1987.

Simon, M.A.: Biopsy of musculoskeletal tumors. J. Bone Joint Surg. 64A:1253–1257, 1982.

Simon, M.A.: Causes of increased survival of patients with osteosarcoma.: Current controversies. J. Bone Joint Surg. 66A:306–310, 1984.

Springfield, D.S.: Bone and soft tissue tumors. In Morissy, R.T. (ed): Pediatric Orthopaedics. Philadelphia, J.B. Lippincott, pp. 325–363, 1990.

Stephenson, R.B., London, M.D., Hankin, F.M., et al.: Fibrous dysplasia: An analysis of options for treatment. J. Bone Joint Surg. 69A:400–409, 1987.

22

Orthopaedic Aspects of Child Abuse

Child abuse continues to be a major social and medical concern in both urban and rural areas, with the incidence steadily increasing in some states. Although most primary care physicians have been well instructed in the clinical recognition of abused children, certain physical and radiographic features of the skeletal system found in child abuse not only can aid in the recognition of this condition but also can clearly establish its diagnosis.

Child abuse is most common in children under 1 year of age and seldom occurs in normal children over 3 years of age. Older children with handicaps, particularly when mental retardation is part of the handicap, can be victims of abuse. Abuse of children affects all socioeconomic levels.

Musculoskeletal injury associated with child abuse occurs by one or more mechanisms. The extremity might be grabbed and twisted, producing a long-bone fracture. Shaking the child may result in rib or vertebral fractures, clavicle fracture, and subdural hematoma. Direct blows to the extremity are less common but also lead to fractures. It has been established that vigorous passive exercise in an infant can lead to similar skeletal abnormality.

The child is typically brought to the hospital emergency room with a history of an injury that resulted from a benign fall at home. Often the parents claim not to have been present when the injury occurred. The history given by each of the parents or caretakers may differ. The child may have been unobserved or may have been playing with siblings.

Typical physical findings include injury to both soft tissues and bone. Bruises, abrasions, burns, or scars from prior injury may be present. If a fracture is present, pain on movement and swelling with crepitance may be noted. The child with inflicted trauma will often appear fearful at the approach of the medical personnel.

Confirmation or suspicion of the diagnosis of child abuse relies heavily on imaging studies used to evaluate the child. In addition to radiographs of the injured extremity, a full radiographic skeletal survey is required. The survey includes radiographs of the skull, spine, ribs, pelvis, and long bones of the upper and lower extremities. If the radiographic findings are inconclusive, a technetium-99 bone scan is indicated, since bones with subtle recent or healed fractures will demonstrate increased isotope uptake, even in areas that appear normal on radiographs. While both the skeletal survey and the bone scan will each have a small percentage of false-negative results, the combination is generally successful in establishing the correct diagnosis.

Several skeletal radiographic features are characteristic of child abuse; some of these findings are more specific than others. A single long-bone fracture occurs more often in child abuse than multiple fractures, although multiple fractures at different stages of healing are the hallmark of child abuse. The humerus, femur, and tibia are most commonly involved. Fractures in the diaphysis occur as transverse or spiral fractures (Figs. 22.1, 22.2). The combination of a skull fracture and an extremity fracture in a young child should always raise the suspicion of abuse. Rib fractures from child abuse occur characteristically posteriorly, at the junction of the rib with the transverse process of the thoracic vertebra (Fig. 22.3). Rib fractures from accidental chest compression or from resuscitation attempts usually occur more laterally.

A curved, incomplete metaphyseal fracture is pathognomonic for child abuse (Fig. 22.4). This metaphyseal fracture radiographically appears to be a "corner fracture" adjacent to the growth plate. However, histologic and postmortem radiographic studies have demonstrated that this fracture is not an avulsion fracture nor a Salter-Harris type II physeal injury but rather is a fracture that occurs through the metaphysis immediately adjacent to the zone of provisional calcification of the growth plate.

Because of this location adjacent to, but not involving, the growth plate, this fracture should not lead to growth disturbances.

Differential Diagnosis of Child Abuse

While there should be a high suspicion of child abuse in the child with radiographic abnormalities consistent with prior or recent trauma, care must be exercised not to overdiagnose child abuse. Several conditions found in the infant and young child need to be included in the radiographic differential diagnosis. In the newborn, prematurity and obstetric trauma are the principal conditions to be considered. In the older infant or toddler, the primary systemic skeletal conditions to consider in the differential diagnosis of child abuse are nutritional abnormalities, infection, osteogenesis imperfecta, and infantile cortical hyperostosis, also known as Caffey's disease.

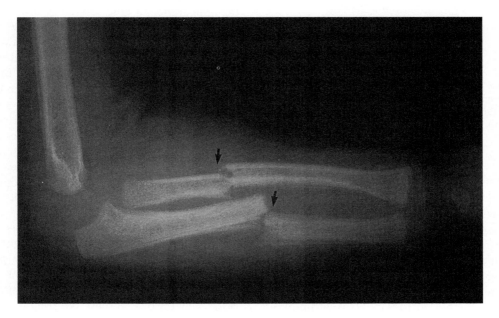

Figure 22.1. Radiograph of the forearm demonstrating transverse fractures of the mid-radius and ulna (*arrows*), partially healed when the child was brought to the hospital. These fractures were caused by child abuse.

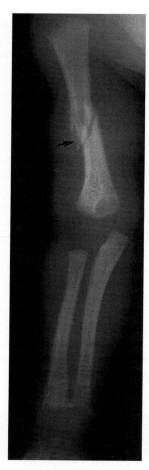

Figure 22.2. Anteroposterior radiograph of the upper extremity showing an oblique midshaft humeral fracture (*arrow*) in child abuse. (Note also the metaphyseal changes in the radius and ulna, indicative of rickets.)

PREMATURITY AND OBSTETRIC TRAUMA

In the newborn period, prematurity and obstetric trauma may be confused with child abuse. Particularly in infants who have had a difficult delivery or who have congenital joint contractures, a fracture that occurred at birth may not be noted until the infant is a few weeks of age. Since new bone formation is visible on radiographs within about 5 days after a fracture in infants, the history of birth trauma should be sought. In the infant, most fractures, including those of the femur, are healed by 4 weeks after the injury, so timing of an injury can be estimated.

Premature infants may be noted to have osteopenic bones and metaphyseal fractures that were not noted clinically. These once-ill infants often have nutritional deficiencies that predispose to injury or infection. Periosteal new bone formation may be seen on radiographs as a result of subclinical injury or infection, and these skeletal lesions may appear to have occurred at various times.

OSTEOGENESIS IMPERFECTA

Osteogenesis imperfecta, known to some as brittle bone disease, is the condition that potentially may be most often confused with child abuse, particularly if the mother or father is not known to have this condition. Because of a defect in type I collagen, children with osteogenesis imperfecta have slender long bones that are prone to fracture. Radiographically, the cortex of the long bones may be noticeably thinner than normal. This same collagen defect produces the appearance of blue sclerae in some, but not all, children with this condition. While the severely affected child may be born with multiple fractures, those less involved will appear with fractures in later infancy or in the toddler stage. Fractures that have occurred at various times can be noted on the radiographs. Children being abused and children with osteogenesis imperfecta may both have diaphyseal fractures, but if a metaphyseal fracture is present, child abuse is more likely the cause. Fractures in children with osteogenesis imperfecta heal at the same rate as normal bone.

The physical findings of osteogenesis imperfecta may be subtle, and the diagnosis may be hard to establish firmly. Both parents should be examined for evidence of this condition and a complete family history of prior generations should be sought. The sclerae of both parents and child need to be examined for a blue tint. On the radiographic skeletal survey, the skull is care-

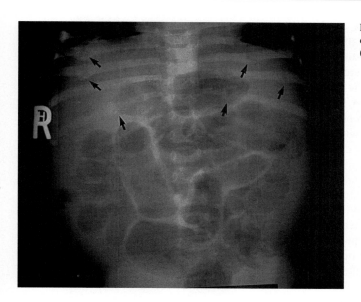

Figure 22.3. A trunk radiograph demonstrates multiple posterior rib fractures (*arrows*) in a baby who had been shaken.

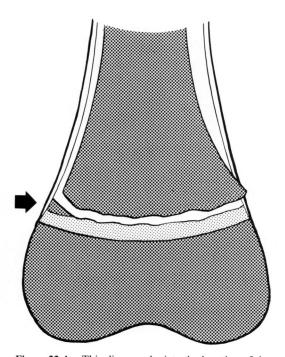

Figure 22.4. This diagram depicts the location of the typical fracture associated with child abuse. This fracture does not involve the growth plate but instead passes through the adjacent metaphysis. The location of this fracture will lead to the radiographic appearance of a "corner fracture."

fully evaluated for wormian bones, a feature of osteogenesis imperfecta, and the appearance of the cortices of the long bones is assessed. While blue sclerae, a positive family history, or specific radiographic findings can establish this diagnosis, all three are frequently absent, in which case periodic reexamination may be the only way to establish a diagnosis. Molecular analysis of the type I collagen in the affected child and the parents can establish the diagnosis of osteogenesis imperfecta in the majority of cases. Although the misdiagnosis of a mild case of osteogenesis imperfecta as child abuse has occasionally resulted in litigation, the chance of unrecognized osteogenesis imperfecta occurring in a infant or toddler with no family history, white sclerae, and no wormian bones on radiographs is slight.

INFANTILE CORTICAL HYPEROSTOSIS

Infantile cortical hyperostosis, or Caffey's disease, is less frequently seen today than it was 2 or 3 decades ago. Clinically, this condition is found in infants before the age of 6 months and presents with irritability, swelling, tenderness, and sometimes redness in the extremities. The face may appear to have become more round in shape, particularly in the jaw region. Radiographs demonstrate an exuberant periosteal new bone reaction involving primarily the diaphysis of the affected bone or bones. Initially this new bone formation may resemble the "onion-skin" appearance seen with Ewing's sarcoma, but this malignancy does not occur in such young children. The mandible is commonly involved and is thought to be the reason for the changes in facial appearance. Once this condition has been differentiated from child abuse, the treatment is periodic physical examination and radiographic evaluation. Biopsy is not needed if the age, physical findings, and radiographic appearance are typical for this condition, which resolves spontaneously over a period of several months without adverse sequelae (Fig. 22.5).

RICKETS

Nutritional abnormalities likewise may mimic the radiographic changes seen in the abused child. Rickets at this age usually results from a nutritional cause. Generally, a dietary history will detect the fact that the child has obtained insufficient vitamin D, commonly because of the parents' dietary preference. It is uncommon for fractures to occur in rickets, but the presence of periosteal new bone and flared metaphyses may mimic the radiographic picture of child abuse. Widening of the growth plate on the radiographs, best seen in the knee region and in the wrist, is characteristic of rickets and should cause this diagnosis to be strongly suspected (Fig. 22.6).

SCURVY

Scurvy may present with swollen extremities that are more symptomatic than with rickets. Scurvy, caused by a deficiency in vitamin C, is rare before 6 months of age. Radiographs may demonstrate nondisplaced fractures and periosteal new bone formation secondary to subperiosteal hem-

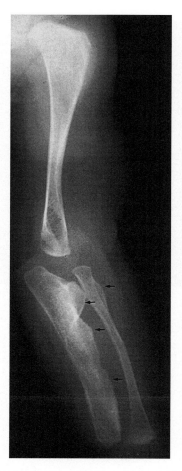

Figure 22.5. Radiograph of a 4-month-old infant showing changes of marked irregular hyperostosis of the ulna (*arrows*) and slight changes in the radius that are characteristic of Caffey's disease.

orrhage, with the radiographic changes often being asymmetrical. This can often be mistaken for the radiographic findings in child abuse (Fig. 22.7).

COPPER DEFICIENCY

Copper deficiency may produce a radiographic picture similar to that seen in abused children. Copper deficiency is rare in full-term infants and in breast-fed children. If nutritional deficiency in copper occurs, the radiographic picture that results consists of osteoporosis, metaphyseal cup-

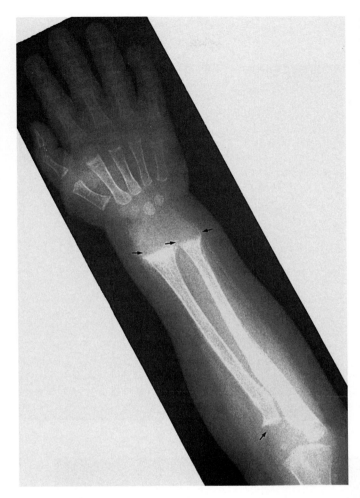

Figure 22.6. Anteroposterior forearm radiograph showing rickets with osteoporosis and widening, fraying, and cupping of the metaphysis (*arrows*). Slight periosteal new bone is present on the ulna.

ping, and spur formation, and possibly fractures, leading to periosteal new bone formation. This diagnosis should be considered only in children with known nutritional deficiency or those receiving prolonged parenteral nutrition.

HYPERVITAMINOSIS A

Hypervitaminosis A produces a radiographic picture of periosteal new bone formation, but it is generally in the diaphyseal region rather than in the metaphysis. The extremities demonstrate pain and swelling in the region of the affected long bones. Usually a dietary history will reveal an in-

creased intake of vitamin A, which will be elevated in serum studies.

CONGENITAL SYPHILIS

Congenital syphilis continues to be seen, especially in urban areas, where an increased incidence has recently been reported. This condition usually presents in the first few months of life and can be confused with child abuse. However, the radiographic lesions of periosteal new bone formation are generally symmetrical (Fig. 22.8). If a radiolucency is noted in the medial aspect of the proximal tibial metaphysis, some consider this pathognomonic for

Figure 22.7.   Scurvy with dramatic periosteal new bone at the sites of subperiosteal hemorrhage (*arrows*).

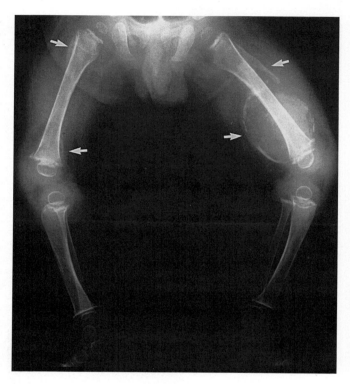

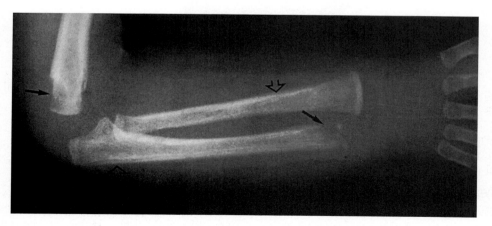

Figure 22.8.   Congenital syphilis leads to radiographic changes of metaphyseal destruction (*arrows*) and periosteal new bone (*open arrow*), as seen in this infant's forearm radiograph.

congenital syphilis. Studies of serum from the child and the mother will confirm this diagnosis.

OSTEOMYELITIS

Osteomyelitis, particularly in the ill neonate, may lead to radiographic findings of periosteal new bone formation. In the older infant or toddler, acute osteomyelitis will produce more systemic findings, and the history of a recent infection can be readily elicited.

SIDE EFFECTS OF MEDICATION

Since periosteal new bone formation is often a primary finding on the radiographs of an abused child, any condition that produces this finding may be confused with child abuse. Periosteal new bone formation can be found in infants being treated with prostaglandin E_2 to maintain patency for a patent ductus arteriosus. This radiographic finding is also seen in children receiving methotrexate therapy for a malignancy or leukemia.

Summary

All of the disorders described in the differential diagnosis are much less common than is child abuse. If the physical and radiographic findings combined with the social circumstances suggest child abuse, this diagnosis must be made.

From the orthopaedic standpoint, there is nothing special about the treatment of fractures sustained from child abuse compared to fractures caused by other mechanisms. However, if child abuse is suspected, it may be necessary to keep the child in the hospital until the social and family situation has improved, even if the fracture itself would not usually warrant an inpatient hospital stay.

If the diagnosis of child abuse is made by the treating physician, a report must be made to an appropriate source that can further investigate the family. In hospitals that have a child abuse team, the child's case should be referred to them. However, in the many hospitals lacking this type of specialized team, the report of child abuse should be made to the police. While reporting child abuse is uncomfortable for many physicians, the failure to do so will endanger the life of the abused child, who may sustain more serious injury the next time abuse occurs.

Suggested Readings

Ablin, D.S., Greenspan, A., Reinhart, M., and Grix, A.: Differentiation of child abuse from osteogenesis imperfecta. Am. J. Roentgenol. 154:1035–1046, 1990.

Dent, J.A. and Patterson, C.R.: Fractures in early childhood: osteogenesis imperfecta or child abuse? J. Pediatr. Orthop. 11:184–186, 1991.

Ellenshein, N.S. and Norris, K.J.: Value of radiologic skeletal survey in the assessment of abused children. Pediatrics 74:1075–1078, 1984.

Jaudes, P.K.: Comparison of radiography and radionuclide bone scanning in the detection of child abuse. Pediatrics 73:166–168, 1984.

King, J., Diefendorf, D., Apthorp, J., et al.: Analysis of 429 fractures in 189 battered children. J. Pediatr. Orthop. 8:585–589, 1988.

Kleinman, P.K., Marks, S.C., Spevak, M.R., et al.: Radiologic contributions to the investigation and prosecution of cases of fatal infant abuse. N. Engl. J. Med. 320:507–511, 1989.

Loder, R.T. and Bookout, C.: Fracture patterns in battered children. J. Orthop. Trauma 5:428–433, 1991.

Merten, D.F. and Carpenter, B.L.: Radiologic imaging of inflicted injury in the child abuse syndrome. Pediatr. Clin. North Am. 37:815–837, 1990.

Silverman, F.: Roentgen manifestations of unrecognized skeletal trauma in infants. Am. J. Roentgenol. 413–426, 1953.

Thomas, S.A., Rosenfield, N.S., Leventhal, J.M., et al.: Long-bone fractures in young children: distinguishing accidental injuries from child abuse. Pediatrics 88:471–476, 1991.

23

Orthopaedic Aspects of Chromosomal, Genetic, and Metabolic Disorders

Several chromosomal, genetic, and metabolic disorders have major effects on the musculoskeletal system. These effects may be on the bone growth through a modification of physeal function or may be on the connective tissue that forms ligaments and tendons. This chapter is not intended to provide a complete listing of these conditions with orthopaedic components but rather to highlight several conditions that the primary care physician has a reasonable chance of seeing in practice.

Conditions with Abnormal Chromosomes

DOWN'S SYNDROME

The most common condition with chromosomal abnormalities is Down's syndrome, which occurs in approximately 1 of each 660 live births. Trisomy 21 is the chromosomal abnormality most often found. Most affected children are born to mothers over the age of 35. Described in 1866 in England by John Down, this syndrome is usually recognizable early in life by the typical facial features, associated with generalized hypotonia.

In addition to the specific orthopaedic problems encountered, there is a generalized retardation in growth in these children. The tibia is particularly affected, and the lower extremities are short compared to the trunk. The final height for most individuals with Down's syndrome is a few inches above or below 5 ft. Motor milestones are delayed, and independent walking commonly occurs between the ages of 2 and 3. Generalized ligamentous laxity is a prominent feature of Down's syndrome and accounts for many of the orthopaedic problems that occur as the child grows. Early recognition and management of these orthopaedic problems is important to maintain mobility, and thus the ability to lead a life of relative independence.

Cervical spine abnormality is common in children with this condition, and flexion and extension lateral cervical spine radiographs are required of these children before they can compete in the Special Olympics. Between 10 and 30% of children with Down's syndrome have more than 5 mm of movement between the anterior aspect of the ring of C1 and the odontoid process of C2 (normal for a preadolescent child is up to 5 mm). This increased atlantoaxial movement may increase the risk of spinal cord compression at this level, and cervical cord myelopathy does occur to varying degrees in 10 to 15% of these "at-risk" children. Even though the majority of children with Down's syndrome do not develop neurologic findings from this laxity, if atlantoaxial laxity has been noted, careful neurologic examination of the extremities must be performed periodically, at least annually. If no neurologic symptoms or signs exist with increased atlantoaxial laxity, avoidance of sports activities in which sudden flexion of the neck may occur, such as in tumbling, gymnastics, and diving, is prudent. If this excessive laxity is associated with a loss of extremity function or if specific evidence of a myelopathy is present, posterior atlantoaxial fusion is needed. If the neurologic abnormalities are of recent onset, return of neurologic function is expected after stabilization surgery has been completed.

In the lower extremity, ligamentous laxity leads to instability at the hip and knee joints. Voluntary or habitual dislocation of the hip(s) is common and initially presents before the age of 10. True congenital dislocation of the hip in Down's syndrome is rare, and this instability usually develops after walking independence has been achieved. This latter instability may be noted on routine examination or may be associated with the child's beginning to limp or refusing to walk. An anteroposterior radiograph of the pelvis will confirm hip subluxation or dislocation, often with an associated acetabular dysplasia. In the younger child, surgical treatment, including both femoral and pelvic osteotomy, is usually needed if hip stability is to be regained, yet later redislocation rates are high. Hip pain from an unstable hip is an important cause of walking difficulties in adults with Down's syndrome.

At least a third of children and adolescents with Down's syndrome will have subluxation or dislocation of the patella. Instability of the patella can lead to sudden falls because of the inability of the quadriceps muscle to extend the knee when walking. If there is no functional problem associated with the patellar hypermobility, no treatment is needed. If marked anterior knee pain, falling, or walking difficulty is present, surgical treatment to realign the patella is recommended, with the knowledge that re-

dislocation may later occur as the repair stretches.

If knee pain is present but findings on knee examination are minimal, the hip should be examined and imaged to eliminate the possibility of the knee pain being referred from the hip.

The primary problems in the feet of patients with Down's syndrome are metatarsus adductus, bunions, and flat feet. The infant or toddler is commonly noted to have metatarsus adductus, generally due to metatarsus primus varus with an increased intermetatarsal angle between the first and second metatarsal shafts. While soft shoes, such as tennis shoes, are easily worn and the feet are asymptomatic during childhood, bunions develop during the teenage and early adult years, often leading to marked foot pain and shoe-fitting problems in later adult life. The flat feet commonly present do not generally require treatment with either orthosis or surgery during the growing years of these patients.

OTHER CHROMOSOMAL SYNDROMES

Prader-Willi syndrome results from an abnormality of the long arm of chromosome 15. Children with this disorder are typically obese and short. Lower-extremity hypotonia and easy tiring are common. The feet and hands are small for the body size, and finger swelling may be seen. Scoliosis is relatively common.

The *fragile X syndrome* is being detected with increasing frequency in mentally retarded males without previously detected chromosomal abnormalities. These patients have delayed motor milestones but do achieve walking ability. The primary orthopaedic abnormalities in these children are in the lower extremities. Flat feet are common, partly due to the lax joints that are characteristic of this condition. Scoliosis or kyphosis during the teenage years is fairly common.

Henry Turner originally described a series of young women with a single X chromosome in 1938. While this condition occurs in approximately one in every 2500 live births, spontaneous abortion is the fate for most with this XO pattern. Orthopaedic features of *Turner's syndrome* include a short neck (easily confused in appearance with Klippel-Feil syndrome), scoliosis during adolescence, growth plate abnormalities that lead to relatively short height, and valgus malalignment of the knee and elbow. Surgical treatment may be needed to realign the lower extremities and to correct severe scoliosis.

Infants with trisomy or an extra chromosome are born with abnormalities of the spine and extremities. While infants with *trisomy 13* and *trisomy 18* often live short lives and generally do not require aggressive orthopaedic care, infants with *trisomy 8* survive and characteristically have orthopaedic problems, which include scoliosis and kyphosis, generalized joint stiffness, and foot deformity.

Infants born with either a deletion or a duplication of a part of one chromosome have a better prognosis than in most trisomy conditions, though mental retardation is a prominent feature. Scoliosis is common in childhood or adolescence, and vertebral malformations may be present at birth. Foot and hand abnormalities are often apparent at birth in these children.

Nearly 100 different chromosomal syndromes have been described to date. While chromosomal abnormalities may be present in a child with a normal appearance, chromosomal analysis is an important part of the evaluation of dysmorphic infants with musculoskeletal abnormalities.

Genetic Conditions

OSTEOGENESIS IMPERFECTA

Osteogenesis imperfecta, sometimes known as brittle bone disease, is characterized by a marked propensity of bones to fracture. The underlying genetic defect involves an abnormality of type I procollagen and collagen. The severity of the osteogenesis imperfecta is dependent on the location of this defect within the genome. The wide heterogeneity of this condition is best explained by the fact that each individual displays the defect at a different genetic locus. Because of this marked heterogeneity, classification into clearly defined groups is difficult.

The most severely involved infants with osteogenesis imperfecta are born with multiple long bone and rib fractures (Fig. 23.1). Respiratory difficulty, present at birth, is related to the rib deformity, and only a small percentage of these infants survive the newborn period. If a severely involved infant does survive, multiple fractures plague the child throughout life and independent walking is rarely achieved.

Infants who are less severely involved have no respiratory difficulties at birth and may have several fractures noted in infancy. Even if no fractures are present at birth, the diagnosis of osteogenesis imperfecta may be established. A positive family history for osteogenesis imperfecta and the presence of blue sclerae may indicate this diagnosis. Helpful radiographic features are the presence of wormian bones on the skull radiograph and identification of healing fractures on extremity films (Fig. 23.2). Molecular analysis of a skin biopsy can establish the presence or absence of abnormal type I procollagen or collagen.

If the infant does not demonstrate blue sclerae (which result from relative transparency of the sclerae because of the collagen defect) and if there is no family history of this disorder, the diagnosis is usually delayed until more than one fracture occurs during infancy or early childhood. Osteogenesis imperfecta, particularly in milder cases, may be confused with child abuse, and the analysis of type I collagen is helpful in differentiating these conditions.

Once the diagnosis of osteogenesis imperfecta is established, the primary orthopaedic attention is directed toward effective

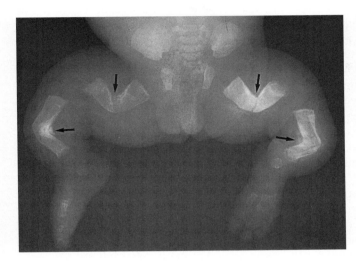

Figure 23.1. Radiograph of the lower extremities of a newborn infant with osteogenesis imperfecta demonstrating multiple fractures (*arrows*) involving the femora and tibiae and accompanied by severe deformity. The early healing of the tibial fractures indicates that the fractures occurred during the intrauterine period.

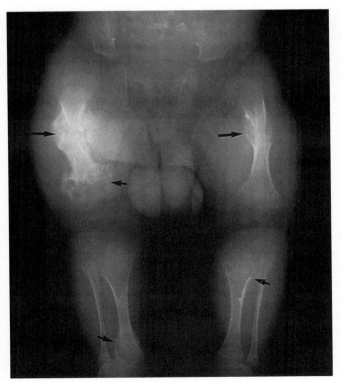

Figure 23.2. Anteroposterior lower-extremity radiograph of the long bones of a 2-month-old child showing multiple fractures (*arrows*), all in various stages of healing. The diagnosis of osteogenesis imperfecta was established.

management of the fractures. While the time for fracture healing is virtually the same for these children as for normal children, angular deformity is a common result of multiple fractures, even when appropriate cast immobilization is performed. Bowing of the lower extremity bones potentiates further bowing as microfractures occur during everyday activity. If progressive angular deformity occurs, surgical realignment of the long bone is needed to permit continued ambulation and reduce the likelihood of repeated fracture. As the child matures, the frequency of fracture decreases.

Orthopaedic care should be directed at the maintenance of walking ability as much as possible. Bone strength is improved by weight bearing, so protective orthoses and surgical realignment can play an important role in permitting continued walking after fracture healing is completed. While fluoride treatment improves the radiographic density of bone in children with this condition, the rate of fracture in children undergoing fluoride treatment is unchanged.

Scoliosis is common in this condition. If the spinal deformity is progressive, treatment by use of a brace is difficult, since the application of the brace may produce rib fracture or further chest wall deformity without controlling the scoliosis. If the scoliosis worsens significantly, spinal instrumentation and fusion is commonly needed to reestablish trunk balance.

The goal of treatment in children with osteogenesis imperfecta is to prevent malalignment of the long bones when fracture reduction is performed, to surgically realign the long bones that have developed deformity, and to allow ambulation if feasible. Aggressive orthopaedic care during childhood will allow greater independence during young adult life, by which time the frequency of fractures decreases considerably.

NEUROFIBROMATOSIS

Although neurofibromatosis is considered to be a spectrum of diseases, von Recklinghausen's neurofibromatosis (NF-1) accounts for about 85% of patients in this disease family. NF-1 is a relatively common disorder, appearing in one of 3000 to 4000 people. While NF-1 is inherited by an autosomal-dominant mode, nearly half of the cases appear as a new mutation.

The diagnosis of NF-1 is based largely on physical findings, though the clinical expression of NF-1 varies dramatically from one child to the next, even within the same family. Multiple (six or more) café au lait spots are present during early childhood but are generally absent at birth. Cutaneous and subcutaneous neurofibromas likewise are absent at birth but increase in number with increasing age. Tumors of the central nervous system, particularly optic nerve glioma, are common in NF-1 but are not present at birth. Unless a large plexiform neurofibroma or a skeletal deformity is identified at birth, the diagnosis of NF-1 is delayed until the cutaneous or neural complications of this disorder are manifested as the child grows older.

The primary musculoskeletal conditions that should alert one to the possible diagnosis of neurofibromatosis are congenital anterolateral bowing of the tibia, localized gigantism of a portion of an extremity, and rapidly progressive kyphoscoliosis in a child under the age of 10.

Congenital bowing of the tibia is of two types, with the convexity anterolateral in one type and posteromedial in the other. Posteromedial bowing is not associated with neurofibromatosis, does not lead to a pathologic fracture, and is expected to remodel with ongoing growth. However, more than half of all infants with anterolateral bowing are affected with neurofibromatosis, even though café au lait spots are absent at birth. Most often the infant is born with the tibia and fibula bowed but intact, though an established pseudoarthrosis can be present at birth. If left untreated, this anterolateral tibial bowing will fracture and develop a pseudoarthrosis when the infant begins to stand or walk (Fig. 23.3A). A

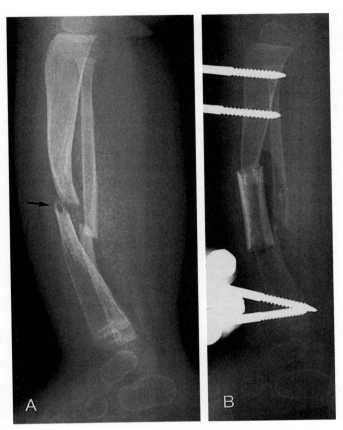

Figure 23.3. A, Lateral tibial radiograph showing a pseudoarthrosis (*arrow*) secondary to the fracture of a bowed tibia in a 1-year-old child with neurofibromatosis. **B,** Lateral tibial radiograph demonstrating the first operative appearance after excision of the pseudoarthrosis and bone graft replacement.

clamshell type of ankle-foot orthosis should be used from the time the diagnosis is made to prevent, or at least delay, this pathologic fracture. Elective osteotomy to straighten this bowing should be avoided, because a pseudoarthrosis will result. If an established pseudoarthrosis of the tibia occurs, surgical treatment is needed to establish union (Fig. 23.3B). At surgery, the pseudoarthrosis site contains hamartomatous tissue, not neurofibromas, even though the association with NF-1 is so strong. Bone healing is notoriously slow at the site of the pseudoarthrosis, even with modern surgical methods, and if bone union cannot be achieved through surgery a below-knee amputation may be the only recourse.

Localized gigantism of a part of one extremity at birth is usually due to the presence of a plexiform neurofibroma. Hyper-pigmented skin may be noted over the affected region. This plexiform neurofibroma may involve one digit or the entire extremity. Marked enlargement of one or more nerves within the lesion is seen at surgery. Some soft-tissue debulking is possible in less extensive neurofibromas. However, when major peripheral nerves are enlarged and involved, the amount of surgical resection that is feasible while still maintaining distal extremity function is limited. When the foot or a single digit is extensively involved, amputation often offers the best chance to restore nearly normal function.

Progressive spinal deformity is a commonly recognized feature of neurofibromatosis. All children with NF-1 should be examined at least annually for early detection of scoliosis. The two primary types of scoliosis present are the dystrophic and the idiopathic forms. Associated with vertebral body erosion by neurofibromas or arachnoid ectasia, the dystrophic type is usually seen in children between the ages of 5 and 10. This spinal deformity is rapidly progressive and is typically associated with localized kyphosis at the same location. Brace treatment is usually ineffective, and anterior and posterior spinal fusion is often needed to prevent the development of severe deformity. If spinal instrumentation is needed, a magnetic resonance (MR) scan of the spine is extremely helpful to detect the location of neurofibromas and assist in surgical planning. If a kyphoscoliosis of the dystrophic type becomes severe, neglected spinal cord compression at the site of deformity will lead to paraplegia.

The idiopathic form of scoliosis tends to occur during later childhood and adolescence and is similar to this type of spinal deformity seen in children and teenagers without neurofibromatosis. Spine radiographs do not demonstrate vertebral erosions. Brace treatment is commonly successful in preventing severe deformity.

Several features of spine radiographs may be indicative of neurofibromatosis, even without scoliosis or kyphosis. Localized neural foramen enlargement may result from a neurofibroma of the nerve root. Scalloping of the posterior vertebral body or partial erosion of a pedicle can mean that an intradural neurofibroma or dural ectasia is present. Thinned, irregular ribs are often seen in the region of neurofibromas. Cervical spine vertebral erosions may lead to cervical instability, a feature of NF-1 that should be evaluated prior to administration of anesthesia for any of the multiple surgical procedures needed in this disease.

Although the orthopaedic features are primarily addressed here, any organ system can be involved in neurofibromatosis. Of particular concern is the susceptibility of this group of children to develop central nervous system tumors. Visual examinations should be routinely performed throughout childhood to allow early detection. Neurosarcoma occurs in at least 5% of patients with neurofibromatosis and should be suspected if a neurofibroma in the extremity becomes painful or grows quickly.

MARFAN'S SYNDROME

An autosomal-dominant disorder associated with very tall individuals, Marfan's syndrome is a well-recognized connective tissue disorder that affects the eyes, the heart and aorta, and the musculoskeletal system. The four primary groups of clinical findings on which this diagnosis is based are eye findings (lens dislocation), valvular and vascular abnormalities (mitral or aortic valve defects or aortic aneurysm), musculoskeletal features (arachnodactyly, scoliosis, sternal deformity, joint hypermobility, and others), and a positive family history. If two or more of these criteria groups are present, the diagnosis of Marfan's syndrome can be made. The use of the term "marfanoid" to describe a tall individual with only the musculoskeletal features should be discouraged.

The child with Marfan's syndrome is tall, often in the 90th percentile for age. Extremities are thin and muscle mass is frequently underdeveloped. The lower body segment is longer than usual in relation to the upper half of the body. The feet are long and thin and usually flat. Arachnodactyly, or spider-like digits, is present in both the hand and foot. Hypermobility of all joints is common. While it is not present at birth, spinal deformity commonly develops with growth. It is clear that regular orthopaedic evaluation is needed for those with Marfan's syndrome.

A young child with Marfan's syndrome may have a delay in walking due to joint hypermobility. In more severely involved children, standing will lead to a marked valgus position of the heel and ankle and a recurvatum and valgus position of the knees. These are not fixed deformities but are a reflection of joint laxity and muscle weakness. As a temporary measure, use of an ankle-foot orthosis may speed the development of walking by stabilizing the ankle and controlling the foot position as hip and knee control develops.

As a general rule, the amount of joint laxity decreases with increasing age. However, during childhood or adolescence, symptoms of joint instability during exercise or athletics may arise, particularly at the knee and the shoulder. Anterior or multidirectional instability of the shoulder is symptomatic during throwing sports or overhead activity. Patellar subluxation may be painful during a wide variety of activities. In this syndrome, a muscle strengthening program should be stressed or the sport causing the pain should be avoided. Surgical treatment for instability of these joints in Marfan's syndrome is less successful than usual, since soft-tissue repairs in Marfan's syndrome tend to stretch out with time, with resultant return of the instability.

From a practical standpoint, parents of children with Marfan's syndrome often have difficulty finding a shoe to fit the child. The foot is long and slender, with a narrow heel that is in valgus with weight bearing. Although orthoses will not lead to stabilization of the connective tissue structures of the foot, use of an orthosis should be tried if the flatfoot is painful. As a side benefit, the orthosis makes it easier to find a shoe that fits. Subtalar fusion is not usually needed to stabilize the hindfoot in these patients.

Chest wall deformity often develops due to the increased rate of growth of the ribs, producing either a pectus carinatum (outward) or pectus excavatum (inward) deformity. Although this is primarily a cosmetic deformity, a pectus excavatum may be a factor in impaired pulmonary or cardiac function if the deformity is severe or if it is associated with marked scoliosis.

Involvement of the spine is probably the most serious musculoskeletal manifestation of Marfan's syndrome. Scoliosis, the most common deformity, first arises between the ages of 5 and 10 years. With the increased growth rate in Marfan's syndrome, progression of scoliosis is often quite rapid. Almost always associated with progressive thoracic scoliosis is a progressive thoracic lordosis that produces restriction of lung function and makes brace treatment less effective in preventing the progression of scoliosis. In selected girls with Marfan's syndrome and scoliosis at a young age, consideration can be given to using estrogen and progesterone to induce early puberty, thus limiting the amount of growth and making the scoliosis easier to control. If curve progression occurs despite bracing, spinal instrumentation and surgery is needed, though surgical complications are more common in Marfan's syndrome than in patients with idiopathic scoliosis.

In the thoracolumbar and lumbar spine, patients with Marfan's syndrome may develop problems as well. Thoracolumbar kyphosis is often noted when sitting during early childhood; though this early kyphosis generally resolves, a structural kyphosis that causes low back pain may appear during adolescence. Severe spondylolisthesis at the lumbosacral junction is more common than usual and should be considered in the presence of low back pain and hamstring tightness. In older teenagers and young adults, dural ectasia or an anterior meningocele may be the cause of low back pain in Marfan's syndrome and produces vertebral erosions similar to those seen in neurofibromatosis.

EHLERS-DANLOS SYNDROMES

More than ten types of connective tissue disorders are included in the family of Ehlers-Danlos syndromes. Inheritance patterns differ among the various types. Specific biochemical defects have been discovered for many of the more rare types. Genetic analysis studies have shown that there appears to be a close relationship between the clinical picture seen and the location of the specific genetic defect, as well as some interrelationship with the genetic defect found in os-teogenesis imperfecta.

Any child with excessive joint hypermo-bility, recurrent dislocations of multiple joints, and excessively lax or fragile skin should be suspected of having a type of Ehlers-Danlos syndrome. In its most mild form, Ehlers-Danlos syndrome may be manifested by joint laxity, for example in a child who can easily place his foot behind his head but is without any discernible skin changes. The elbows and knees can be hy-perextended and the fingers and thumb ap-pear "double-jointed." Skin changes asso-ciated with Ehlers-Danlos syndrome may range from mild hyperextensibility to the extremes of the circus "rubber-man." Commonly, scars spread easily and assume the classic "cigarette-paper" appearance. In more severe cases, the skin is extremely fragile and is easily bruised.

The primary orthopaedic concern is re-lated to the joint instability present in vary-ing degrees. Walking may be delayed until muscular control of the joints improves. Dislocation or subluxation may occur at any joint, though commonly involved joints in-clude the shoulder, knee, hip, and thumb regions.

Recurrent subluxation of the patella or the shoulder are treated during childhood with muscle strengthening to allow muscu-lar control to substitute for the ligament and capsular laxity. For mildly affected individ-uals, return to athletic participation is often possible once strength is improved and symptoms have resolved, but the choice of appropriate sports must be individualized.

Surgical repair by tightening the lax con-nective tissue structures, as with Marfan's syndrome, is frequently unsuccessful. A pa-tellar knee support is useful in some pa-tients, but muscle strengthening should be the primary initial mode of treatment for symptoms of joint subluxation. If hip insta-bility occurs, muscle strengthening is not ef-fective and surgical care, including femoral and pelvic osteotomy, is needed. Recurrent

dislocations at the base of the thumb will impede the ability to grip objects; fusion of the unstable joint is effective in improving hand function.

NAIL-PATELLA SYNDROME

Nail-patella syndrome is manifested by abnormal nails, absent or hypoplastic patel-lae, elbow dysplasia, and the finding of iliac horns on the pelvic radiograph. Inheritance is by autosomal-dominant means, and life expectancy is essentially normal.

The primary orthopaedic finding in the upper extremity is a flexion contracture of the elbows, associated with radial head dis-location during childhood. Forearm rotation is usually somewhat impaired. Radiographs demonstrate hypoplasia of the lateral hu-meral condyle and posterior dislocation of the radial head. Surgical treatment has not produced an improvement in elbow motion.

In the lower extremity, the knee is pri-marily involved. The patellae are absent or hypoplastic. Subluxation or dislocation of the rudimentary patellae is common, and the quadriceps muscle is underdeveloped. This patellar instability causes the child to walk with the knee slightly flexed and the foot externally rotated for stability. If the patella is dislocated in the child, surgical re-alignment is indicated.

The interesting pathognomonic finding of iliac horns on the anteroposterior pelvic ra-diograph will confirm the diagnosis of nail-patella syndrome. Projecting posteriorly from the iliac wing, these horns are often palpable on physical examination but cause no symptoms or disability.

MULTIPLE HEREDITARY EXOSTOSES

Inherited as an autosomal-dominant trait, this disorder is characterized by the presence of osteochondromas or exostoses at the metaphyseal region of most long bones, in addition to similar exostoses in the vertebrae and pelvis. These exostoses are not noted at birth but appear in early childhood.

The initial physical findings are of bony projections palpable adjacent to virtually all the joints. Radiographs demonstrate broad-based osteochondromas projecting from the metaphyseal regions of many long bones (Fig. 23.4). Because a cap of cartilage sits on the end of each osteochondroma, the lesion often appears larger on examination than is demonstrated on the radiograph.

All osteochondromas cannot and should not be removed surgically. As normal growth of the child occurs, the osteochondromas will also increase in size. The most common reasons for surgical treatment are pain over an osteochondroma, interference by the osteochondroma with normal long bone growth, or a disproportionate increase in the size of the lesion. Growth disturbance by these osteochondromas occurs most often in the forearm, hand, or lower leg. If angular deformity of a long bone occurs, realignment osteotomy of the affected bone is performed at the same time as the osteochondroma resection. Malignant degeneration of osteochondromas can occur in adults with the formation of a chondrosarcoma in the cartilage cap of the osteochondroma. A sudden increase in the size of a painful lesion should be treated with surgical excision.

SKELETAL DYSPLASIAS

Well over 100 types of skeletal dysplasia have been described, each affecting the long bones and the spine a little differently. When faced with evaluating an infant or older child who has short stature or disproportionate body segments, the differential diagnosis can be narrowed significantly by physical examination and radiographs.

Possible distinguishing facial features should first be evaluated. When looking at the extremities and trunk, is this a short-trunk or short-limb type of dwarfism? If the limbs are short, is the shortening in the proximal segment (rhizomelia), in the middle segment (mesomelia), or in the hand and foot (acromelia)? On radiographs of the extremities, is the dysplasia mainly in the epiphyses or in the metaphyses? On the an-

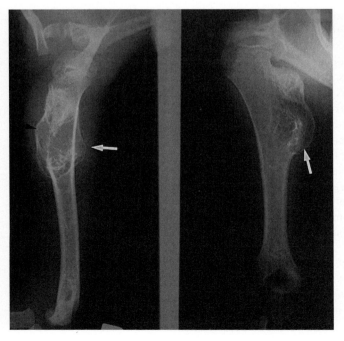

Figure 23.4. An osteochondroma (*arrows*) is projecting from the proximal humerus of a 4-year-old child with multiple hereditary exostoses. The growth abnormality of the humerus is related to disproportionate growth of the osteochondroma.

teroposterior and lateral spine radiographs, are the vertebral bodies flattened or are there any anterior projections from the vertebral body? With the facts gleaned from this examination and radiographs, combined with a careful family history, a "short list" of possible diagnoses is usually readily reached. Since the natural history of the musculoskeletal problems varies significantly between syndromes, obtaining the correct diagnosis before treatment proceeds is important. The opinion of a medical geneticist should be sought for diagnostic confirmation and for counseling of the family.

Achondroplasia

The most common of the skeletal dysplasias, achondroplasia is recognizable at birth. The infant has a short-limbed, rhizomelic form of dwarfism with characteristic facial features of frontal bossing and depression of the nasal bridge. Inheritance is autosomal dominant. Paternal age over 40 is associated with a higher risk of a spontaneous mutation leading to an achondroplastic child. While the exact genetic defect remains undefined, the skeletal effect is an impairment of enchondral ossification, leading to decreased longitudinal growth of the long bones.

Respiratory difficulties and sleep apnea occur in the young child with achondroplasia, especially during the first year. Upper-airway compromise may result from the midface hypoplasia or small thoracic cage size due to hypoplastic ribs. Compression of the cervical spinal cord at the foramen magnum may lead to apnea or flaccidity. Although the foramen magnum enlarges relative to the spinal cord as growth proceeds, surgical decompression of the spinal cord may be necessary to improve respiratory function.

Hypotonia is commonly present at birth and for the first several months of life. Motor milestones are usually delayed and independent walking is often not achieved until 18 months of age or later. It is not known exactly why this hypotonia is present, but some believe the foramen magnum compression may play a role. As a result of this hypotonia, when the infant with achondroplasia sits, kyphosis of the thoracolumbar spine is present. Initially this is a flexible kyphosis that resolves in over 90% as standing and walking are achieved, but progressive thoracolumbar kyphosis may persist in some children. If significant thoracolumbar kyphosis is still present by age 5 or 6, spinal fusion surgery is indicated to prevent worsening.

While kyphosis persists in only a relatively small number of children with achondroplasia, all achondroplastic children are born with spinal stenosis. Even at the time of birth, the anteroposterior lumbar spine radiograph will demonstrate narrowing of the interpediculate distances, a feature of this disorder that can be used to help confirm the diagnosis. The anteroposterior diameter of the spinal canal is relatively normal, but the interpediculate distance of the lumbar spinal canal measures only about half of the normal size. Although the stenosis is most marked in the lumbar spine, the cervical and thoracic spinal canals are also somewhat smaller than normal.

As a result of this spinal stenosis, compression of the cauda equina or the spinal cord is relatively common in achondroplasia. Signs and symptoms of spinal claudication are most common, occurring anytime after the mid-teen years, when degenerative disc changes produce even more stenosis. The patient will note weakness and sensory changes in the lower extremities when standing or walking, with relief obtained by flexing the lumbar spine through squatting or bending forward. Bladder and bowel control may be affected.

If neurologic findings are persistent, an MR scan is obtained to evaluate the levels and degree of stenosis. If the MR study confirms cauda equina or spinal cord compression, multilevel decompressive laminectomy is needed to prevent progressive neurologic loss.

Although spinal canal stenosis is the primary musculoskeletal feature of achondroplasia that interferes with function, angular deformity of the lower extremities may also affect walking ability. Genu varum (bowed legs) is common, secondary to overgrowth of the fibula relative to the tibia (Fig. 23.5). While essentially all with achondroplasia have some bowing of the legs, only about 50% will require treatment, which consists of a realignment tibial osteotomy. Bracing is not effective for this bowing because of

the marked ligamentous laxity usually present at the knee (Fig. 23.6).

Lengthening of the lower extremities of achondroplastic children by 20 to 35 cm to attain heights of a little over 5 ft has recently been extensively practiced in Europe and the former Soviet Union. The time needed to lengthen the femur and tibia bilaterally by this amount (as well as the humerus in the upper extremity) is between 2 and 3 years, and complications are relatively common. Nonetheless, unaffected parents of children with achondroplasia often inquire about the role of lengthening in this condition. Compared with other skeletal

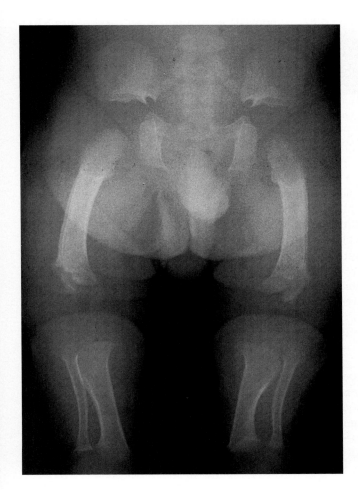

Figure 23.5. This lower-extremity anteroposterior radiograph of an infant with achondroplasia demonstrates the fibular overgrowth and typical flattened appearance of the ilia.

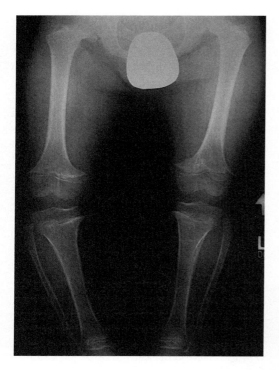

Figure 23.6.   Standing anteroposterior radiograph of a 9-year-old boy with achondroplasia demonstrating bowing of the right leg greater than the left. Osteotomy of the tibia corrected this bowing.

dysplasias and congenital limb deficiencies, lengthening of bones in achondroplasia is somewhat easier because of the redundancy of soft-tissue structures present in children with achondroplasia. While leg lengthening in achondroplasia can be achieved, the exact role for this procedure remains to be determined. If leg lengthening is attempted, sustained support and cooperation of both the child and the family are required.

Spondyloepiphyseal Dysplasia

The two main types of spondyloepiphyseal dysplasia (SED) are SED congenita and SED tarda. Short stature is a prominent feature of SED congenita, and the diagnosis of this condition can be made at birth. SED tarda, on the other hand, is usually diagnosed during late childhood or early adolescence, since final height is over 5 ft. SED congenita is inherited by an autosomal-dominant mode (though most cases are new mutations), while the mode of inheritance for SED tarda is X-linked recessive.

Physical features of a child with SED congenita include short limbs (but with normal-sized hands), short trunk with a tendency toward a pectus carinatum, and a flat-appearing face. Cleft palate is relatively common. Angular deformity of the lower extremities frequently develops during the first few years of childhood. Regular ophthalmologic check-ups are needed during childhood, as retinal detachment often occurs in this syndrome. Hearing loss is also a feature of SED congenita.

Atlantoaxial instability with odontoid hypoplasia is common at an early age in SED congenita and may be at least part of the cause of delayed motor milestones frequently seen in this condition. If walking is delayed significantly, flexion and extension lateral cervical spine radiographs are used to evaluate instability at the atlantoaxial level, though delayed ossification of the vertebrae may make accurate measurement difficult. If there is sufficient concern that atlantoaxial instability may be present, an MR study with the neck flexed is valuable in assessing the extent of possible spinal cord compression. If instability and spinal cord compression are demonstrated, posterior occipitoaxial fusion is recommended. Commonly, following the atlantoaxial stabilization surgery, upper- and lower-extremity function will improve significantly.

The trunk of these children is short due to the platyspondylia uniformly seen in the thoracic and lumbar spine (Fig. 23.7). Further trunk shortening can occur as a result of progressive scoliosis, for which brace treatment is first attempted, with spinal fusion surgery reserved for those in whom scoliosis continues to progress despite use of a brace.

In the lower extremities, progressive coxa vara and genu varum or genu valgum are the most common orthopaedic problems

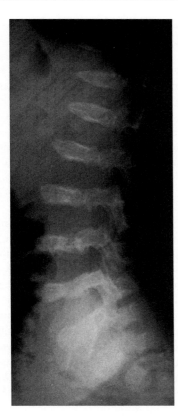

Figure 23.7. This lateral spinal radiograph of a child with spondyloepiphyseal dysplasia demonstrates the characteristic platyspondylia with marked uniform flattening and irregularity of the vertebrae.

encountered. Hip radiographs will confirm delayed ossification of the femoral head, and serial radiographs will demonstrate a progressive varus deformity of the hip. Valgus osteotomy of the proximal femur is commonly used to restore a more normal position of the hip, but patients with SED congenita often require total hip arthroplasty as young adults. Angular deformity in the region of the knee and ankle is treated by realignment osteotomy.

The tarda form of spondyloepiphyseal dysplasia is not recognizable at birth but is usually diagnosed when the child or adolescent is evaluated for either short stature or hip pain. Although these boys are usually taller than 5 ft, they are shorter than unaffected family members, mainly because of a shortened trunk. Radiographs of the spine are remarkable primarily for platyspondylia. Low back pain may be present during adolescence and adult life.

The primary orthopaedic problem with SED tarda is premature degenerative arthritis of the hips. Pain is usually present during the teenage years. Hip radiographs demonstrate changes consistent with degenerative arthritis, including narrowing of the joint cartilage space and osteophyte formation on the femoral head. Nonsteroidal anti-inflammatory medication is initially effective, but total hip arthroplasty is usually needed in early adult life to obtain pain relief and to preserve function.

Diastrophic Dysplasia

Although diastrophic dysplasia is rare, orthopaedic manifestations are the primary features of this disorder. It is inherited in an autosomal-recessive manner. The clinical findings are sufficiently characteristic to allow this diagnosis to be made at birth.

Physical findings at birth that are typical of this disorder include short-limb dwarfism, severe clubfeet, joint contractures, limited movement of the fingers, and a "hitchhiker's thumb" deformity. About half of these infants have a cleft palate. Within a few weeks after birth, the ears become swollen, with later scarring of the ear cartilage leading to a "cauliflower ear" appearance.

The clubfeet are very rigid and require surgical correction, usually during the first year of life. Walking is possible even without clubfoot correction but is facilitated after plantigrade feet have been achieved. Progressive hip deformity occurs with gradual subluxation, and corrective osteotomy is often needed.

Spinal involvement is a major component of diastrophic dysplasia. Cervical spine kyphosis is common in young children with this disorder and often resolves without active treatment. However, if cervical kyphosis progresses, cervical spine fusion is needed to prevent spinal cord compression. Scoliosis occurs in about 70% of these patients, but only about half of these need treatment, which usually consists of spinal fusion after progression of the scoliosis has been detected.

Multiple Epiphyseal Dysplasia

Inherited as an autosomal-dominant trait, multiple epiphyseal dysplasia has two primary manifestations: hip abnormalities and mild short stature. Height is above the third percentile and is greater than the other skeletal dysplasias. Unless a clear family history has already been established, the diagnosis is not made at birth and is often delayed until the child begins to develop hip pain.

Hip pain often initially occurs between the ages of 5 and 10 years. Radiographs of the hip, as well as of the knee and shoulder, will demonstrate epiphyses that appear slightly flattened but otherwise normal. In some cases, avascular necrosis of the femoral epiphysis is present in addition to the epiphyseal dysplasia; therefore it is easy to confuse this condition with Legg-Perthes disease of the hip. Whenever someone has what appears to be bilateral Legg-Perthes disease, further radiographic evaluation of other long-bone epiphyses is needed to rule out or confirm the diagnosis of multiple epiphyseal dysplasia. If synovitis of the hip occurs, restriction of activity is needed until hip movement improves. If radiographs demonstrate changes in the femoral head consistent with avascular necrosis, the author advocates brace treatment as would be done with Legg-Perthes disease. Nonetheless, any patient with multiple epiphyseal dysplasia is apt to require a total hip arthroplasty during early or middle adult life to relieve hip pain from premature degenerative arthritis of the hip.

Metabolic Disorders
HYPOPHOSPHATEMIC RICKETS

Hypophosphatemic rickets, also known as vitamin D-resistant rickets, is transmitted in a X-linked dominant manner and is the most common form of rickets seen in the United States today. The genetic defect that leads to rickets is an abnormality in phosphate resorption in the proximal renal tubules that leads to hyperphosphaturia.

If a family history of this disorder is known, the diagnosis can be made at the time of birth, since hypophosphatemia is present at that time even though the clinical features of rickets do not occur until later. Boys with this disorder will develop obvious rickets in early childhood and are of relatively short final stature. On the other hand, though affected girls have hypophosphatemia, the clinical picture of rickets varies significantly from minimal to severe.

In infancy, serum studies are used to make this diagnosis. Serum calcium is normal or slightly low, serum phosphate is low, and serum alkaline phosphatase is elevated, especially later when the clinical picture of rickets is more apparent. Urine phosphate levels are elevated. Administration of physiologic amounts of vitamin D or its derivatives does not produce a response.

As the child becomes older, typical skeletal changes of rickets (of any cause) become obvious, particularly in boys. Bowing of the lower extremities is more common than are knock-knees. Joints may appear swollen and enlarged, sometimes with restriction of movement. Short stature becomes more apparent as the child ages since longitudinal bone growth is diminished.

Plain radiographs will demonstrate the skeletal changes well. The most typical finding is widening and fraying of the physis at the end of all the long bones, associated with angulation or bowing of the tibia and femur in the lower extremity. This physeal widening is seen best in rapidly growing bones, such as around the knee, wrist, and shoulder, and is produced by inadequate calcification in the zone of provisional calcification of the physis, resulting in a widening of the uncalcified zone of hypertrophy (Fig. 23.8). Widening or cupping of the metaphyses is seen at the joints that appear clinically enlarged. Periodic radiographic assessment of the width of the physis is useful to gauge the skeletal response to medical treatment.

While the mainstay of treatment is medical care with replacement phosphate and, in some, a form of vitamin D, realignment osteotomy of the bowed tibia and/or femur is needed if angular deformity is sufficiently severe. The need for repeated osteotomy during the years of growth is unfortunately

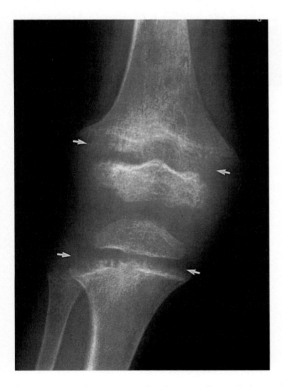

Figure 23.8. Anteroposterior knee radiograph in a child with hypophosphatemic rickets shows marked widening, cupping, and fraying of the poorly calcified physes of the femur and tibia (*arrows*).

fairly common in boys with this disorder. If surgical realignment is to be successful, careful medical control of the rickets is needed postoperatively to allow for appropriate calcification of the healing bone that forms at the osteotomy site. Because cast immobilization and bed rest are often part of postosteotomy care, these children require close evaluation for hypercalcemia that may develop as a result of the immobilization.

MUCOPOLYSACCHARIDOSES

In the family of disorders known as the mucopolysaccharidoses, seven different types have so far been described, each being characterized by a deficiency in a specific enzyme that results in abnormal accumulation of mucopolysaccharides. These types of mucopolysaccharidosis (MPS) are Hurler's syndrome (type I MPS), Scheie's syndrome (type IS MPS), Hunter's syndrome (type II MPS), Sanfilippo's syndrome (type III MPS), Morquio's syndrome (type IV MPS), Maroteaux-Lamy syndrome (type VI MPS), and β-glucuronidase deficiency (type VII MPS). Hunter's syndrome is transmitted by X-linked recessive means, while all the other syndromes are transmitted by autosomal-recessive inheritance.

Throughout this group of disorders, orthopaedic problems occur primarily in the spine and the lower extremities. Thoracolumbar kyphosis and upper cervical spine instability are the most common spinal abnormalities, while angular deformity, hip maldevelopment, and joint stiffness are seen in the lower extremities.

However, several of the MPS syndromes do not require much orthopaedic care. Sanfilippo's syndrome (type III MPS) usually has little or no skeletal involvement. Hurler's syndrome (type I MPS) does include thoracolumbar kyphosis and joint stiffness, but death often occurs during early to midchildhood from cardiopulmonary causes, making orthopaedic care unnecessary (Fig. 23.9). Children with Scheie's syndrome

Figure 23.9. **A,** Skeletal changes are common in Hurler's syndrome. This chest radiograph shows the characteristic wide, spatulate ribs. **B,** A radiograph of the arm of a child with Hurler's syndrome shows widened, poorly modeled long bones and markedly widened metacarpals and phalanges. The normal trabecular pattern has been replaced.

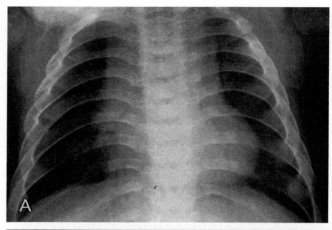

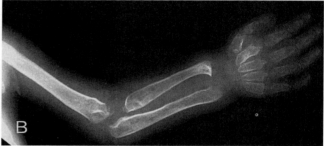

(type IS MPS) may have genu valgum, but walking ability is lost in later childhood and death commonly occurs during the teenage years. Those with Hunter's syndrome (type II MPS), if survival past the teenage years occurs, are likely to develop degenerative hip disease, but orthopaedic treatment during childhood is minimal.

Patients with either Maroteaux-Lamy syndrome (type VI MPS) or β-glucuronidase deficiency (type VII MPS) may require orthopaedic surgery. Both syndromes produce thoracolumbar kyphosis that may progress, as well as joint stiffness associated with radiographic abnormalities in the epiphyseal regions. Children with type VI MPS may develop radiographic changes in the hips that are similar to those seen in Legg-Perthes disease. Children with type VII MPS can develop a progressive lateral hip subluxation or dislocation that should be treated surgically in an attempt to delay

degenerative changes. Angular deformity, especially genu valgum, may require realignment osteotomy if this deformity interferes with walking.

Morquio's Syndrome

Among all the mucopolysaccharidoses, Morquio's syndrome (type IV MPS) leads to the largest number of orthopaedic problems, with all of these children requiring some form of orthopaedic care to the spine or lower extremities. While the child appears normal at birth, skeletal changes begin to be apparent before 2 years of age. Thoracolumbar kyphosis is noted clinically and lateral spinal radiographs demonstrate anterior projections from the center of the vertebral bodies (Fig. 23.10). (If these radiographic changes are noted prior to the clinical diagnosis of Morquio's syndrome, the vertebral appearance may be misconstrued as being congenital kyphosis.) Genu valgum

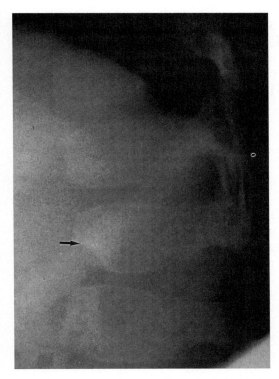

Figure 23.10. Lateral spine radiograph of a child with Morquio's syndrome showing anterior beaking of the L1 vertebral body (*arrow*).

compression and is a common cause for a decrease in the walking ability of these patients during late childhood or early adolescence. Rather than ascribing a change in walking ability to the genu valgum deformity, the neck should be carefully evaluated with lateral flexion and extension cervical spine radiographs to detect abnormal movement at the C1-C2 level. An MR study with the neck in both a flexed and an extended position will demonstrate the level and degree of spinal cord compression present. If atlantoaxial instability is found, occipitoaxial posterior fusion is indicated and will often lead to an improvement in neurologic function of the extremities.

appears early and persists or worsens during mid-childhood, at times requiring corrective osteotomy of the tibia.

As the child with Morquio's syndrome grows, deformity of the thoracic cage, with a prominent pectus carinatum, becomes obvious. In addition, subluxation of the hips with resultant development of misshapen femoral heads occurs, leading to premature degenerative arthritis and the need for total joint arthroplasty in early adult life.

Of all the musculoskeletal problems encountered in Morquio's syndrome, however, odontoid hypoplasia and atlantoaxial instability is potentially the most serious. Occurring in a large percentage of patients with Morquio's syndrome, this upper cervical instability will lead to spinal cord

Suggested Readings

Crawford, A.H., Jr. and Bagamery, N.: Osseous manifestations of neurofibromatosis in childhood. J. Pediatr. Orthop. 6:72-88, 1986.

Davidson, R.G.: Atlantoaxial instability in individuals with Down syndrome: a fresh look at the evidence. Pediatrics 81:857-865, 1988.

Ferris, B., Walker, C., Jackson, A., and Kirwan, E.: The orthopaedic management of hypophosphataemic rickets. J. Pediatr. Orthop. 11:367-373, 1991.

Gertner, J.M. and Root, L.: Osteogenesis imperfecta. Orthop. Clin. North Am. 21:151-162, 1990.

Goldberg, M.J.: The Dysmorphic Child: An Orthopedic Perspective. Raven Press, New York, 1987.

Jones, K.L.: Smith's Recognizable Patterns of Human Malformation, 4th ed., W.B. Saunders, Philadelphia, 1988.

Mankin, H.J.: Rickets, osteomalacia, and renal osteodystrophy. An update. Orthop. Clin. North Am. 21: 81-96, 1990.

Nicolletti, B., Kopits, S.E., Ascani, E. and McKusick, V.A. (eds): Human Achondroplasia: A Multidisciplinary Approach. Plenum, New York, 1988.

Pueschel, S.M. and Scola, F.H.: Atlantoaxial instability in individuals with Down syndrome: epidemiologic, radiographic, and clinical studies. Pediatrics 80:555-560, 1987.

Tsipouras, P. and Ramirez, F.: Genetic disorders of collagen. J. Med. Genet. 24:2-8, 1987.

Wynne-Davies, R., Hall, C.M., and Apley, A.G.: Atlas of Skeletal Dysplasias. Churchill-Livingstone, Edinburgh, 1985.

24

The Young Athlete

Athletic activity is an integral part of the lives of many young people. Whether engaging in organized or playground sports or in physical education at school, children and teenagers nearly daily play games in which they are physically active. As a part of these sports activities, injuries of the musculoskeletal system can and do occur on a regular basis. The treatment of a large number of musculoskeletal injuries has already been presented in earlier chapters of this book, and this treatment of specific injuries remains essentially the same whether the injury is incurred during athletic activities or from some other traumatic cause. What makes athletic injuries somewhat different is the philosophy of care that not only deals with the injury but also aims at an early return to sports participation.

Treating injured young athletes is different than treating musculoskeletal injuries in a child or adolescent. The development of the field of sports medicine has provided much valuable information on conditioning and injury prevention and has resulted in a twofold focus for injury management in these young athletes: not only to treat the orthopaedic problem but also to return the athlete to sports participation as quickly as safely possible. A prescription by a physician to stop all athletic activities for several weeks or months is not likely to be accepted by parents and children who have become exposed to the role of sports medicine in high-performance professional and college athletics.

The primary-care physician plays a part

in the care of these young athletes in several ways. Primary-care physicians provide treatment to young patients injured during sports participation almost on a daily basis. A physician may provide preparticipation physical examinations for the local school. Some schools seek on-the-field physician coverage for games. Regardless of the setting in which interaction with young athletes occurs, the primary-care physician should keep in mind this goal of young athletes to return to their sport as soon as is safely possible.

Preparticipation History and Physical Examination

The review of the health status of the aspiring young athlete has two primary purposes: to detect current health problems and to determine if there are substantial risks for either musculoskeletal injury or sudden death if the child engages in sports participation. Ideally, this review occurs as a part of an annual physical examination by the primary-care physician, but annual physical examinations are not widely used by teenagers. Because of this, the requirement for a health status review prior to sports participation serves the alternate purpose of forcing teenagers to undergo medical evaluation.

The required frequency for the preparticipation evaluation varies widely among school districts. While annual evaluations in the primary-care physician's office remains the ideal, it is generally not practical for the school to provide annual evaluations for all students participating on athletic teams. As a compromise, it is acceptable to require one evaluation in junior high school and another in high school for all prospective athletes. Annual evaluations may be required for athletes who sustained a significant injury in the prior year or who have risk factors for cardiac disorders.

The prior medical history is one of the most productive parts of the preparticipation evaluation. History of past injury is key, particularly of injuries that required temporary cessation of sports participation. A history of fainting or dizziness during sports activity is an important feature to note, as this may indicate an underlying cardiac disorder. A family history of sudden unexpected death in a teenager or young adult should be sought. Often the history is better able to identify those at risk for sudden death during sports activity than is electrocardiography, which cannot practically be performed on all prospective young athletes.

Whether performed in the physician's office or as a part of a group examination in the school, the physical examination should include a brief general examination (including blood pressure, visual acuity, heart, lungs, and abdomen) and a more detailed orthopaedic examination. The orthopaedic examination is designed to detect any musculoskeletal features that increase the risk of injury, such as limitation of movement of the spine or peripheral joints, muscle atrophy, or joint instability. Table 24.1 lists the major features of the basic orthopaedic screening examination for young athletes.

If an abnormality is found on the preparticipation physical examination, several options are available. Significant orthopaedic findings should lead to a referral to an orthopaedist for more thorough evaluation. Muscle atrophy that has persisted from a prior injury can be treated with strengthening exercises, and the child can return to sports participation after strength is re-

Table 24.1.
Basic Orthopaedic Sports Screening Examination

Area of Examination	Desired Finding
General	Body habitus
	Gait, absence of limp
	Symmetry of extremities, both muscles and leg lengths
Neck	Chin up and down, ear to shoulder, chin to shoulder
Shoulder	Full range of motion
	Stability at glenohumeral joint
	Strength of deltoid and rotator cuff to hold arm abducted; no pain
	Nontender acromioclavicular joints
Elbow	Painless, full flexion and extension
	Full forearm supination/pronation
Wrist and hand	Normal wrist flexion and extension
	Normal finger motion, grasp strength
	Absence of finger deformity
Back	Scoliosis, kyphosis absent
	No excessive hamstring tightness or back pain during forward bend, fingertips to floor with knees straight
Hip	Symmetrical movement between hips, especially internal rotation
	Normal Trendelenburg test
Knee	No effusion
	Collateral and cruciate ligament stability
	No patellar pain
	Adequate quadriceps strength
	No tibial tubercle tenderness
Ankle	Plantarflexion and dorsiflexion equal bilaterally
	No instability in inversion
	Toe-walk and heel-walk (leg strength)
Foot	No foot deformity, especially pes cavus
	Normal pain-free subtalar movement (tarsal coalition)
	No heel pain or tenderness

gained. While many of the mild abnormalities found can be managed by a good conditioning and stretching program, other findings, such as limitation of neck motion, preclude safe participation in collision sports or wrestling, and other sports options need to be pursued. The majority of abnormal findings on these orthopaedic screening examinations will not be serious enough to require avoidance of all sports activities.

The physician should help guide those with physical limitations to find an appropriate sport and must be sensitive to the needs of the young individuals when advising what should or should not be pursued.

Sports and the Preschool Child

While organized sports have much to offer older children and teenagers, sports for preschool children should have a different emphasis. In 1992, the Committee on Sports Medicine and Fitness of the American Academy of Pediatrics published recommendations for this age group. Because participation in organized sports relies not only on motor skills development but also on the ability to interact with coaches and teammates as well as the ability to follow instructions, children are not generally ready for team sports until after the age of 6. Notwithstanding possible limitations for organized sports, it is recommended that all preschool children regularly participate in physical activity, as a much preferable option to watching television. In this age group, sports activity should be enjoyable, with an emphasis on participation, with a by-product being the improvement of individual motor skills in that sport. Conditioning is not an appropriate primary focus at this age. There is no evidence that physical training during these preschool years will lead to improved sports performance in subsequent years, and children sooner or later follow the same general sequence of skill acquisition (such as running, kicking, throwing, hopping, and catching a ball), though the time for this skill acquisition may vary among individuals by a year or two.

Training the Young Athlete

The response of children to exercise is different than the response seen in older adolescents and in adults. Methods used in adults to increase endurance, strength, and flexibility need to be modified, especially in younger children, since the young child's body is unable to respond in the same way as the adult's to the stress of these activities.

Maximum oxygen uptake, or Vo_2max, is generally regarded as the best single indicator of aerobic fitness. Normally, in growing girls, the Vo_2max increases until puberty, while in boys this maximum oxygen uptake continues to increase even after puberty. It appears in studies of children between the ages of 6 and 18 that the weight-adjusted Vo_2max is similar to that found in adults. It is more difficult to improve the Vo_2max in children than in adults. What appears to be an improvement in aerobic capacity is often due more to the effects of a rapid growth spurt than to the training itself. Despite this weight-adjusted aerobic capacity being similar for children as for adults, energy expenditure for some endurance sports has been noted to be higher in the young child than in the adult.

On the other hand, anaerobic capacity is definitely limited in the growing child compared to the adult, even when using weight-adjusted measurements. The exact cause of this inability of children to use muscle glycogen and produce lactate as efficiently as adults when responding to exercise is unclear but may be related to a lower level of phosphofructokinase activity in the child. This diminished anaerobic capacity is not a big problem, because children have the ability to make quick cardiopulmonary adjustments in response to increases in intensity of activity. The limited anaerobic capacity, however, should be known by those designing training programs for children, because intense exercise threshold training is not recommended for children and does not produce the same beneficial effects on endurance that it has in adults.

The use of strength training during childhood has been controversial. Although strength training in adult athletes helps performance and reduces the risk of injury, similar results in prepubertal children have not been documented. In 1983, the American Academy of Pediatrics issued a statement indicating that weight training had minimal benefit in prepubertal individuals and that weight lifting as a sport should be avoided by preadolescents due to a high injury rate. Several subsequent reports have now convincingly demonstrated that prepubescent children can make substantial strength gains through a properly designed program. If used, this strength-training program should be carefully supervised and should consist of some form of resistance training, with much less reliance on weight training than in older teenagers or adults. Although bone scans after resistance training have not demonstrated apparent physeal changes, the possibility of damage to the growth plate from repetitive impact remains a potential problem with strength training in the prepubertal individual.

Flexibility training in children has been largely ignored due to the fact that children are naturally more flexible than teenagers and adults. Generally, females are more flexible than males of the same age. Flexibility appears to begin to decrease in the prepubertal period and continues to slowly decrease throughout life. Joint mobility can be enhanced by stretching exercises, especially of the low-force, long-duration type. Although improved flexibility may improve sports performance in some sports, the most acknowledged benefit of flexibility training is the avoidance of injury. While a period of stretching exercises prior to athletic activities appears to be beneficial for all children and adolescents, not all muscles can be stretched every day, and specific exercises need to be tailored to the needs of the individual young athlete and the sport being played.

In any conditioning program for young athletes, an additional feature that must be considered is the different manner in which a child dissipates heat engendered by exercise. Children perspire less than adults despite having a greater number of sweat glands. At puberty, a higher level of perspiration is produced by each gland. Children also produce more heat with comparable exercise and have a less efficient means to convey this heat from the muscle to the skin. In addition, because of a higher ratio of surface area to body mass, when the ambient temperature is warm, heat loss becomes more difficult for children. Heat loss becomes even harder if the skin is fully covered by a team uniform.

Although the child's body is not as efficient as the adult's in eliminating excess body heat from exercise, children do perspire. The electrolytes lost in the perspiration are generally compensated for by internal electrolyte shifts, so the major loss to the body from perspiration is body water. During all practice sessions and games, young athletes must be assured free access to water. Cool water, rather than electrolyte solutions, is the best replacement for water lost through perspiration during exercise. Because the ability to perspire varies among individuals, weighing athletes before and after conditioning sessions will identify those with excessive water losses (3% of body weight or more). If large water losses are seen during conditioning, rehydration is mandatory before practice is resumed.

Excessive heat production with exercise may produce a variety of symptoms, ranging from cramps to coma and death. Usually affecting the calf muscles and the hamstrings, cramps are most common in prepubertal children and obese individuals and are thought to be due to dehydration and excessive heat. In heat exhaustion, nausea and vomiting are common along with dizziness and an elevated body temperature. Treatment of heat exhaustion consists of cessation of exercise and rehydration, either orally or intravenously. Heat stroke is the most serious heat illness and is characterized by disorientation, seizures, or coma. Perspiration and peripheral vasodilation are present but the body temperature is above 106°F. Heat stroke is a medical emergency that leads to death if not treated quickly with ice packs, intravenous fluids, and quick transport to a hospital.

It is clear that the body of a young athlete can respond positively to various types of training regimens. However, in establishing goals for these training programs for the growing child, it is essential to keep in mind the limitations of the body of the prepubertal child in responding to certain training stimuli. Having fun, playing with peers, and learning the skills of sports remain the most important components of sports participation in the young athlete rather than a rigorous physical training program, which is more appropriate after puberty.

Sports Injury Evaluation and Management On and Off the Field

To the young athlete, the most important question to be answered by the physician in the evaluation of an acute sports injury is "when can I go back to play?" To answer this question reasonably, it is necessary to know what anatomic structures have been injured, the severity of the injury, and the risk of further injury if the sport continues to be played.

ON THE FIELD

It is important for the team physician to have access to basic first-aid supplies and resuscitation equipment. The equipment available should be checked prior to the start of the game to ensure that needed supplies are present. It is helpful for the physician to know who will contact an ambulance if one is needed.

When an injury occurs during a game, the examination on the field obviously focuses on the injured area. If the injury is to the upper extremity, the athlete is walked to the sidelines for a more complete examination. If a lower-extremity injury is present, the exact region of pain is localized by the athlete. Visual inspection for deformity is quickly completed. If obvious deformity,

indicating a displaced fracture, is present, the leg should be splinted before moving the athlete from the field. If instability is present, the athlete should be assisted off the field without having to bear weight on the injured leg. Once on the sidelines, a more thorough examination is performed.

Special precautions are needed when a young athlete is unconscious or has a suspected spinal injury. If the child is unconscious and not breathing, basic resuscitation is needed at once. If the child is unconscious but is breathing regularly and has a good pulse, the neck should be stabilized prior to transport off the field to the hospital. If the child has been hit on the head and has been transiently unconscious, he or she should be taken to the sidelines where questions are asked to determine the state of consciousness. If pain is present in the neck, the athlete should be questioned about tingling or numbness in the arms or legs. If the neck is tender in the midline posteriorly, the neck should be splinted prior to transporting the athlete or placing him or her in an upright position. Back pain, if the result of contact during the playing of a collision sport, should also be treated as if a compression fracture or similar injury has occurred, and the athlete should be transported on a back board to the sidelines.

On the sidelines, a thorough orthopaedic examination of the injured area is essential, away from the focus of the spectators. The site of pain or swelling is noted. Careful notation of any ligament instability of the knee or ankle is important and will be useful later for the orthopaedist, since the best examination of an injured joint is in the first few minutes after injury, before a significant hematoma and local edema have developed. The key question to answer at this time is whether or not the injured child athlete can safely return to the game.

Playability can sometimes be easy to determine. If the child has been unconscious or has altered mental status, if knee or ankle instability is present, or if neck or back pain is present, all these clearly indicate that return to the sport that day is unsafe and unwise. However, most injuries to the extremities are less severe, involving more minor injuries to the ligaments and muscles. A word of caution should be noted once again here: if there is any tenderness over the physis, rather than over a ligament or muscle, a fracture of the growth plate should be suspected, and further play should not be allowed that day and until orthopaedic and radiographic evaluation has been completed.

A rough grading of the degree of ligament or muscle injury is possible. *Mild or first-degree ligament sprains* involve only a few ligament fibers, are associated with only mild pain and tenderness, and are associated with no instability. *Second-degree or moderate sprains* have a larger number of fibers disrupted, with accordingly more pain and tenderness, but gross instability is absent. In first- and second-degree sprains, typically in the ankle, pain is worse a few hours after the injury than it is immediately following the injury. *Third-degree or severe sprains* are complete tears of the ligament and are associated with greater pain and obvious joint instability.

Strains, or tearing of muscle fibers, are often even harder to quantitate than are injuries to ligaments. The degree of injury is usually more apparent several hours after the injury than at the initial examination. With a *grade I muscle strain*, a small number of muscle fibers are torn and pain is mild. Pain will be slightly greater when the muscle is contracted against resistance. In a *grade II muscle strain*, pain is greater and any attempt to contract the muscle against resistance leads to immediate pain, causing an apparent weakness of the injured muscle. A *severe or grade III muscle strain* is a total rupture of the muscle and is uncommon in the child athlete. In teenagers, this rupture is most often seen at the musculotendinous junction; surgical repair is the treatment of choice.

While moderate and severe ligament sprains and muscle strains disqualify the child or teenager from returning to the game that day, some children with mild ligament or muscle injuries can safely continue playing. Before permitting the child to return to the game, however, the physician should have the athlete perform some of the movements needed for the sport in question, such as running and cutting or jumping on the injured leg. If these movements can be performed satisfactorily, a return to the game can be considered. If an ankle sprain is deemed to be mild, taping can be useful in preventing a mild ankle injury from becoming a more severe injury when the athlete returns to the game.

OFF THE FIELD OR IN THE OFFICE

When an injured child athlete is examined away from the playing field, it is useful to obtain as accurate a history as possible of how the injury occurred. Has this type of injury occurred previously? Did the child try to walk after the injury or was weight bearing impossible? Did the pain and difficulty walking become more marked several hours after the injury? If bone injury is present, immediate weight bearing is usually avoided, while ligament or muscle injuries are commonly more painful several hours later than at the time of the injury.

A focused but complete examination of the injured area must be performed, searching for the primary area of tenderness and pain with palpation and relating this to the physician's knowledge of the anatomical structures in this region. If a ligament injury is present, gentle stressing of the joint may demonstrate instability, but if the injury has occurred several hours previously the pain may be too marked to allow an adequate stability assessment. In these situations, aseptic aspiration of the knee or ankle hematoma and injection of 0.5% lidocaine into the joint will often facilitate the joint examination and detect instability not previously noted. If joint instability is present, a radiograph of the injured joint is necessary to look for physeal or osteochondral fractures.

The ankle is the most commonly injured lower-extremity joint in athletes. Most ankle sprains are from excessive inversion, with the lateral ligaments injured. There are three major lateral ankle ligaments: anterior talofibular, calcaneofibular, and posterior talofibular. The anterior talofibular ligament is the most commonly injured of these; when it is injured, tenderness is present just anterior to the lateral malleolus. If there is tenderness just caudal to the tip of the lateral malleolus, the calcaneofibular ligament is injured. If tenderness is present anterior to the medial malleolus, the deltoid ligament has been injured. If tenderness is present over both the lateral and medial ligaments, the sprain is more severe and requires a longer time to heal.

The initial treatment for an ankle ligament sprain is the application of ice to decrease the amount of local hemorrhage and edema formation. The ice will also provide some degree of local pain relief. Periodic use of cold packs or ice should be continued for at least 24 hours after the initial injury. The injured extremity should be elevated to decrease the amount of localized swelling. A compression dressing is often also used to diminish edema. Weight bearing should be avoided initially by the use of crutches.

With an ankle sprain, the time to return to sports activity obviously depends on the severity of the ligament tear. If the initial hemorrhage and edema can be controlled, recovery is quicker. When the initial pain has resolved, active range-of-motion exercises are used to maintain dorsiflexion and plantarflexion and to diminish leg muscle atrophy. Since pain is present mainly with inversion, the use of a stirrup-type ankle splint will protect the young athlete from inverting and everting the foot while still permitting up and down movements of the foot at the ankle. Return to sports participation is possible when pain is absent with ankle movement, both passively and while running. Taping the ankle or wearing a stirrup or air-filled splint is often done to prevent recurrence of ankle sprains once healing is attained.

Knee ligament sprains have to be treated more conservatively than ankle ligament sprains. Even with a first-degree or mild knee ligament sprain, play should not be resumed on the same day. This is partly because playing with an injured knee ligament presents a significant risk of increasing the severity of the injury and partly because taping or bracing to protect against further injury is not as effective with the knee as it is with the ankle. Second-degree knee ligament sprains generally require a period of cast immobilization, and third-degree sprains most often are treated with surgical repair. Although use of a knee brace may be needed after a severe knee injury to allow a return to sports participation, the use of prophylactic knee braces to prevent initial knee injuries in football has not been efficacious.

Muscle injuries are commonly more painful a few hours after the tear has occurred than at the initial time of injury, so pain is often marked by the time these injuries are seen in the office. The degree of muscle tearing can sometimes be quantitated by the amount of passive motion lost in the adjacent joint. For example, the quadriceps is a common region of muscle tearing or hematoma. Mild muscle injuries allow passive knee flexion to past 90°, while more severe injuries correlate with greater limitation of knee flexion. The more the motion of the adjacent joint is limited, the longer the child will have to refrain from sports activity. Generally, muscle hematomas or tears respond to early application of ice, rest, and gradual return to increased motion of the adjacent joints. If, after a muscle injury, the range of motion of the adjacent joint is not improving and pain in the muscle is increasing instead of declining, it is possible that myositis ossificans is developing. A radiograph may demonstrate some calcification of the muscle hematoma, but not before 1 week after the injury. If this diagnosis is made, physical therapy or attempts to improve joint range of motion are stopped until tenderness is absent from the muscle, at which stage therapy for joint motion and muscle strengthening is reinstituted.

For any soft-tissue injury, be it muscle, ligament, or tendon, ice is used for the first 24 to 48 hours after the injury to decrease the local hemorrhage and edema. Thereafter, heat treatments, either wet or dry, are useful to help "loosen up" the injured area as rehabilitation is started. Ice treatments are often helpful after rehabilitation workouts to decrease reactive swelling and pain. After any of these injuries, return to sports participation needs to be delayed until pain is absent, joint motion is essentially normal, and muscle strength has returned to nearly normal, otherwise the risk of reinjury is high; reinjury will result in even further restriction of sports participation.

Taping in Sports

In most athletes, young or old, taping performs two primary functions: prevention of injury and treatment of a ligament or muscle injury. This is accomplished by the tape limiting one or more planes of movement of the joint being treated. Rigid immobilization is not achieved with tape, but relative restriction of movement, effectively augmenting the function of the joint ligaments, is feasible. The most common use of prophylactic taping is at the ankle, with the tape usually applied to limit inversion of the foot at the ankle.

A few general taping principles are of importance. The ligament should always be supported in the shortened position; if protecting an ankle from inversion, the foot should be held everted as the tape is applied from the medial to the lateral side. The area of tape application must be dry and preferably free of body hair to allow for tape adhesion. A skin adherent, such as benzoin,

should be used. Most tape should be applied by overlapping tape strips, not wrapping circumferentially. Continuous circumferential tape wrapping is discouraged, as it impairs distal limb circulation as well as venous return, and will result in increasing pain for the athlete during sports activity.

Taping can be used to help protect any joint from moving into a position of higher risk of injury. However, the ankle joint is the area for which protection from injury through taping has been demonstrated to be the most effective, so the method of taping an ankle to prevent recurrent inversion sprains is explained here. The athlete's foot is held off the table in neutral dorsiflexion and in mild eversion. Tape of 1 inch or 1½ inch width is used. A nearly circumferential strip of tape is placed just proximal to the level of the fifth metatarsal head, and a similar anchor strip is placed at the mid-distal calf, near the level of the lower end of the gastrocnemius muscle bellies. Several (usually five or six) stirrup tape strips are applied beginning on the medial side of the distal calf, coursing under the sole of the foot, and ending on the lateral calf. All these tapes should overlap to some degree. The heel is then locked in place with tape straps that begin laterally, cross anteriorly over the front of the distal tibia just above the medial malleolus, continue across the heel cord, pass distal to the lateral malleolus onto the lateral calcaneus and under the sole of the foot, and finally end on the top of the medial forefoot. A few of these straps are applied with the foot slightly everted to hold the heel in place. Additional figure-of-eight straps are applied to complete the ankle wrap. If the deltoid ligament on the medial side needs to be protected, the foot is held in slight inversion (instead of eversion) as the same tape straps are applied.

Probably the most simple and common use of taping to protect from injury is the so-called "buddy taping" of the fingers, following an injury to one of the interphalangeal joints. Generally, the index and long fingers work smoothly as a unit, while the ring and little fingers work synchronously. These then are the combinations of buddy-taping that should be used following finger dislocations or ''jammed fingers'' to allow the child to continue playing with less risk of reinjury.

Suggested Readings

Bar-Or, O.: Pediatric Sports Medicine for the Practitioner: From Physiologic Principles to Clinical Applications. Springer-Verlag, New York, 1983.

Committee on Sports Medicine and Fitness, American Academy of Pediatrics: Fitness, activity, and sports participation in the preschool child. Pediatrics 90: 1002–1004, 1992.

Ellison, A.E., ed.: Athletic Training and Sports Medicine. American Academy of Orthopaedic Surgeons, Park Ridge, Ill., 1984. (Provides good illustrations of taping techniques.)

Reider, B.: Sports Medicine: The School-Age Athlete. W.B. Saunders, Philadelphia, 1991.

Smith, N.J., ed.: Sports Medicine: Health Care for Young Athletes. American Academy of Pediatrics, Evanston, Ill., 1983.

Smith, N.J.: Common Problems in Pediatric Sports Medicine. Year Book Medical Publishers, Chicago, 1989.

Sullivan, J.A. and Grana, W.A., eds: The Pediatric Athlete. American Academy of Orthopaedic Surgeons, Park Ridge, Ill., 1990.

Index

Page numbers in italics indicate figures; those followed by "t" indicate tables.